CRRN Exam Study Guide

All-in-One CRRN Review + 450 Practice Questions with In-Depth Explanation for the Certified Rehabilitation Registered Nurse Exam

Jacqueline Gordon
© 2023-2024
Printed in USA.

Disclaimer:

Table of Contents

Why do you need to be CRRN Certified?

➢ Firstly, being CRRN certified validates your expertise in the domain, enabling you to stand out among your peers and gain professional recognition. It showcases your commitment to continuous learning and staying updated with the latest advancements in the field.

➢ Additionally, the CRRN certification signifies your ability to deliver safe and high-quality care to patients. This can enhance patient trust and satisfaction, and lead to improved patient outcomes.

➢ Furthermore, the CRRN certification sets you apart in the job market, making you a sought-after candidate. Many employers prioritize hiring CRRN certified candidates due to the added confidence in their skills and knowledge.

➢ Lastly, obtaining the CRRN certification can open up opportunities for career advancement and higher salaries. Many healthcare organizations value the expertise and dedication of CRRN certified candidates and may offer increased responsibilities and compensation packages accordingly.

<u>Willing to Join Our Author Panel?</u>

Dear,

We would like to invite you to join our 'Panel Of Authors'.

First of all, Thank you for your hard work and dedication to your patients. We know that the hours are long and the workload is demanding, but you do it with grace and dignity. Your compassion is evident in the way you treat your patients, and we are grateful for all that you do.
We believe that your expertise and experience will be a valuable contribution to our books. Our goal is to provide valuable content that helps our readers to step forward in their career development. This is a unique opportunity to share your expertise with others in need and help shape their future.

The requirements for joining our panel of authors are as follows:

- A minimum experience of 8 years
- Proper certification from a renowned organization
- Good writing and teaching skills
- Enthusiasm in sharing knowledge

If you meet these requirements and are interested in joining our panel, please send us your resume along with a writing sample for our review to **propublisher@zohomail.com**.

We would be happy to have you on board!
We are happy that our panel of authors can provide the best content because they are experienced and passionate in their own field. We would love for you to join our panel of authors and help us continue to provide quality content for our readers. You will also be able to connect with other experts in your domain from around the world and build a network of support. Undoubtedly, this will be a great opportunity for you to make a difference in your profession.

Thank You.

Why is this book the right choice for you to clear the CRRN Exam?

Latest Study Guide:

If you are looking for an up-to-date study guide for the CRRN Exam, then look no further than this book. This book provides everything you need to know to ace the exam with tons of practice questions to help you prepare. This book is also constantly updated to ensure that it always covers the latest information on the exam as per the outline provided.

CRRN ® TEST CONTENT OUTLINE

1. Nursing Models and Theories
2. Functional Health Patterns
3. The Function of the Rehabilitation Team and Transitions of Care
4. Legislative, Economic, Ethical, and Legal Issues

Experienced Set of Authors:

There are many reasons to choose this book over others, but one of the most important is that it is written by experienced authors who are CRRN Certified. The authors of this book have a wealth of experience in taking and passing exams, and we have used our knowledge to create a study guide that is comprehensive and easy to follow.

With our experienced authors and comprehensive coverage, our book is the best way to prepare for this important test.

Detailed rationale for the answer:

We provide an in-depth explanation for each question, so you can understand not only the correct answer but also why it is correct. This book also gives you an ample amount of practice to help you feel confident on exam day.

Similar Question Format as that in the actual exam:

One of the most important features of this book is that the questions and answers follow the same pattern as the actual exam. This is extremely important because you need to be familiar with the format of the exam to do well on it.

Fine Tunes your thinking:

Going through the questions, answers and explanations repeatedly will sharpen your thinking and understanding ability. This will help you to understand the root of the question in the CRRN Exam and make the right selection of the answer.

Clear and Concise:

This CRRN Prep is written in simple language and is not overly technical. This sets this book apart from other study materials because when you are studying for the CRRN Exam, you need to be able to understand the material without getting bogged down in details. This book will help you do just that. This combination of easy-to-understand language and practical testing will help you be successful on the CRRN exam.

Magical Steps to Pass the CRRN Exam with Ease:

1. Belief: You must believe that you can pass the CRRN exam with ease. This belief will help you stay focused and motivated throughout your studies. We help build your confidence by giving you the feel of attending virtual exams in our book, making you familiar with the type of questions that will be asked in the exam, and giving you a thorough idea about all the topics.

2. Visualization: Visualize yourself passing the CRRN exam with flying colors. This will help you stay positive and focused on your goal. Taking multiple tests and solving various questions will help improve your positivity and confidence. We try our best to improve your positivity.

3. Study: Make sure to study all the material thoroughly. Quality Learning is more important than Quantity Learning. Time yourself when you take tests and try to complete them within the stipulated time.

4. Practice: The more you practice the more is the chance of passing the exam. By doing this, you will get a feel for the types of questions that will be asked and how to best answer them. We have an abundant number of questions for you to practice.

5. Relax: On the day of the exam, make sure to relax and stay calm. This will help you think more clearly and perform at your best.

Smart Learning with Trust in Yourself will make Success knock at your door! All the Best!

CRRN GUIDE

1 Nursing Models and Theories:

Nursing models and theories play a crucial role in the field of rehabilitation nursing. These models and theories provide a framework that guides and supports the practice of rehabilitation registered nurses. They help in organizing and understanding the complex nature of patient care and enable nurses to provide effective interventions.

One important nursing model is the Holistic Model of Nursing, which emphasizes the need to consider the physical, emotional, social, and spiritual aspects of a patient's well-being during rehabilitation. This model helps rehabilitation nurses to address the comprehensive needs of their patients and develop individualized care plans.

Another significant theory is the Self-Care Theory by Dorothea Orem, which focuses on empowering patients to take an active role in their own rehabilitation process. Rehabilitation nurses apply this theory by assessing patients' abilities and providing education and support to enhance their self-care skills.

Furthermore, the Theory of Adaptation by Callista Roy is relevant in rehabilitation nursing, as it guides nurses in helping patients adapt to their functional limitations and achieve their maximum potential.

Additionally, the Biopsychosocial Model is essential in rehabilitation nursing, as it acknowledges the interplay of biological, psychological, and social factors in a patient's overall functioning and recovery.

1.1 Task 1: Understand nursing models and theories as a framework for rehabilitation nursing practice.:

In rehabilitation nursing practice, understanding nursing models and theories is essential for providing a framework of care. These models and theories guide nurses in delivering comprehensive and effective rehabilitation interventions to patients.

One important nursing model is the Roy Adaptation Model, which focuses on assessing patients' adaptive responses to their environment and implementing interventions to promote adaptation and enhance overall well-being.

Another significant theory is the Self-Care Deficit Theory developed by Dorothea Orem, which emphasizes patients' ability to care for themselves and the nurse's role in facilitating self-care through education and support.

Additionally, the Psychosocial Rehabilitation Model focuses on addressing the psychological and social aspects of rehabilitation, such as coping skills, self-esteem, and reintegration into the community.

Understanding these models and theories allows rehabilitation registered nurses to provide individualized care plans, collaborate with interdisciplinary teams, and evaluate patient outcomes effectively. By utilizing these frameworks, nurses can optimize the rehabilitation process and improve patients' quality of life.

1.1.1 Knowledge of:

Knowledge of nursing models and theories is essential for rehabilitation registered nurses to provide effective care. These models and theories serve as frameworks for understanding and guiding nursing practice in the rehabilitation setting.

Firstly, nurses must have a solid understanding of models such as the biopsychosocial model, which recognizes the interconnectedness of biological, psychological, and social factors in a patient's health. This model helps nurses address the multifaceted needs of rehabilitation patients.

Furthermore, knowledge of theories like self-efficacy theory and the transtheoretical model of change allows nurses to support patients in setting rehabilitation goals and overcoming obstacles. These theories emphasize the importance of patient empowerment and motivation in achieving successful rehabilitation outcomes.

Additionally, rehabilitation registered nurses should be familiar with the nursing process, including assessment, planning, implementation, and evaluation. This systematic approach ensures comprehensive and individualized care for patients undergoing rehabilitation. This knowledge enables them to provide holistic care, support patient empowerment, and facilitate successful rehabilitation outcomes.

1.1.1.1 Nursing theories and models significant to rehabilitation (e.g., King, Rogers, Neuman, Orem):

In the field of rehabilitation nursing, several nursing theories and models have been developed to provide a framework for practice. These theories assist rehabilitation registered nurses in understanding and addressing the unique needs of their patients.

One such theory is the King's Theory of Goal Attainment, which emphasizes the importance of setting mutually agreed-upon goals between the nurse and the patient. By collaboratively identifying and working towards these goals, the rehabilitation nurse can provide effective care and promote patient empowerment.

Another influential theory is Rogers' Science of Unitary Human Beings, which focuses on the interconnectedness of individuals with their environment. According to this theory, rehabilitation nurses should strive to create a supportive and healing environment that facilitates the patient's recovery.

The Neuman Systems Model views the patient as an open system influenced by stressors. Rehabilitation nurses using this model assess the patient's stressors and develop interventions to promote adaptation and stability.

Lastly, Orem's Self-Care Deficit Theory highlights the importance of patients' ability to perform self-care activities. Rehabilitation nurses using this theory help patients identify and develop the skills necessary for self-care and independence.

These nursing theories and models play a significant role in guiding rehabilitation nursing practice by providing a framework for assessment, intervention, and evaluation. By incorporating these theories into their practice, rehabilitation registered nurses can provide holistic and patient-centered care to promote optimal health and well-being.

1.1.1.2 Rehabilitation standards and scope of practice:

Rehabilitation standards and scope of practice are crucial for Rehabilitation Registered Nurses (RRNs) in providing effective care. These standards define the qualifications and responsibilities of RRNs in the field of rehabilitation nursing. They encompass a wide range of aspects such as clinical skills, ethical guidelines, and professional behavior. RRNs must adhere to these standards to ensure safe and high-quality care for their patients.

The scope of practice for RRNs includes assessing and diagnosing patients, developing and implementing individualized care plans, and evaluating the outcomes of interventions. They collaborate with interdisciplinary healthcare teams and provide education to patients and their families. RRNs also play a vital role in promoting health and preventing complications.

Additionally, RRNs need to stay updated with the latest evidence-based practices, technological advancements, and legal regulations related to rehabilitation nursing. They must continuously enhance their knowledge and skills through professional development activities and maintaining a commitment to lifelong learning.

By following these standards and embracing the scope of practice, RRNs contribute significantly to optimizing the functional abilities, independence, and overall well-being of their patients.

1.1.1.3 Nursing process (i.e., assessment, diagnosis, outcomes identification, planning, implementation, evaluation):

The nursing process is a systematic framework that guides registered nurses in providing quality care to their patients. It consists of several essential steps: assessment, diagnosis, outcomes identification, planning, implementation, and evaluation.

During the assessment phase, the nurse collects information about the patient's health history, current condition, and any related factors that may impact their rehabilitation journey. This helps in identifying the patient's needs and defining their overall goals.

The next step is diagnosis, where the nurse analyzes the collected data to make a professional judgment about the patient's condition. This helps in identifying the specific problems or potential complications that the patient might face during their rehabilitation process.

Outcomes identification involves setting measurable goals in collaboration with the patient and their loved ones. These goals are specific, realistic, and achievable within a certain time frame.

Planning is the stage where the nurse develops a comprehensive care plan that outlines the strategies and interventions needed to achieve the identified goals. This plan is individualized and takes into account the patient's unique needs and preferences.

The implementation phase involves carrying out the planned interventions, which can include administering medications, providing therapies, and educating the patient and their family.

Finally, the evaluation phase assesses the effectiveness of the interventions implemented. The nurse monitors the patient's progress, compares it to the desired outcomes, and adjusts the care plan accordingly.

The nursing process is crucial for rehabilitation registered nurses as it provides a structured approach to delivering patient-centered care and ensures continuity throughout the rehabilitation process. By following these steps, nurses can effectively identify, plan, and implement appropriate interventions to help patients achieve their rehabilitation goals.

1.1.2 Skill in:

Skill in: Assessment, communication, critical thinking, problem-solving, collaboration, and cultural competence.

Assessment involves evaluating the physical, emotional, and cognitive status of patients to determine their rehabilitation needs. Good communication skills are essential for effectively communicating with patients, their families, and the interdisciplinary team. Critical thinking is required to analyze information and make informed decisions about patient care. Problem-solving skills are necessary to address challenges and overcome barriers to rehabilitation. Collaboration with other healthcare professionals is crucial for providing coordinated and comprehensive care. Cultural competence is important for understanding and respecting the values, beliefs, and customs of diverse patient populations. These skills enable rehabilitation nurses to deliver high-quality care, promote patient autonomy, and optimize patient outcomes.

1.1.2.1 Applying nursing models and theories:

Applying nursing models and theories is crucial for Rehabilitation Registered Nurses in their practice. These frameworks provide a systematic approach to care, help in understanding patients' needs, and guide decision-making.

Nursing models, such as the Roy Adaptation Model or the Orem Self-Care Model, help nurses in assessing patients and planning interventions. These models consider various factors that influence a patient's health, including physical, psychological, social, and environmental aspects.

Theories, such as the Health Belief Model or the Transtheoretical Model, assist nurses in understanding patients' behaviors and motivations. These theories can be utilized to promote lifestyle changes, compliance with treatment plans, and overall well-being.

By applying nursing models and theories, Rehabilitation Registered Nurses can tailor their care plans to meet the specific needs of each patient, enhance patient outcomes, and improve the overall quality of care provided.

1.1.2.2 Applying rehabilitation scope of practice:

Applying rehabilitation scope of practice is a crucial aspect of the role of a Rehabilitation Registered Nurse. It involves understanding and utilizing nursing models and theories as a framework for rehabilitation nursing practice. This enables the nurse to provide holistic care to patients and help them achieve their maximum level of functioning and independence.

One important aspect of applying rehabilitation scope of practice is understanding different nursing models and theories that guide rehabilitation nursing. These models and theories provide a foundation for assessing, planning, implementing, and evaluating care plans for patients undergoing rehabilitation.

Additionally, the Rehabilitation Registered Nurse must have a comprehensive understanding of the scope of practice in rehabilitation nursing. This includes knowledge on evidence-based practices, understanding the multidisciplinary team approach, and collaborating with other healthcare professionals to provide coordinated and individualized care for patients.

Furthermore, the nurse must have the skills to assess and identify the unique needs of each patient, develop appropriate goals, and implement interventions to promote functional recovery. They also focus on educating patients and their families about self-care and rehabilitation strategies to facilitate a smooth transition to their home environment.

1.1.2.3 Applying the nursing process:

Applying the nursing process is a critical aspect of rehabilitation nursing practice. The nursing process is a systematic framework that guides nurses in delivering patient-centered care. It consists of five steps: assessment, diagnosis, planning, implementation, and evaluation.

During the assessment phase, the rehabilitation registered nurse collects and analyzes patient data to identify their needs. This involves gathering information about their medical history, current condition, and functional abilities.

Next, the nurse diagnoses the patient's problems based on the assessment findings. This helps create an individualized care plan.

In the planning phase, the nurse collaborates with the patient, their family, and the interdisciplinary team to set goals and develop a comprehensive plan of care.

The implementation phase involves executing the care plan through interventions such as providing medications, performing treatments, and coordinating therapies.

Lastly, the nurse evaluates the outcomes of the interventions and modifies the care plan accordingly.

Applying the nursing process ensures that rehabilitation registered nurses provide holistic, evidence-based, and patient-centered care to promote optimal health and independence.

1.2 Task 2: Incorporate relevant research, nursing models, and theories into individualized patient-centered rehabilitation care.:

Task 2 involves incorporating relevant research, nursing models, and theories into individualized patient-centered rehabilitation care as a Rehabilitation Registered Nurse. This entails using evidence-based practices, established nursing models, and theories to develop individualized care plans for patients undergoing rehabilitation. By incorporating research, nurses can stay informed about the latest advancements and best practices in rehabilitation care. Nursing models, such as the Patient-Centered Care Model, can guide nurses in providing holistic care that considers each patient's unique needs and preferences. Theories, such as the Health Belief Model or the Self-Care Theory, can provide a theoretical framework for understanding patients' behaviors and promoting their active involvement in their own rehabilitation. Overall, this task helps ensure that rehabilitation care is patient-centered, evidence-based, and tailored to meet each individual's specific needs and goals.

1.2.1 Knowledge of:

Knowledge of: Nursing Models and Theories

As a Rehabilitation Registered Nurse, it is important to have a solid understanding of nursing models and theories. These frameworks provide a structure for delivering individualized patient-centered rehabilitation care. Familiarity with various nursing models, such as the Roy Adaptation Model or the Orem Self-Care Deficit Theory, helps guide the decision-making process in providing appropriate care for patients. Each model has its own set of concepts and assumptions that can be applied to assess, plan, implement, and evaluate patient needs. These models also emphasize the importance of considering the holistic needs of patients, including their physical, emotional, and psychosocial well-being. By integrating nursing theories into practice, Rehabilitation Registered Nurses can ensure that care is evidence-based, patient-centered, and promotes optimal health outcomes.

1.2.1.1 Evidence-based research:

Evidence-based research is a crucial aspect of nursing practice, particularly in the field of rehabilitation. It involves the systematic gathering and analysis of relevant research findings to inform decision-making and improve patient care. By utilizing evidence-based research, Rehabilitation Registered Nurses can provide individualized and patient-centered care that is based on the best available evidence. This approach helps nurses stay up-to-date with the latest advancements in rehabilitation, ensures that interventions are effective and safe, and enhances overall patient outcomes. Evidence-based research also enhances the credibility and reliability of nursing practice as it relies on scientific evidence rather than personal opinions or assumptions. Nurses can access a wide range of evidence from various sources, such as peer-reviewed journals, research databases, and clinical guidelines. They must critically appraise the evidence, considering its validity, applicability, and relevance to the specific patient population or clinical context. By incorporating evidence-based research into their practice, Rehabilitation Registered Nurses can enhance the quality of care and promote positive rehabilitation outcomes.

1.2.1.2 Nursing theories and models significant to rehabilitation (e.g., King, Rogers, Neuman, Orem):

In the field of rehabilitation nursing, various nursing theories and models play a significant role in providing individualized patient-centered care. Some of the noteworthy theories and models include those developed by King, Rogers, Neuman, and Orem.

Imogene King's Theory of Goal Attainment focuses on the interaction between the nurse and patient to establish mutually agreed-upon goals, with the aim of achieving optimal health outcomes. This theory emphasizes the importance of communication and collaboration in the rehabilitation process.

Martha Rogers' Science of Unitary Human Beings emphasizes a holistic approach to nursing care, considering the individual as an integral part of the environment. Rogers' theory encourages nurses to consider the interconnectedness between the physical, psychological, and social aspects of the patient's rehabilitation journey.

Betty Neuman's Systems Model centers around the idea that individuals are in constant interaction with their environment, and focuses on the impact of stressors on health and wellness. This model guides rehabilitation nurses in assessing and managing stressors that may hinder the patient's progress.

Dorothea Orem's Self-Care Deficit Nursing Theory emphasizes the importance of promoting self-care abilities in patients. In a rehabilitation setting, this theory guides nurses in identifying and addressing the patient's deficits in self-care, while simultaneously empowering them to take an active role in their own rehabilitation process.

By incorporating these nursing theories and models into their practice, rehabilitation registered nurses can provide patient-centered care that addresses the unique needs and goals of each individual. This ensures a comprehensive and effective approach to rehabilitation and facilitates positive outcomes for patients.

1.2.1.3 Nursing process (i.e., assessment, diagnosis, outcomes identification, planning, implementation, evaluation):

The nursing process is a systematic approach used by Rehabilitation Registered Nurses to provide individualized patient-centered care. It consists of several key steps including assessment, diagnosis, outcomes identification, planning, implementation, and evaluation.

Assessment involves gathering information about the patient's health status, including their physical, emotional, and social well-being. This helps the nurse identify the patient's needs and determine appropriate care interventions.

Diagnosis involves analyzing the data collected during assessment to identify the patient's health problems and potential complications. This helps the nurse establish priorities and develop a care plan.

Outcomes identification involves setting measurable goals and outcomes in collaboration with the patient, family, and healthcare team. This helps ensure that the care provided is focused on achieving specific outcomes and promoting the patient's well-being.

Planning involves developing a comprehensive care plan that addresses the patient's needs, goals, and preferences. This may include interventions such as medication administration, therapeutic exercises, or healthcare education.

Implementation involves carrying out the care plan and providing the necessary interventions to promote the patient's rehabilitation and recovery. This may involve coordinating care with other healthcare professionals and ensuring the patient's comfort and safety.

Evaluation involves assessing the effectiveness of the care provided and determining if the desired outcomes have been achieved. This helps the nurse make any necessary adjustments to the care plan and ensure that the patient's needs are being met. By following this process, nurses can ensure that the care provided is comprehensive, individualized, and focused on promoting the patient's rehabilitation and well-being.

1.2.1.4 Related theories and models (e.g., developmental, behavioral, cognitive, moral, personality, caregiver development and function):

Related theories and models play a crucial role in shaping the practice of a Rehabilitation Registered Nurse. These theories and models provide a framework for understanding and addressing the needs of individual patients in a holistic and patient-centered manner.

Developmental theories offer insights into the different stages of human growth and development, allowing nurses to tailor their interventions accordingly. Behavioral theories focus on observable behaviors and how they can be modified through reinforcement or punishment. Cognitive theories explore the mental processes involved in learning, problem-solving, and decision-making.

Moral theories examine ethical principles and guide nurses in making ethically sound choices in their practice. Personality theories help nurses understand how individual differences in personality can influence patient behavior and response to rehabilitation therapies.

Caregiver development and function models emphasize the importance of supporting and empowering caregivers in their role, recognizing the impact they have on patient outcomes.

By incorporating these theories and models into their practice, Rehabilitation Registered Nurses can provide individualized care that addresses the specific needs and goals of each patient and promotes their overall well-being and rehabilitation.

1.2.1.5 Rehabilitation standards and scope of practice:

Rehabilitation standards and scope of practice are crucial aspects of the role of a Rehabilitation Registered Nurse. These standards refer to the guidelines and criteria that nurses must adhere to when providing rehabilitation care to patients. The scope of practice outlines the specific tasks and responsibilities that nurses can perform within the field of rehabilitation. It includes activities such as assessing patients' functional abilities, developing individualized care plans, implementing therapeutic interventions, and evaluating patient progress. Key components of rehabilitation standards and scope of practice include ensuring patient safety, promoting collaboration with other healthcare professionals, and maintaining professional competence through continuous learning. By following these standards and understanding their scope of practice, Rehabilitation Registered Nurses can provide effective and patient-centered care to support individuals in their recovery journey.

1.2.1.6 Patient-centered care:

Patient-centered care is a fundamental component of rehabilitation nursing practice. It focuses on tailoring care to meet the individual needs and preferences of each patient. This approach recognizes that patients are unique and have their own goals and values that should guide their care. In patient-centered care, the patient is actively involved in their own healthcare decisions, and their input is considered and respected. This involves establishing a therapeutic relationship with the patient, promoting open communication and trust. Rehabilitation nurses use various nursing models and theories to guide their practice in delivering patient-centered care. These models and theories help nurses assess the patient's needs, plan and implement care, and evaluate outcomes. Nursing models and theories such as the Roy Adaptation Model or the Orem's Self-Care Deficit Theory provide frameworks that help nurses understand the complex and dynamic nature of rehabilitation care. By incorporating relevant research, nursing models, and theories into their practice, rehabilitation registered nurses can ensure they provide individualized patient-centered care that promotes optimal recovery and well-being.

1.2.2 Skill in:

Skill in: Rehabilitation Registered Nurses (RN) must possess a variety of skills to provide effective patient-centered care. These skills include communication, critical thinking, assessment, and collaboration. RNs need to effectively communicate with patients, their families, and interdisciplinary teams to ensure coordinated care. Furthermore, critical thinking skills are crucial for problem-solving and decision-making in complex rehabilitation cases. Accurate assessment skills enable RNs to identify patients' needs, develop individualized care plans, and evaluate outcomes. Collaboration with physicians, therapists, and other healthcare professionals is essential to provide comprehensive rehabilitation care. RNs must also be familiar with nursing models and theories to guide their practice, such as the Roy Adaptation Model or the Neuman Systems Model. Overall, these skills empower Rehabilitation RNs to optimize patient outcomes and enhance their quality of life.

1.2.2.1 Incorporating evidence-based research into practice:

Incorporating evidence-based research into practice is a crucial aspect of being a Rehabilitation Registered Nurse. It involves integrating new findings and studies into the care of individual patients. By using evidence-based research, nurses can optimize patient outcomes and provide high-quality, patient-centered rehabilitation care.

To incorporate evidence-based research into practice, nurses must stay current with the latest research in their field. They can access peer-reviewed journals, attend conferences, and participate in continuing education programs. By staying informed, nurses can make informed decisions and provide the best possible care to their patients.

One important aspect of incorporating evidence-based research is the use of nursing models and theories. These frameworks provide a systematic approach to care and help guide decision-making. Nurses can use models and theories to assess patient needs, develop individualized care plans, and evaluate the effectiveness of interventions. By staying up-to-date with the latest research, utilizing nursing models and theories, and applying evidence-based practice, nurses can provide the highest level of care to their patients.

1.2.2.2 Applying nursing models and theories:

When it comes to providing individualized patient-centered rehabilitation care as a Rehabilitation Registered Nurse, incorporating relevant research, nursing models, and theories is crucial. By utilizing these frameworks, nurses can enhance their decision-making processes and improve patient outcomes.

Nursing models such as the Person-Centered Nursing Framework or the Self-Care Theory help guide nurses in assessing and addressing the holistic needs of their patients. These models emphasize the importance of the patient's unique perspective, promoting a collaborative approach to care.

By considering relevant research findings, nurses can stay informed about evidence-based practices and interventions that have been proven effective in rehabilitation. This helps ensure that care provided aligns with the best available evidence, optimizing patient progress and recovery.

Overall, applying nursing models and theories in rehabilitation care allows the Rehabilitation Registered Nurse to tailor interventions to the individual needs of their patients, empowering them to achieve their full potential and improve their quality of life.

1.2.2.3 Applying rehabilitation scope of practice:

Applying the rehabilitation scope of practice is a crucial aspect of providing individualized patient-centered care as a Rehabilitation Registered Nurse. This involves incorporating relevant research, nursing models, and theories into the rehabilitation process. By doing so, nurses can ensure that patients receive the most effective and evidence-based care possible.

One important aspect of applying the rehabilitation scope of practice is understanding and implementing various nursing models and theories. These frameworks provide a systematic approach to understanding patient needs and tailoring care plans accordingly. Examples of nursing models that can be incorporated include the Neuman Systems Model, the Roy Adaptation Model, and the Health Promotion Model. These models help nurses to assess and address the physical, psychological, and social aspects of a patient's rehabilitation journey.

In addition to nursing models, incorporating relevant research into practice is essential for providing high-quality rehabilitation care. By staying up-to-date with the latest evidence, nurses can ensure that their interventions align with best practices and optimize patient outcomes. This may involve reviewing published research studies, attending conferences and workshops, and collaborating with interdisciplinary teams to share knowledge.

When applying the rehabilitation scope of practice, it is important to remember that each patient is unique and their care should be individualized. This means considering the patient's goals, preferences, and values when developing and implementing the rehabilitation plan. By doing so, Rehabilitation Registered Nurses can provide patient-centered care that promotes not only physical recovery but also emotional well-being and overall quality of life.

1.2.2.4 Applying the nursing process:

Applying the nursing process is a crucial skill for Rehabilitation Registered Nurses (RRNs) to provide individualized patient-centered care. This process involves five key steps: assessment, diagnosis, planning, implementation, and evaluation.

During the assessment phase, RRNs gather information about the patient's health status, needs, and preferences. This includes physical, emotional, and social aspects. The diagnosis step involves identifying actual or potential health problems based on the assessment findings.

In the planning phase, RRNs develop a care plan that addresses the identified problems and sets goals for rehabilitation. This plan considers patient preferences, evidence-based research, and relevant nursing models and theories.

In the implementation step, RRNs put the plan into action, providing the necessary treatments, therapies, and interventions. They also coordinate with other healthcare professionals to ensure comprehensive care.

Lastly, the evaluation stage assesses the effectiveness of the interventions and the progress made towards the patient's goals. This step helps RRNs modify the care plan as needed to optimize outcomes.

By applying the nursing process, RRNs can provide holistic and individualized care, promoting the rehabilitation and well-being of their patients.

2   Functional Health Patterns:

Functional Health Patterns is a framework used in healthcare to evaluate an individual's overall health and well-being. It assesses various aspects of a person's health, including their physical, emotional, cognitive, social, and spiritual well-being. This holistic approach helps healthcare professionals, such as Rehabilitation Registered Nurses, understand the individual's unique health needs and develop a personalized care plan.

The Functional Health Patterns framework consists of 11 different categories, each focusing on a specific aspect of health. These categories include health perception and management, nutritional-metabolic, elimination, activity-exercise, sleep-rest, cognitive-perceptual, self-perception-self-concept, role-relationship, sexuality-reproductive, coping-stress tolerance, and values-beliefs.

By evaluating each of these patterns, Rehabilitation Registered Nurses can identify potential areas of concern, provide appropriate interventions, and support individuals in achieving optimal health and well-being. This comprehensive approach helps promote independence, functionality, and quality of life for patients in rehabilitation settings.

2.1   Task 1: Apply the nursing process to optimize the restoration and preservation of the patient's health and holistic well-being across the lifespan.:

Task 1: Apply the nursing process to optimize the restoration and preservation of the patient's health and holistic well-being across the lifespan.

As a Rehabilitation Registered Nurse, one of the key responsibilities is to apply the nursing process to ensure the best possible outcomes for patients. This involves a systematic approach to assess, diagnose, plan, implement, and evaluate patient care.

In terms of restoration and preservation of health, the nurse must first assess the patient's physical, emotional, and psychological well-being. This includes gathering information about their medical history, current symptoms, and any limitations or challenges they may face.

Next, the nurse will use this information to diagnose the patient's health status and identify any areas of concern or potential risks. This may involve working with other healthcare professionals to coordinate care and develop a comprehensive treatment plan.

Once a plan is in place, the nurse will implement the necessary interventions to address the patient's specific needs. This may include administering medications, providing education and support, and coordinating therapies or treatments.

Throughout the process, the nurse must continually evaluate the effectiveness of the interventions and make adjustments as needed. This ensures that the patient's health and well-being are continually optimized and that any changes in their condition are properly addressed.

By applying the nursing process, Rehabilitation Registered Nurses can play a vital role in supporting the restoration and preservation of their patients' health and holistic well-being across the lifespan.

2.1.1 Knowledge of:

As a Rehabilitation Registered Nurse, it is essential to have a strong knowledge base on various aspects of the nursing process to optimize the restoration and preservation of the patient's health and holistic well-being across the lifespan. This includes understanding the steps involved in the nursing process, such as assessment, diagnosis, planning, implementation, and evaluation. The nurse should be knowledgeable about different health patterns and how they relate to the overall functioning of the patient. This includes topics like sleep and rest, activity and exercise, nutrition, cognitive and sensory perception, self-perception, and relationships. Additionally, the nurse should be well-informed about the appropriate interventions and treatments for each health pattern, as well as any necessary referrals and resources available to facilitate the patient's rehabilitation journey. Having comprehensive knowledge in these areas allows the Rehabilitation Registered Nurse to provide optimal care and support to patients during their recovery process.

2.1.1.1 Physiology and management of health, injury, acute and chronic illness, and adaptability:

Physiology and management of health, injury, acute and chronic illness, and adaptability are crucial areas in the field of nursing, specifically for Rehabilitation Registered Nurses. Understanding the physiological processes that underlie health, injury, illness, and adaptability is essential for providing optimal care. This knowledge enables nurses to assess patients' conditions, identify any deviations from normal physiology, and develop effective management plans.

In terms of health, nurses need to have a comprehensive understanding of how different body systems function and interact harmoniously to maintain homeostasis. They should be able to monitor vital signs, perform physical assessments, interpret laboratory results, and recognize signs and symptoms indicating health or compromised health. Additionally, Rehabilitation Registered Nurses must be knowledgeable about preventive measures to promote health, such as patient education and lifestyle modifications.

When it comes to injury, nurses should have a solid understanding of the pathophysiology of common injuries, including fractures, sprains, and strains. This knowledge allows them to assess the extent of damage, administer appropriate interventions, and provide comprehensive care throughout the recovery process.

Regarding acute and chronic illnesses, nurses must possess expertise in the underlying physiology of various diseases and conditions. This knowledge helps them recognize the signs and symptoms, assess the severity, and implement appropriate interventions for acute illnesses like infections, cardiovascular events, and respiratory distress. For chronic illnesses such as diabetes, hypertension, and asthma, nurses need to understand the long-term impact on the body and how to effectively manage symptoms, prevent complications, and promote self-care.

Finally, adaptability refers to the ability of the body to respond and adjust to different internal and external stimuli. Nurses must be familiar with the physiological mechanisms involved in adaptation processes, such as the stress response, immune system responses, and compensation mechanisms for organ failure. By understanding these mechanisms, nurses can recognize when the body is under stress or unable to adapt and intervene accordingly. By understanding the underlying physiological processes, nurses can effectively assess patient conditions, design appropriate management plans, and promote holistic well-being.

2.1.1.2 Pharmacology (e.g., antispasmodics, anticholinergics, antidepressants, analgesics):

Pharmacology plays a crucial role in the field of nursing, especially for Rehabilitation Registered Nurses. It involves the study of various medications and their effects on the body. A wide range of drugs are utilized in rehabilitation settings to optimize patient health and well-being.

One important class of medications used by these nurses are antispasmodics, which help to relieve muscle spasms and reduce pain. Anticholinergics are another group of drugs that inhibit the action of acetylcholine, promoting relaxation and reducing symptoms such as excessive sweating or urinary incontinence.

Antidepressants are commonly prescribed in rehabilitation to manage depression and improve mood. They work by balancing certain chemicals in the brain. Analgesics, or pain relievers, are also crucial in rehabilitation nursing to alleviate pain and enhance patient comfort.

It is essential for Rehabilitation Registered Nurses to have a deep understanding of pharmacology, as it allows them to safely administer medications and monitor patient responses. This knowledge helps optimize the restoration and preservation of patient health across the lifespan.

2.1.1.3 Rehabilitation standards and scope of practice:

Rehabilitation standards and scope of practice refer to the guidelines and boundaries that govern the role and responsibilities of a Rehabilitation Registered Nurse. These standards ensure that nurses have a clear understanding of their duties and limitations in providing care to patients throughout the lifespan.

Some key aspects of rehabilitation standards and scope of practice include assessing and evaluating patients' health conditions, developing personalized care plans, and implementing evidence-based interventions to promote optimal health and well-being.

Rehabilitation nurses are also responsible for coordinating interdisciplinary care, educating patients and their families on self-care techniques, and advocating for patients' rights and needs.

Furthermore, rehabilitation standards and scope of practice encompass ethical considerations, cultural competence, and the importance of ongoing professional development to maintain competencies in the field.

2.1.1.4 Technology (e.g., smart devices, internet sources, personal response devices, telehealth, adaptive and advanced equipment):

Technology has greatly impacted the field of healthcare and rehabilitation nursing. Smart devices, such as smartphones and wearable fitness trackers, provide patients with the ability to monitor their health and track their progress. These devices allow for real-time communication and data collection, allowing healthcare professionals to make more informed decisions. Internet sources provide an abundance of information regarding various medical conditions, treatment options, and rehabilitation techniques. Personal response devices, such as emergency call buttons and fall detection systems, ensure the safety and well-being of patients. Telehealth services allow for remote monitoring and virtual consultations, reducing the need for in-person visits and increasing access to healthcare. Adaptive and advanced equipment, such as prosthetics and assistive technology, enhance independence and functional abilities for individuals with disabilities. Overall, technology in healthcare has transformed the way rehabilitation nurses provide care, resulting in improved patient outcomes and holistic well-being.

2.1.1.5 Alterations in sexual function and reproduction:

Alterations in sexual function and reproduction refer to the changes and issues that occur in these areas of a person's health. As a Rehabilitation Registered Nurse, it is essential to understand and address these concerns to optimize the patient's restoration and preservation of health.

One aspect to consider is the impact of certain medical conditions or surgeries on sexual function. For example, patients with spinal cord injuries may experience changes in sensation or function related to sexual activity. Other conditions like diabetes or hormonal disorders can also affect reproductive health.

Addressing alterations in sexual function and reproduction requires a comprehensive approach. It involves assessing the patient's sexual history, discussing concerns or changes in sexual function, and providing education and support. This may involve collaborating with other healthcare professionals such as urologists or gynecologists.

Additionally, it is crucial to consider the emotional and psychological aspects of sexual health. Patients may experience feelings of frustration or embarrassment related to changes in sexual function. Providing a supportive and non-judgmental environment is essential in promoting holistic well-being. By taking a comprehensive and holistic approach, nurses can support patients in managing and optimizing their sexual health.

2.1.2 Skill in:

As a Rehabilitation Registered Nurse, having skills in various areas is essential for optimizing the restoration and preservation of a patient's health and holistic well-being across their lifespan. Some important skills for a Rehabilitation Registered Nurse include:

1. Assessment: This involves gathering comprehensive data about the patient's physical, mental, and emotional condition to develop an individualized care plan.
2. Communication: Effectively communicating with patients, their families, and other healthcare team members is crucial for coordinating care and providing education.
3. Clinical judgment: Using critical thinking skills to analyze assessment data, identify problems, and make appropriate clinical decisions.
4. Collaboration: Working collaboratively with an interdisciplinary team to ensure a holistic and integrated approach to patient care.
5. Patient education: Providing patients with information and resources to promote independence, self-care, and overall well-being.
6. Advocacy: Serving as a patient advocate by ensuring their rights and preferences are respected and advocating for their needs within the healthcare system.

These skills are vital for Rehabilitation Registered Nurses to provide high-quality care and support to patients in their journey towards health and wellness.

2.1.2.1 Assessing health status and health practices:

Assessing health status and health practices is a crucial component of a Rehabilitation Registered Nurse's role in optimizing the restoration and preservation of a patient's health and holistic well-being across the lifespan. This process involves gathering comprehensive information about a patient's overall health, including physical, mental, and emotional aspects. By conducting assessments, nurses can identify any existing health conditions, determine the patient's current health status, and evaluate their health practices.

Subtopics that fall under assessing health status include collecting a patient's medical history, performing physical examinations, and utilizing diagnostic tests. Nurses must inquire about the patient's lifestyle habits, such as exercise routines, dietary choices, and tobacco or alcohol consumption, to evaluate their health practices. Understanding a patient's health status and practices allows nurses to create individualized care plans and provide appropriate interventions to promote optimal health outcomes. Through this process, nurses gather information to understand a patient's current health status, identify any existing health conditions, and evaluate their health practices in order to formulate appropriate care plans and interventions.

2.1.2.2 Teaching interventions to manage health and wellness:

Teaching interventions to manage health and wellness are crucial for Rehabilitation Registered Nurses in optimizing the restoration and preservation of the patient's health and holistic well-being across the lifespan. These interventions focus on empowering patients with the knowledge and skills necessary to take control of their own health and make informed decisions.

One important aspect of teaching interventions is educating patients about their specific health conditions and how to manage them effectively. This may involve teaching them about their medications, providing guidance on healthy lifestyle choices, and demonstrating self-care techniques.

Additionally, teaching interventions can also involve educating patients about preventive measures to maintain overall health and wellness. This may include teaching about the importance of regular exercise, proper nutrition, stress management, and maintaining a healthy weight.

Moreover, Rehabilitation Registered Nurses play a vital role in teaching patients and their families about the potential risks and complications associated with their health conditions. They provide support and guidance on how to prevent these complications and manage them if they occur. By equipping patients with the necessary knowledge and skills, these interventions empower them to actively participate in their own care and achieve and maintain their health goals.

2.1.2.3   Using rehabilitation standards and scope of practice:
Using rehabilitation standards and scope of practice is crucial for Rehabilitation Registered Nurses to optimize the restoration and preservation of a patient's health and holistic well-being across the lifespan. To achieve this, nurses must adhere to established guidelines and professional standards in their daily practice. These standards ensure that the care provided is safe, effective, and evidence-based. Rehabilitation nurses are responsible for assessing the patient's condition, developing individualized care plans, implementing interventions, and evaluating the outcomes. They collaborate with other healthcare professionals, patients, and their families to ensure a comprehensive approach to care. Rehabilitation nurses utilize their skills in areas such as physical therapy, occupational therapy, speech therapy, and psychological support to address the patient's unique needs. Additionally, they must stay up-to-date with advancements in rehabilitation practices and technology to enhance patient outcomes. By following the rehabilitation standards and scope of practice, nurses can play a vital role in facilitating the recovery and well-being of their patients.

2.1.2.4   Using technology:
The use of technology in nursing is becoming increasingly important in optimizing patient care. Technology has the potential to enhance the restoration and preservation of a patient's health and holistic well-being across their lifespan. There are several ways in which technology can be utilized in the nursing process.
One aspect is the use of electronic health records (EHRs) to store and access patient information efficiently. EHRs improve communication among healthcare providers and help track patient progress. Another important use of technology is the implementation of telehealth services, which allow patients to receive care remotely. This is particularly valuable for patients who have difficulty accessing healthcare due to geographical barriers or physical limitations.
Medical devices and equipment, such as advanced imaging machines and robotics, also play a crucial role in rehabilitation nursing. These technologies assist in diagnosing conditions, monitoring patients, and providing specialized treatments. In addition, technology can support patient education by providing access to reliable health information and resources. Increased utilization of technology in nursing practice can lead to improved patient outcomes and more efficient healthcare delivery.

2.1.2.5   Assessing goals related to sexuality and reproduction:
Assessing goals related to sexuality and reproduction is an important aspect of the nursing process for a Rehabilitation Registered Nurse. This involves understanding and addressing the patient's sexual and reproductive health needs to optimize their overall well-being.
When assessing these goals, the nurse must consider factors such as the patient's age, medical history, cultural and religious beliefs, and current health status. They must also approach these discussions with sensitivity and respect for the patient's privacy.
Subtopics to consider when assessing goals related to sexuality and reproduction may include discussions about family planning, contraception, sexually transmitted infections (STIs), fertility concerns, sexual function, and relationships. It is crucial for the nurse to provide accurate and evidence-based information, support the patient in making informed decisions, and refer them to appropriate resources or specialists if needed.
By addressing the patient's goals related to sexuality and reproduction, the Rehabilitation Registered Nurse can help promote their overall health and well-being.

2.2   Task 2: Apply the nursing process to promote optimal psychosocial patterns and coping and stress management skills of the patients and caregivers.:
As a Rehabilitation Registered Nurse, it is important to apply the nursing process to promote optimal psychosocial patterns and coping and stress management skills of both patients and caregivers. This involves assessing the psychosocial needs of individuals and their ability to cope with stress. It is crucial to identify any psychosocial patterns, such as depression or anxiety, that may hinder their rehabilitation process. By understanding their coping mechanisms, nurses can provide appropriate interventions and support. This can include providing education on stress management techniques, encouraging social support networks, and offering therapeutic activities. Additionally, nurses should ensure that caregivers are equipped with the necessary skills and resources to cope with the demands of caregiving. Overall, by addressing psychosocial patterns and providing coping and stress management skills, rehabilitation nurses can enhance the overall well-being and outcomes of patients and caregivers.

2.2.1   Knowledge of:
As a Rehabilitation Registered Nurse, having knowledge of psychosocial patterns, coping skills, and stress management is crucial in promoting optimal patient and caregiver outcomes. Understanding these concepts allows nurses to provide comprehensive care and support to individuals facing physical and emotional challenges.
Knowledge of different psychosocial patterns helps nurses assess and address patients' mental health and emotional well-being. This includes understanding how patients cope with stress and identifying factors that may impact their ability to manage daily activities. By recognizing psychosocial patterns, nurses can develop personalized interventions to promote positive coping strategies.
Additionally, having knowledge of stress management techniques equips nurses to guide patients in effectively managing stressors related to their rehabilitation journey. This may involve teaching relaxation techniques, providing resources for support groups, or assisting in creating adaptive coping mechanisms.
By applying the nursing process, Rehabilitation Registered Nurses can support patients and caregivers in developing and maintaining optimal psychosocial patterns and coping skills, ultimately enhancing their overall rehabilitation experience.

2.2.1.1   Community resources (e.g., face-to-face support groups, internet, respite care, clergy):
Community resources, such as face-to-face support groups, the internet, respite care, and clergy, play a crucial role in promoting optimal psychosocial patterns and coping skills for patients and caregivers. Face-to-face support groups provide a valuable opportunity

for individuals to connect with others who are facing similar challenges, share experiences, and receive emotional support. The internet offers a wide range of resources, such as online support groups, forums, and educational materials, which can be accessed conveniently from anywhere. Respite care services provide temporary relief to caregivers, allowing them to recharge and maintain their own well-being. Clergy members often offer spiritual guidance and support, which can be comforting for individuals navigating difficult times. Utilizing these community resources can enhance the overall psychosocial well-being of patients and caregivers, promoting effective coping strategies and stress management skills.

2.2.1.2 Coping and stress management strategies for patients and support systems:

Coping and stress management strategies are crucial for patients and their support systems during the rehabilitation process. Patients often experience high levels of stress and anxiety due to the challenges they face, such as physical limitations and lifestyle changes. It is important for the rehabilitation registered nurse to provide the necessary support and guidance to help patients cope effectively with their stress.

One effective strategy is providing education and information about the rehabilitation process, as well as teaching stress management techniques such as deep breathing and relaxation exercises. Additionally, providing emotional support and creating a safe and supportive environment can help patients feel more comfortable and less stressed.

Support systems, including family members and friends, also play a vital role in assisting patients with coping. It is important to involve them in the rehabilitation process and provide them with resources and support, such as counseling or support groups, to help them manage their own stress and better support the patient. The rehabilitation registered nurse should prioritize providing education, emotional support, and resources to help patients effectively manage their stress and improve their overall well-being.

2.2.1.3 Cultural diversity:

Cultural diversity is an important aspect in the field of nursing, especially for Rehabilitation Registered Nurses. It refers to the presence of multiple cultures and ethnicities within a healthcare setting. Nurses need to have knowledge of cultural diversity to provide optimal care to patients and their caregivers.

Understanding cultural diversity enables nurses to respect and value different beliefs, practices, and traditions of individuals from various cultures. It helps in fostering effective communication and building trust with patients and their families.

Nurses should be aware of cultural norms, values, and customs to ensure culturally competent care. This includes being sensitive to dietary preferences, religious practices, and language barriers. Additionally, nurses should be familiar with cultural health beliefs that may influence a patient's decision-making process and treatment choices.

Cultural diversity also encompasses the consideration of socioeconomic factors, such as income levels and social support systems, as these can impact an individual's health outcomes and coping mechanisms.

By embracing cultural diversity, Rehabilitation Registered Nurses can promote optimal psychosocial patterns and enhance the coping and stress management skills of both patients and caregivers from diverse cultural backgrounds. This ultimately leads to improved patient outcomes and satisfaction in the rehabilitation process.

2.2.1.4 Physiology of the stress response:

The physiology of the stress response is a complex system involving the hypothalamus, pituitary gland, and adrenal glands. When a person experiences stress, the hypothalamus releases a hormone called corticotropin-releasing hormone (CRH), which signals the pituitary gland to release adrenocorticotropic hormone (ACTH). ACTH then stimulates the adrenal glands to release cortisol, the primary stress hormone. cortisol triggers several physiological changes, such as increased heart rate and blood pressure, enhanced mental alertness, and the suppression of non-essential bodily functions like digestion. The stress response also activates the sympathetic nervous system, which increases adrenaline production and contributes to the fight-or-flight response. Chronic stress can negatively impact a person's health, leading to conditions like heart disease, depression, and weakened immune function. It is important for rehabilitation registered nurses to understand the physiology of stress in order to effectively promote coping and stress management skills in patients and caregivers.

2.2.1.5 Safety concerns regarding harm to self and others:

When dealing with patients in rehabilitation settings, safety concerns regarding harm to oneself and others are of paramount importance. As a Rehabilitation Registered Nurse, it is crucial to have a thorough understanding of this topic. This knowledge helps in implementing appropriate strategies to promote patient and caregiver safety. One aspect of this topic is identifying potential risks, such as aggressive or impulsive behaviors from patients, which could harm themselves or others. Another aspect involves assessing the patient's mental health status and identifying any signs of self-harm or suicidal ideation. It is also important to recognize environmental factors that may contribute to safety concerns, such as inadequate supervision or lack of safety measures in the facility. Consequently, as a nurse, it is necessary to educate patients and caregivers on safety precautions, implement appropriate interventions like close monitoring and supervision, and collaborate with interdisciplinary teams to ensure the overall well-being of all involved.

2.2.1.6 Technology for self-management:

Technology for self-management is an important aspect of promoting optimal psychosocial patterns and coping skills for patients and caregivers. This topic focuses on how technology can assist individuals in managing their own health and well-being.

One subtopic in this area is the use of mobile applications, which allow patients to track their symptoms, medication schedules, and exercise routines. These apps can help individuals stay organized and adhere to their treatment plans.

Another subtopic is the use of wearable devices, such as fitness trackers or smartwatches, which can monitor vital signs and provide real-time feedback on activity levels, heart rate, and sleep quality. These devices enable patients to monitor their own health and make informed decisions about their lifestyle choices.

Additionally, telehealth and telemedicine technologies allow patients to have virtual consultations with healthcare professionals, reducing the need for in-person visits and improving access to care. This can be particularly beneficial for patients in rural areas or those with mobility issues. By utilizing mobile apps, wearable devices, and telehealth technologies, individuals can better manage their health and improve their overall well-being.

2.2.1.7 Theories (e.g., developmental, coping, stress, grief and loss, self-esteem, role, relationship, interaction):

As a Rehabilitation Registered Nurse, having knowledge of various theories related to psychosocial patterns, coping, stress management, and other aspects is crucial for promoting the optimal well-being of patients and caregivers. These theories help us understand and address different psychosocial challenges that individuals may face during the rehabilitation process.

Developmental theories assist us in recognizing and supporting the unique needs and abilities of individuals at different stages of life. Coping theories help us understand how individuals adapt and manage stressors in their lives, while stress theories provide insight into the effects of stress and ways to mitigate its impact.

Grief and loss theories help us understand the emotional and psychological responses to loss, guiding us in providing appropriate support during times of bereavement. Self-esteem theories shed light on how individuals perceive and value themselves, helping us promote a positive self-image in our patients.

Role and relationship theories enable us to identify the dynamics within families and communities, allowing us to facilitate healthy interactions and support systems. Interaction theories highlight the importance of effective communication and mutual understanding between patients, caregivers, and healthcare professionals.

By integrating these theories into our practice, we can enhance our ability to provide comprehensive care and support to individuals undergoing rehabilitation, enabling them to develop effective coping mechanisms and manage stress while promoting their psychosocial well-being.

2.2.1.8 Types of stress and stressors:

Types of stress can be categorized into acute stress, episodic acute stress, and chronic stress. Acute stress is a response to immediate pressure or demand that lasts for a short period of time. Episodic acute stress occurs when individuals experience repeated episodes of acute stress, leading to a constant state of high stress levels. Chronic stress is a long-term stress that persists over a prolonged period of time.

Stressors can be classified into different types as well. Environmental stressors include physical factors such as noise, temperature, and pollution. Psychological stressors include factors like workload, financial problems, and relationship issues. Physiological stressors are related to physical conditions like illness or injury. Social stressors involve conflicts, competition, and social pressures. Lastly, cognitive stressors pertain to one's thoughts, beliefs, and perceptions.

Understanding the various types of stress and stressors is crucial for rehabilitation registered nurses to effectively assess and manage patients' psychosocial patterns and coping mechanisms. By recognizing and addressing these stressors, nurses can support patients and caregivers in developing effective stress management skills and promoting optimal psychological well-being.

2.2.1.9 Stages of grief and loss:

The stages of grief and loss are important concepts that rehabilitation registered nurses should be familiar with. Grief and loss can be experienced by patients and their caregivers in various situations, such as the loss of physical abilities or independence due to a disability or illness.

The stages of grief, as originally described by Elisabeth K�bler-Ross, include denial, anger, bargaining, depression, and acceptance. These stages are not necessarily linear and can be experienced in varying degrees and orders.

Understanding these stages can help nurses provide appropriate support and interventions to promote optimal psychosocial patterns and coping skills. It is important for nurses to validate and acknowledge patients' feelings, provide a safe space for expression, and offer resources for grief counseling or support groups if needed.

Additionally, nurses can help patients and caregivers develop healthy coping mechanisms and stress management skills. This can include teaching relaxation techniques, encouraging realistic goal setting, and promoting self-care activities.

Overall, having knowledge of the stages of grief and loss allows rehabilitation registered nurses to effectively support patients and caregivers on their journey towards acceptance and adjustment.

2.2.1.10 Individual roles, relationships, and alterations (e.g., cultural, environmental, societal, familial, gender, age):

Individual roles, relationships, and alterations are crucial factors to consider when promoting optimal psychosocial patterns and coping skills in patients and caregivers as a Rehabilitation Registered Nurse. Understanding the cultural, environmental, societal, familial, gender, and age-related influences on an individual's life is essential for providing tailored care.

Cultural factors shape an individual's beliefs, values, and behaviors. Being aware of cultural norms and practices helps in establishing effective communication and building trust. Environmental factors, such as living conditions and access to resources, influence an individual's well-being and coping abilities. Socioeconomic status and community support are significant determinants in psychosocial functioning.

Familial relationships play a vital role in an individual's recovery. Assessing the dynamics, support systems, and communication patterns within the family is essential in facilitating positive outcomes. Additionally, understanding gender roles and expectations can help address potential barriers or challenges to psychological well-being.

Age-related factors impact an individual's coping strategies. Pediatric patients require a developmentally appropriate approach, while geriatric patients may have unique challenges associated with aging. Adapting interventions to meet the specific needs of each age group is crucial.

Considering these individual roles, relationships, and alterations allows the Rehabilitation Registered Nurse to provide holistic care that addresses the diverse psychosocial needs of both patients and caregivers.

2.2.1.11 Psychosocial disorders (e.g., substance abuse, anxiety, depression, bipolar, PTSD, psychosis):

Psychosocial disorders refer to a range of mental health conditions that affect an individual's thoughts, emotions, and behaviors. Some common examples include substance abuse, anxiety, depression, bipolar disorder, post-traumatic stress disorder (PTSD), and psychosis.

As a Rehabilitation Registered Nurse, it is essential to possess knowledge of these disorders to effectively promote optimal psychosocial patterns and coping skills for both patients and caregivers. This involves applying the nursing process, which includes assessment, diagnosis, planning, implementation, and evaluation.

Assessment involves gathering information about the patient's psychosocial history, symptoms, and current coping strategies. Diagnosis includes identifying the specific disorder or disorders present and understanding their impact on the individual's functioning. After completing the assessment and diagnosis, a plan can be developed to address the patient's needs. This may include individual or group therapy sessions, medication management, stress management techniques, and referrals to other healthcare professionals. Implementing the plan involves providing interventions and support to help the patient achieve optimal psychosocial well-being.

As a Rehabilitation Registered Nurse, it is essential to regularly evaluate the effectiveness of interventions and modify the plan as needed. This involves regularly communicating with the patient, monitoring their progress, and adjusting the treatment plan accordingly.

By applying the nursing process, Rehabilitation Registered Nurses can play a crucial role in promoting optimal psychosocial patterns and helping patients and caregivers develop effective coping and stress management skills.

2.2.1.12 Traditional and alternative modalities (e.g., medications, healing touch, botanicals, spiritual, mindfulness, self-care):

In the field of rehabilitation nursing, it is essential for Rehabilitation Registered Nurses to have knowledge of traditional and alternative modalities to effectively promote optimal psychosocial patterns and coping skills for patients and caregivers.

Traditional modalities often include medications prescribed by healthcare providers to manage various conditions and symptoms. These medications can help alleviate pain, reduce anxiety, and improve overall well-being.

Alternative modalities, on the other hand, offer different approaches to promote healing and well-being. Healing touch is a modality that involves using gentle touch or energy therapy to help reduce pain, anxiety, and stress. Botanicals, such as herbal supplements or essential oils, are also utilized for their potential healing properties. Spiritual practices, including prayer or meditation, can provide solace and emotional support.

Mindfulness and self-care techniques are important tools for patients and caregivers to cope with stress and manage their physical and mental health. Practicing mindfulness involves being present in the moment and focusing on one's thoughts and emotions. Engaging in self-care activities, such as exercising, getting enough rest, and engaging in hobbies, can help individuals maintain their overall well-being. This knowledge will enable them to provide comprehensive care and support to patients and caregivers, promoting optimal psychosocial patterns and enhancing coping and stress management skills.

2.2.2 Skill in:

As a Rehabilitation Registered Nurse, having skill in promoting optimal psychosocial patterns and coping and stress management skills of patients and caregivers is crucial. This skill involves effectively applying the nursing process to facilitate a positive overall patient experience during their rehabilitation journey.

One important aspect of this skill is the ability to assess the psychosocial needs of patients and caregivers. This includes understanding their emotional and mental well-being, identifying stressors, and recognizing coping mechanisms. By assessing their individual needs, the nurse can provide targeted support and interventions.

Another aspect of this skill is the ability to develop and implement appropriate interventions to promote psychosocial well-being. This may involve providing emotional support, teaching coping strategies, facilitating communication, and promoting relaxation techniques. Furthermore, the Rehabilitation Registered Nurse should also possess communication and counseling skills to effectively engage with patients and caregivers. This includes active listening, empathy, and the ability to provide education and guidance.

Overall, having skill in promoting optimal psychosocial patterns and coping and stress management is essential for a Rehabilitation Registered Nurse to support the overall well-being of patients and caregivers during the rehabilitation process.

2.2.2.1 Assessing potential for harm to self and others:

Assessing the potential for harm to self and others is a crucial aspect of a Rehabilitation Registered Nurse's role in promoting optimal psychosocial patterns and coping skills of patients and caregivers. This assessment involves evaluating the patient's mental state, behavior, and any risk factors that may contribute to self-harm or harm directed towards others. The nurse should observe signs of depression, anxiety, aggression, or suicidal thoughts and evaluate the patient's access to weapons or harmful substances.

Additionally, assessing the social support system and identifying any history of violent behavior is also essential. Subtopics within this topic may include evaluating the patient's self-esteem, impulse control, and stress management techniques. By thoroughly assessing these potential risks, the nurse can develop appropriate interventions and create a safe environment for the patient and those around them.

2.2.2.2 Assessing the ability to cope and manage stress:

Assessing the ability to cope and manage stress is crucial in the field of Rehabilitation Nursing. As a Rehabilitation Registered Nurse, you need to have the skills to evaluate and support patients and caregivers in developing effective coping mechanisms and stress management techniques. This includes recognizing signs of stress and understanding the impact it can have on overall health and recovery.

To accurately assess stress levels and coping abilities, you can employ various methods such as patient interviews, observation, and standardized assessment tools. By exploring a patient's psychosocial patterns and asking open-ended questions, you can gain insights into their stressors, support systems, and current coping strategies. Additionally, it is important to consider cultural, spiritual, and personal beliefs that may influence their coping abilities.

By identifying stress triggers and evaluating coping skills, you can collaborate with patients and caregivers to develop personalized interventions. This may involve providing education on stress management techniques, encouraging self-care practices, and facilitating access to support networks. Moreover, you can continuously monitor their progress and make adjustments accordingly. By evaluating stress levels, understanding coping strategies, and implementing appropriate interventions, you can promote optimal psychosocial patterns and enhance the overall well-being of patients and caregivers.

2.2.2.3   Facilitating appropriate referrals:

Facilitating appropriate referrals is an important aspect of a Rehabilitation Registered Nurse's role in promoting optimal psychosocial patterns and coping skills for patients and caregivers. It involves identifying the specific needs of the individual and connecting them with appropriate healthcare professionals or resources.

One key aspect of facilitating appropriate referrals is having a thorough understanding of the patient's condition and the available services. This includes knowledge of different specialists, therapists, and support groups that can address the patient's specific needs. By having this knowledge, the nurse can make informed recommendations for referrals.

Communication is also crucial in facilitating appropriate referrals. The nurse needs to effectively communicate with the patient, caregivers, and other healthcare professionals to ensure that everyone is on the same page and understands the reason for the referral. This includes providing relevant information, such as medical history, symptoms, and goals of the referral.

In addition, the nurse needs to consider factors such as accessibility and affordability when making referrals. This includes ensuring that the recommended services are accessible to the patient and that they can afford them. If necessary, the nurse may need to explore alternative options or assist with finding financial assistance.

Overall, facilitating appropriate referrals requires knowledge, effective communication, and consideration of accessibility and affordability. By ensuring that patients and caregivers are connected with the right resources, a Rehabilitation Registered Nurse can promote optimal psychosocial patterns and coping skills.

2.2.2.4   Implementing and evaluating strategies to reduce stress and improve coping (e.g., biofeedback, cognitive behavioral therapy, complementary alternative medicine, pharmacology):

Implementing and evaluating strategies to reduce stress and improve coping is essential in the field of rehabilitation nursing. One approach to achieving this is through the use of biofeedback, which is a technique that allows individuals to monitor and gain control over their own physiological responses. By providing real-time feedback on things like heart rate, blood pressure, and muscle tension, biofeedback can help patients learn how to better manage their stress levels.

Cognitive-behavioral therapy (CBT) is another effective strategy for reducing stress and improving coping skills. This form of therapy focuses on identifying and changing negative thought patterns and behaviors that contribute to stress. By helping patients develop healthier and more adaptive ways of thinking and behaving, CBT can lead to significant improvements in stress management and coping abilities.

Complementary alternative medicine (CAM) approaches, such as acupuncture, yoga, and meditation, can also be beneficial in reducing stress and enhancing coping skills. These practices promote relaxation, mindfulness, and overall well-being, which can have a positive impact on mental and emotional health.

In some cases, pharmacological interventions may be necessary to address severe stress and anxiety. Medications such as anti-anxiety agents or antidepressants can help regulate neurotransmitters in the brain and alleviate symptoms of stress. However, it is important to carefully evaluate the potential risks and benefits of pharmacological interventions, taking into account individual patient factors and preferences.

Overall, the implementation and evaluation of strategies to reduce stress and improve coping are crucial components of the rehabilitation nursing process. By utilizing techniques like biofeedback, CBT, CAM approaches, and pharmacology when appropriate, rehabilitation nurses can support patients and caregivers in achieving optimal psychosocial patterns and enhancing their stress management skills.

2.2.2.5   Using therapeutic communication:

Using therapeutic communication is an essential skill for Rehabilitation Registered Nurses when promoting optimal psychosocial patterns and coping strategies for patients and caregivers. This communication technique involves actively listening, providing empathy, and using therapeutic interventions to establish trust and rapport with individuals in order to facilitate their emotional and mental well-being.

Therapeutic communication helps nurses to establish a safe and non-judgmental environment, which encourages patients and caregivers to express their thoughts and feelings. By employing effective communication skills, nurses can assess and address their patients' psychosocial needs, identify stressors, and develop appropriate coping strategies. This approach also helps nurses to enhance patient education, promote shared decision-making, and improve patient outcomes.

Some key aspects of using therapeutic communication are active listening, validating feelings, providing support and reassurance, promoting empathy and understanding, addressing barriers to communication, and using non-verbal cues effectively. Incorporating these techniques into practice can help Rehabilitation Registered Nurses foster positive relationships, empower patients and caregivers, and enhance overall psychosocial well-being.

2.2.2.6   Assessing and promoting self-efficacy, self-care, and self- concept:

Assessing and promoting self-efficacy, self-care, and self-concept are crucial aspects of the nurse's role in promoting optimal psychosocial patterns, coping, and stress management skills in patients and caregivers.

Self-efficacy refers to a person's belief in their ability to successfully complete a task or achieve a goal. The nurse can assess self-efficacy by evaluating the patient's confidence in managing their health conditions and performing self-care activities. This assessment can guide the development of personalized interventions to enhance self-efficacy, such as providing education, setting realistic goals, and offering support.

Self-care involves the activities individuals engage in to maintain their physical and emotional well-being. As a rehabilitation registered nurse, it is essential to assess the patient's self-care practices and identify any barriers or challenges they may face. Promoting self-care may involve teaching patients effective self-care strategies, providing resources, and collaborating with the interdisciplinary team to ensure a comprehensive care plan.

Self-concept refers to an individual's perceptions, beliefs, and thoughts about themselves. It influences one's self-esteem, self-worth, and overall mental health. Nurses can assess self-concept by engaging in therapeutic communication, actively listening, and observing the patient's behavior and verbal cues. Promoting a positive self-concept involves providing emotional support, offering validation, and fostering positive relationships.

By assessing and promoting self-efficacy, self-care, and self-concept, rehabilitation registered nurses can empower individuals to effectively cope with stress, manage their health, and foster psychosocial well-being.

2.2.2.7 Accessing supportive team resources and services (e.g., psychologist, clergy, peer support, community support):

Accessing supportive team resources and services is crucial in promoting optimal psychosocial patterns and coping skills for patients and caregivers in rehabilitation nursing. These resources include psychologists, clergymen, peer support, and community support. Psychologists play a vital role in helping individuals manage and overcome psychological issues related to their rehabilitation journey. They provide counseling and therapeutic interventions to address emotional challenges. Clergy members offer spiritual support and guidance, helping patients and caregivers find solace and strength through faith. Peer support groups enable individuals to connect with others who have similar experiences, fostering a sense of belonging and understanding. Community support services provide additional assistance and resources, such as financial aid, housing, and transportation. These services create a comprehensive network of support, ensuring that patients and caregivers receive the necessary assistance throughout their rehabilitation process.

2.2.2.8 Promoting strategies to cope with role and relationship changes (e.g., patient and caregiver counseling, peer support, education):

Promoting strategies to cope with role and relationship changes in the context of rehabilitation nursing involves various interventions aimed at supporting both patients and caregivers. Patient and caregiver counseling is an essential component of this approach, providing a safe space for individuals to express their feelings, concerns, and fears. Peer support groups can also be beneficial, allowing patients and caregivers to connect with others who have experienced similar challenges. Education plays a crucial role in equipping patients and caregivers with the necessary knowledge and skills to navigate role and relationship changes effectively. This education may include information on managing stress, adapting to new routines, and promoting healthy communication. By implementing these strategies, rehabilitation registered nurses can help patients and caregivers cope with the changes they face, ultimately promoting optimal psychosocial patterns and enhancing their overall well-being.

2.2.2.9 Including the patient and caregiver in the plan of care:

Including the patient and caregiver in the plan of care is essential for a Rehabilitation Registered Nurse. This ensures that both individuals actively participate in their own healthcare journey. By involving the patient and caregiver, the nurse can gather important information about the patient's needs, preferences, and goals. This collaboration allows for a more personalized and effective care plan. It also promotes a sense of empowerment and ownership in the patient and caregiver, as they become active participants in decision-making and goal-setting. Additionally, involving the caregiver can improve continuity of care and support for the patient during their rehabilitation process. The nurse should assess the patient's and caregiver's understanding of the care plan, provide education and resources as needed, and regularly evaluate and adjust the plan as necessary. Overall, active inclusion of the patient and caregiver in the plan of care enhances the quality of care and promotes positive outcomes.

2.2.2.10 Incorporating cultural awareness and spiritual values in the plan of care:

Incorporating cultural awareness and spiritual values in the plan of care is an essential aspect of providing holistic and patient-centered care as a Rehabilitation Registered Nurse. Understanding and respecting cultural beliefs, practices, and values can positively impact patient outcomes and promote effective communication with patients and their families.
One important aspect is recognizing the influence of culture on a patient's health beliefs and preferences. This requires acknowledging and respecting cultural diversity, and adapting care plans accordingly. This may involve providing culturally appropriate foods, accommodating religious practices, or facilitating communication with interpreters.
Additionally, incorporating spiritual values ensures that patients' spiritual needs are addressed. This could involve providing opportunities for prayer or meditation, facilitating visits from religious leaders, or involving spiritual guidance in the decision-making process.
By incorporating cultural awareness and spiritual values into the plan of care, Rehabilitation Registered Nurses can foster a supportive and inclusive environment for patients and their families. This approach promotes patient autonomy, trust, and improved health outcomes.

2.2.2.11 Promoting positive interaction among patients and caregivers:

Promoting positive interaction among patients and caregivers is crucial for the holistic care and well-being of individuals receiving rehabilitation services. As a Rehabilitation Registered Nurse, it is important to foster a supportive environment where patients and caregivers can effectively communicate and work together towards their goals.
To promote positive interaction, nurses should encourage open and clear communication between patients and caregivers. This can include providing education on effective communication strategies, such as active listening and empathy. Additionally, nurses can facilitate family meetings or support groups, where patients and caregivers can share their experiences and learn from one another.
Promoting teamwork and collaboration is another essential aspect of positive interaction. Nurses should encourage patients and caregivers to actively participate in care planning and decision-making processes. This can help foster a sense of ownership and empowerment, leading to better outcomes and improved overall satisfaction.
Furthermore, nurses should address any potential conflicts or disagreements that may arise between patients and caregivers. This may involve facilitating open discussions, providing mediation if necessary, and offering emotional support to both parties. By creating a supportive environment, nurses can contribute to the overall well-being and success of their patients and their caregivers.

2.2.2.12 Task 3: Apply the nursing process to optimize the patient's functional ability.:

Task 3: Apply the nursing process to optimize the patient's functional ability involves several important aspects. The nursing process includes five steps: assessment, diagnosis, planning, implementation, and evaluation.
During the assessment phase, the Rehabilitation Registered Nurse gathers information about the patient's current functional abilities, including their physical, cognitive, and emotional status. This information helps identify potential areas of improvement.

Next, the nurse diagnoses the patient's functional limitations and potential barriers to achieving optimal functionality. This involves analyzing the assessment data and identifying specific areas that need attention.

With the diagnosis in mind, the nurse then develops a comprehensive plan to address the patient's functional goals. This plan includes setting specific and measurable objectives, outlining interventions and resources needed, and establishing a timeline for achieving the goals.

The implementation phase involves executing the planned interventions, such as providing physical therapy, occupational therapy, and counseling services. The nurse closely monitors the patient's progress and adjusts the plan as needed.

Lastly, the nurse evaluates the effectiveness of the interventions and the patient's functional improvement. This information helps guide further interventions or adjustments to the plan. This involves assessing the patient's current functionality, diagnosing limitations, planning interventions, implementing the plan, and evaluating outcomes.

2.2.3   Knowledge of:

As a Rehabilitation Registered Nurse, it is important to have a comprehensive understanding of the topic of "Knowledge of" under the broad topic of "Task 3: Apply the nursing process to optimize the patient's functional ability, Functional Health Patterns."

This topic encompasses various aspects that are crucial for a Rehabilitation Registered Nurse to be proficient in. Firstly, understanding the anatomy and physiology of the human body is essential. This includes knowledge of the musculoskeletal, neurological, and cardiopulmonary systems.

Additionally, knowledge of common illnesses and injuries that require rehabilitation is vital. This includes conditions such as strokes, spinal cord injuries, amputations, and joint replacements.

Furthermore, it is important to have knowledge of various techniques and interventions used in rehabilitation, such as therapeutic exercises, mobilization, and assistive devices. Understanding the principles of safe body mechanics and proper positioning is also crucial.

Moreover, having knowledge of the psychological and emotional aspects of rehabilitation is important. This includes understanding the impact of illness or injury on a patient's mental health and providing appropriate support and counseling.

2.2.3.1   Anatomy, physiology, and interventions related to musculoskeletal, respiratory, cardiovascular, and neurological function:

Anatomy, physiology, and interventions related to musculoskeletal, respiratory, cardiovascular, and neurological function are essential aspects of a Rehabilitation Registered Nurse's knowledge. Understanding the structure and function of the musculoskeletal system helps in identifying and addressing issues related to bones, joints, and muscles. Respiratory function involves the study of breathing and the management of conditions like asthma or chronic obstructive pulmonary disease. The cardiovascular system's anatomy and physiology provide insights into heart function and circulation, assisting in the treatment of conditions like hypertension or heart failure. Knowledge of neurological function is crucial in assessing and managing disorders like stroke or traumatic brain injuries. Interventions related to these functions encompass various approaches such as exercises, therapeutic modalities, medications, and patient education. Overall, applying the nursing process to optimize patients' functional abilities requires a deep understanding of anatomy, physiology, and implementing appropriate interventions targeted at the musculoskeletal, respiratory, cardiovascular, and neurological systems.

2.2.3.2   Assistive devices and technology (e.g., mobility aids, orthostatic devices, orthotic devices):

Assistive devices and technology play a crucial role in optimizing a patient's functional ability during rehabilitation. These devices include mobility aids such as canes, walkers, and wheelchairs, which help individuals with mobility impairments to move around independently. Orthostatic devices, like standing frames and tilt tables, assist patients in maintaining an upright position and preventing orthostatic hypotension. Orthotic devices, such as braces and splints, provide support and alignment to body parts affected by injury or disability.

These assistive devices and technologies are designed to improve the patient's overall functional health pattern by promoting independence, enhancing mobility, and preventing further complications. By utilizing these devices, rehabilitation registered nurses can help patients regain their independence, improve their mobility, and increase their overall quality of life. It is important for nurses to assess the patient's specific needs, educate them about the proper use of assistive devices, and monitor their progress to ensure optimal outcomes. By incorporating assistive devices and technology into the nursing process, Rehabilitation Registered Nurses can effectively optimize the functional ability of their patients.

2.2.3.3   Clinical signs of sensorimotor deficits:

Clinical signs of sensorimotor deficits refer to the physical manifestations observed in patients with impaired sensory and motor functions. These deficits can occur due to various health conditions such as stroke, spinal cord injury, traumatic brain injury, or peripheral neuropathy.

These signs may include muscle weakness or paralysis, decreased coordination, loss of sensation, reduced range of motion, altered gait or balance, difficulty with fine motor skills, and impaired reflexes. Patients may also experience pain, tingling, or numbness in the affected areas.

Assessment of sensorimotor deficits involves conducting comprehensive evaluations to identify specific deficits and their impact on the patient's functional abilities. This includes testing muscle strength, coordination, sensation, balance, and reflexes. Observing the patient's ability to perform daily activities assists in determining the extent of impairment and planning appropriate rehabilitation interventions.

Effective management of sensorimotor deficits requires a multidisciplinary approach involving collaboration between rehabilitation registered nurses, physical therapists, occupational therapists, and other healthcare professionals. Treatment strategies may include therapeutic exercises, assistive devices, adaptive techniques, and education to promote optimal functional ability and independence. Close monitoring and follow-up are essential to track progress and make necessary adjustments to the rehabilitation plan.

2.2.3.4   Activity tolerance and energy conservation:

Activity tolerance and energy conservation are important considerations in optimizing a patient's functional ability during rehabilitation. Activity tolerance refers to the amount and intensity of physical activity a patient can safely perform without experiencing excessive fatigue or discomfort. It is crucial to assess and monitor activity tolerance to tailor an individualized exercise program that promotes gradual progression and prevents overexertion.

On the other hand, energy conservation techniques are strategies used to minimize energy expenditure during daily activities. This involves teaching patients to pace their activities, prioritize tasks, and use energy-efficient body mechanics. By conserving energy, patients can maintain and increase their ability to perform essential tasks while minimizing fatigue and avoiding excessive stress on their bodies.

By implementing both activity tolerance assessment and energy conservation techniques, rehabilitation registered nurses can help patients regain and maintain their highest level of functional ability. This holistic approach takes into account the individual's physical condition and limitations, promoting a safe and effective rehabilitation process.

2.2.3.5   Pharmacology (e.g., antispasmodics, anticholinergics, antidepressants, analgesics):

Pharmacology plays a crucial role in the field of rehabilitation nursing. It involves the study of various medications and their effects on the body's systems. There are several types of drugs commonly used in rehabilitation nursing, including antispasmodics, anticholinergics, antidepressants, and analgesics.

Antispasmodics are drugs that help relieve muscle spasms and cramps. They work by directly relaxing the muscles, thereby reducing pain and improving mobility. These medications are often prescribed to patients with conditions such as spasticity, multiple sclerosis, or spinal cord injuries.

Anticholinergics are medications that block the action of acetylcholine, a neurotransmitter involved in muscle contractions. They are primarily used to treat conditions such as overactive bladder or urinary incontinence by relaxing the bladder muscles.

Antidepressants are commonly prescribed to patients experiencing symptoms of depression or anxiety. They work by balancing certain chemicals in the brain, improving mood, and alleviating psychological distress.

Analgesics, also known as pain relievers, are drugs that reduce or eliminate pain. They can be categorized into two types: non-opioid analgesics (such as acetaminophen and nonsteroidal anti-inflammatory drugs) and opioid analgesics (such as morphine and oxycodone). These medications are frequently used to manage pain during rehabilitation and promote better functional mobility.

As a rehabilitation registered nurse, it is crucial to have a solid understanding of pharmacology so that appropriate medications can be administered to optimize the patient's functional ability. By accurately assessing the patient's needs and collaborating with other healthcare professionals, nurses can ensure that the right medications are prescribed and monitor their effectiveness and potential side effects. This knowledge enables nurses to provide holistic care and enhance the patient's overall rehabilitation experience.

2.2.3.6   Safety concerns (e.g., falls, burns, skin integrity, infection prevention):

As a Rehabilitation Registered Nurse, it is crucial to have knowledge about safety concerns that may arise during the patient's rehabilitation process. These concerns include falls, burns, skin integrity, and infection prevention. Falls pose a significant risk, especially for patients with mobility issues. It is essential to assess and implement fall prevention strategies, such as using bed alarms and assisting patients with mobilization. Burns can occur due to hot substances, electrical equipment, or improper use of heating pads. Monitoring the environment for potential burn hazards and providing education on proper usage can help prevent burns. Maintaining skin integrity is vital to prevent pressure ulcers and skin breakdown. Regular repositioning, proper hygiene, and adequate nutrition are crucial in promoting skin health. Additionally, infection prevention measures, such as hand hygiene, proper wound care, and use of personal protective equipment, are essential to prevent secondary complications. By addressing these safety concerns, Rehabilitation Registered Nurses can optimize the patient's functional ability and promote a safe and successful rehabilitation journey.

2.2.3.7   Self-care activities (e.g., activities of daily living, instrumental activities of daily living):

Self-care activities refer to the tasks that individuals perform daily to take care of themselves and maintain their functional ability. These activities encompass both basic activities of daily living (ADLs) and instrumental activities of daily living (IADLs). ADLs include tasks such as eating, bathing, dressing, grooming, toileting, and transferring. On the other hand, IADLs involve more complex activities like managing finances, meal preparation, housekeeping, and transportation.

As a Rehabilitation Registered Nurse, it is crucial to have a comprehensive understanding of self-care activities to optimize a patient's functional ability. Assessing a patient's ability to perform these tasks independently or with assistance is essential to create an individualized care plan. This plan may involve providing education and training, recommending assistive devices, or collaborating with other healthcare professionals.

By addressing and supporting the patient's self-care activities, Rehabilitation Registered Nurses can facilitate the patient's independence and improve their overall quality of life. Moreover, optimizing self-care abilities can also contribute to the patient's ability to live in their preferred environment and reduce the need for institutional care.

2.2.4   Skill in:

As a Rehabilitation Registered Nurse, having the skill in optimizing the patient's functional ability is crucial. This skill involves the ability to thoroughly assess the patient's current functional status and identify areas for improvement. The nurse must be skilled in using various assessment tools and techniques to evaluate the patient's overall physical, cognitive, and emotional capabilities. Additionally, the nurse should have knowledge about different therapeutic interventions and exercises that can enhance the patient's functional abilities. This includes knowing how to perform and teach range of motion exercises, strength training, balance training, and coordination exercises. Furthermore, the nurse should have the ability to create personalized care plans and set realistic goals for the patient's rehabilitation journey. By utilizing this skill effectively, the nurse can help patients regain their independence and improve their quality of life.

2.2.4.1   Assessing and implementing interventions to prevent musculoskeletal, respiratory, cardiovascular, and neurological complications (e.g., motor and sensory impairments, contractures, heterotrophic ossification, aspiration, pain):

When working as a Rehabilitation Registered Nurse, assessing and implementing interventions to prevent complications in patients is a crucial part of optimizing their functional ability. This involves assessing and addressing potential musculoskeletal, respiratory, cardiovascular, and neurological complications that may arise. For example, the nurse must evaluate for motor and sensory impairments, contractures, heterotrophic ossification, aspiration, and pain.

To prevent musculoskeletal complications, the nurse may implement range of motion exercises and promote proper body alignment. Respiratory complications can be prevented by encouraging deep breathing and coughing techniques. Cardiovascular complications can be mitigated by monitoring vital signs and promoting physical activity as tolerated. Neurological complications, such as sensory impairments, may require specialized assessments and interventions.

Preventing contractures and heterotrophic ossification involves positioning the patient properly and implementing range of motion exercises. To address aspiration, the nurse may evaluate swallowing function and recommend modified diets or feeding techniques. Managing pain may require a multi-modal approach, including pain assessments and appropriate pain management strategies. Through a comprehensive nursing process, their focus is on optimizing the patient's functional ability and overall well-being.

2.2.4.2 Assessing, implementing, and evaluating interventions for self- care ability and mobility:

In the field of rehabilitation nursing, it is crucial for registered nurses to assess, implement, and evaluate interventions to enhance the self-care ability and mobility of their patients.

Assessment entails gathering information about the patient's functional ability and current limitations. This may involve obtaining a comprehensive health history, conducting physical examinations, and utilizing standardized assessment tools. The information collected guides the development of personalized care plans.

Implementation of interventions involves the selection and application of appropriate strategies to improve self-care ability and mobility. This may include teaching patients self-care techniques, facilitating exercises, providing assistive devices, and collaborating with other healthcare professionals.

Evaluation is an ongoing process to determine the effectiveness of the interventions implemented. Nurses need to monitor the patient's progress, reassess their functional ability, and make adjustments to the care plan as necessary.

Overall, the goal is to optimize the patient's functional ability, ensure safety and independence, and support their overall well-being.

2.2.4.3 Implementing safety interventions (e.g., sitters, reorientation, environment, redirection, non-behavioral restraints):

Implementing safety interventions is an important aspect of optimizing a patient's functional ability, which is essential for rehabilitation registered nurses. These interventions include the use of sitters, reorientation, modifying the environment, redirection, and non-behavioral restraints.

Sitters are trained individuals who stay with patients to ensure their safety and prevent falls or other accidents. They provide constant supervision and assistance as needed.

Reorientation techniques help patients regain their cognitive function and orientation to time, place, and person. This may involve reminding them of their surroundings, providing visual cues, and engaging them in meaningful activities.

Modifying the environment involves removing potential hazards and ensuring a safe and secure space. This includes adjusting lighting, securing furniture, and providing handrails or grab bars.

Redirection techniques are used to redirect a patient's attention away from potentially harmful behaviors or actions. This may involve engaging them in conversation, offering activities or hobbies they enjoy, or providing sensory stimulation.

Non-behavioral restraints are used as a last resort to ensure patient safety when all other interventions have failed. These restraints should be used only when absolutely necessary and in accordance with ethical guidelines.

Overall, implementing safety interventions plays a crucial role in optimizing a patient's functional ability and ensuring their well-being throughout the rehabilitation process.

2.2.4.4 Using technology and assistive devices (e.g., mobility aids, pressure relief devices, informatics, assistive software):

Using technology and assistive devices are integral components in optimizing a patient's functional ability in rehabilitation nursing. These devices include mobility aids such as wheelchairs, crutches, and walkers, which help individuals with impaired mobility to regain their independence. Pressure relief devices are also essential to prevent pressure ulcers and promote healing in patients who are bedridden or have limited mobility. Informatics plays a crucial role in improving patient care, as it allows for better documentation, communication, and coordination among healthcare providers. Assistive software, on the other hand, enhances the patient's ability to perform certain tasks and promotes independence in areas such as communication, cognitive functioning, and self-care. By incorporating technology and assistive devices, rehabilitation registered nurses maximize their patients' functional abilities, promote autonomy, and improve overall patient outcomes.

2.2.4.5 Teaching interventions to prevent complications of immobility (e.g., skin integrity, DVT prevention):

Teaching interventions to prevent complications related to immobility are crucial in optimizing a patient's functional ability during rehabilitation. One important aspect of this topic is focusing on maintaining skin integrity. Immobility often leads to the development of pressure ulcers, which can result in significant discomfort and complications. Therefore, education regarding regular repositioning, adequate nutrition, and appropriate wound care is essential.

Another significant concern is the prevention of deep vein thrombosis (DVT). Prolonged immobility increases the risk of blood clots forming in the deep veins, which can be life-threatening if they travel to the lungs. Teaching interventions encompass promoting early mobility, utilizing compression stockings, and educating patients on recognizing signs and symptoms of DVT.

Overall, teaching interventions to prevent complications of immobility in the realms of skin integrity and DVT prevention are crucial for rehabilitation registered nurses. By providing education, healthcare professionals can empower patients to actively participate in their care and maintain optimal functional ability.

2.2.4.6 Task 4: Apply the nursing process to optimize management of the patient's neurological and other complex medical conditions.:

Task 4 focuses on the application of the nursing process to optimize the management of patients with neurological and other complex medical conditions. This process involves several key steps to ensure comprehensive care.

Firstly, the nurse assesses the patient's condition, including their neurological function and other medical issues. This assessment helps identify any neurologic impairments or complex medical needs that require attention.

Next, the nurse develops a care plan based on the assessment findings. This plan includes goals and interventions tailored to address the patient's specific needs.

The nurse then implements the care plan, providing the necessary treatments and interventions to manage the patient's neurological and other complex conditions. This may involve administering medications, monitoring vital signs, providing emotional support, and facilitating therapies.

Throughout the process, the nurse continuously evaluates the patient's progress and adjusts the care plan accordingly.

By following this systematic approach, the nurse can optimize the management of the patient's neurological and complex medical conditions. This ensures that the patient receives holistic and individualized care to promote their overall well-being and recovery.

2.2.5   Knowledge of:

A Rehabilitation Registered Nurse should possess a comprehensive understanding of the topic 'Knowledge of:' in order to effectively optimize the management of a patient's neurological and other complex medical conditions. This knowledge encompasses various key aspects that are vital for the nurse's practice.

One important aspect is an understanding of the nursing process, which involves a systematic approach to patient care. This process includes assessment, diagnosis, planning, implementation, and evaluation.

In terms of neurological conditions, the nurse should be knowledgeable about the anatomy and physiology of the nervous system. This includes understanding the different regions and functions of the brain, spinal cord, and peripheral nerves.

The nurse should also be well-versed in the signs and symptoms of neurological disorders such as stroke, traumatic brain injury, and spinal cord injuries.

Furthermore, it is crucial for the nurse to have a good grasp of the principles of rehabilitation, including strategies for promoting functional independence, managing pain, preventing complications, and facilitating the patient's adaptation to their condition.

Other important areas of knowledge include pharmacology, as the nurse needs to be familiar with the medications commonly used in the management of neurological conditions, and the application of evidence-based practice in order to provide the best possible care to the patient.

2.2.5.1   Measurement tools (e.g., Rancho Los Amigos, Glasgow, Mini Mental State Examination, ASIA, pain analog scales):

Measurement tools play a crucial role in the assessment and management of patients with neurological and complex medical conditions in rehabilitation nursing. These tools help to objectively measure and track the patient's progress and functional abilities throughout their rehabilitation journey.

One commonly used measurement tool is the Rancho Los Amigos Scale, which assesses the cognitive function and level of consciousness of patients with acquired brain injuries. Another tool, the Glasgow Coma Scale, is used to assess the level of consciousness in patients with neurological conditions.

The Mini Mental State Examination is a cognitive screening tool that helps evaluate a patient's cognitive function, such as memory and attention. The ASIA (American Spinal Injury Association) impairment scale is used to assess and classify the extent and severity of spinal cord injuries.

Additionally, pain analog scales are used to assess the intensity and severity of pain experienced by patients. These scales involve the patient self-reporting their pain level on a numerical or visual representation.

By utilizing these measurement tools, rehabilitation registered nurses can effectively monitor the progress and outcomes of their patients, tailor their treatment plans, and optimize the management of their neurological and complex medical conditions.

2.2.5.2   Neuroanatomy and physiology (e.g., cognition, judgment, sensation, perception):

Neuroanatomy and physiology are crucial aspects for a Rehabilitation Registered Nurse to understand in order to effectively manage patients with complex medical conditions. Cognition refers to the mental processes involved in gaining knowledge and understanding. Judgment refers to the ability to make decisions based on available information. Sensation and perception involve the way we interpret and make sense of the stimuli around us.

Neuroanatomy focuses on the structure and organization of the nervous system, including the brain, spinal cord, and nerves. Physiology, on the other hand, deals with the functioning of these structures and how they contribute to cognition, judgment, sensation, and perception.

For instance, cognition is influenced by various brain regions, such as the frontal lobe, which is responsible for reasoning and problem-solving, and the hippocampus, which is involved in memory formation. Judgment is influenced by the prefrontal cortex, which manages decision-making and impulse control. Sensation and perception rely on sensory areas of the cerebral cortex, such as the visual cortex for processing visual information and the auditory cortex for processing sound.

By understanding the neuroanatomy and physiology of these processes, Rehabilitation Registered Nurses can better assess and support patients with neurological conditions, implement appropriate treatment plans, and enhance their overall rehabilitation outcomes.

2.2.5.3   Pain (e.g., receptors, acute, chronic, theories):

Pain is a complex phenomenon that can be categorized into two main types: acute and chronic. Acute pain is often the result of injury or surgery and is typically short-lived. Chronic pain, on the other hand, persists over a long period of time and may be caused by conditions such as arthritis or nerve damage.

Pain is detected by specialized nerve endings called pain receptors, also known as nociceptors. These receptors are found throughout the body and respond to various stimuli, such as pressure, temperature, and chemical changes.

Different theories attempt to explain how pain is experienced and processed by the body. The gate control theory suggests that pain signals are regulated by a "gate" mechanism in the spinal cord, which can be influenced by other factors such as emotions or distractions. The neuromatrix theory proposes that pain is a complex experience influenced by sensory, cognitive, and emotional factors.

As a Rehabilitation Registered Nurse, understanding the mechanisms of pain, such as receptors and theories, is crucial in optimizing the management of patients' neurological and other complex medical conditions. By assessing and addressing their pain needs, nurses can improve patients' overall well-being and facilitate their rehabilitation process.

2.2.5.4 Pharmacology (e.g., antispasmodics, anticholinergics, antidepressants, analgesics):

Pharmacology, a vital aspect of nursing practice, encompasses the use of medications to treat various medical conditions. In the context of rehabilitation nursing, specific drug classes such as antispasmodics, anticholinergics, antidepressants, and analgesics are commonly used to optimize patient care. Antispasmodics, like baclofen, help alleviate muscle spasms and rigidity often seen in neurological conditions. Anticholinergics, such as benztropine, can be used to manage tremors and rigidity in Parkinson's disease. Antidepressants, like selective serotonin reuptake inhibitors (SSRIs) or tricyclic antidepressants (TCAs), may address mood disorders and neuropathic pain. Furthermore, analgesics like opioids or nonsteroidal anti-inflammatory drugs (NSAIDs) aid in managing pain experienced by patients. Understanding the pharmacokinetics, adverse effects, and interactions of these medications is crucial for the rehabilitation registered nurse to provide optimal care. Consequently, it is imperative for nurses to continuously update their knowledge and collaborate with other healthcare professionals to ensure safe and effective medication management.

2.2.5.5 Safety concerns (e.g., seizure precautions, fall precautions, impaired judgment):

The topic of safety concerns in the context of neurological and complex medical conditions involves various aspects that need to be considered by Rehabilitation Registered Nurses. One important safety concern is seizure precautions, which involves implementing measures to reduce the risk of seizures and ensuring patient safety during a seizure episode. This may include creating a safe environment, educating patients and caregivers about seizure management, and administering medications as prescribed.

Another safety concern is fall precautions, particularly for patients with impaired mobility or balance. Nurses should assess the patient's risk of falling, implement appropriate preventive measures such as bed alarms or assistive devices, and regularly monitor and evaluate the effectiveness of these precautions to ensure patient safety.

Additionally, impaired judgment is a critical safety concern that may be present in patients with neurological or other complex medical conditions. Nurses should closely assess patients' cognitive functioning and decision-making abilities, and take necessary steps to protect them from harm, such as providing supervision, removing potential hazards, and involving family or caregivers in the care plan.

2.2.5.6 Medical equipment and technology (e.g., LVAD, assisted ventilation):

Medical equipment and technology play a crucial role in optimizing the management of patients with neurological and other complex medical conditions in rehabilitation nursing. One important area is the use of LVADs (Left Ventricular Assist Devices) for patients with severe heart failure. LVADs are mechanical pumps that help the heart pump blood throughout the body. They can provide temporary support while waiting for a heart transplant or as a permanent solution.

Assisted ventilation is another key aspect. It involves the use of ventilators to support patients who are unable to breathe adequately on their own. This technology delivers oxygen and removes carbon dioxide, supporting respiratory function.

Rehabilitation registered nurses must have knowledge and skills in operating and monitoring the use of these medical technologies. They need to understand the indications, contraindications, and potential complications associated with LVADs and assisted ventilation. They also play a vital role in educating patients and their families about these devices and providing necessary support and care. By staying up-to-date with advancements in medical equipment and technology, rehabilitation nurses can optimize patient outcomes and contribute to their overall well-being.

2.2.5.7 Central lines, ports, and catheters (e.g., triple lumen, hemodialysis):

Central lines, ports, and catheters are medical devices commonly used in the management of complex medical conditions in patients. They serve as a means to access the circulatory system for various purposes such as administration of medications, fluids, or blood products, as well as monitoring of central venous pressure. Triple lumen catheters are often used for hemodialysis, allowing blood to be filtered and cleansed when the kidneys are unable to perform this function adequately. These devices are generally inserted by trained healthcare professionals using strict sterile techniques to minimize the risk of infection. Nurses play a crucial role in the care and maintenance of central lines, ports, and catheters, ensuring proper flushing, dressing changes, and monitoring for complications such as infection or clotting. The knowledge and skills required for their management are essential for rehabilitation registered nurses to optimize patient outcomes.

2.2.6 Skill in:

As a Rehabilitation Registered Nurse, it is crucial to possess various skills to effectively manage the patient's neurological and other complex medical conditions. These skills include:

1. Assessment: The ability to conduct thorough assessments of a patient's condition, including physical, cognitive, and psychological factors.
2. Planning: Developing goal-oriented and individualized care plans based on the patient's needs and collaborating with the interdisciplinary team.
3. Implementation: Carrying out interventions and therapies to promote the patient's functional abilities, such as mobility exercises, cognitive training, and pain management.
4. Evaluation: Regularly assessing the effectiveness of interventions and adapting the care plan accordingly.
5. Communication: Effectively communicating with patients, families, and healthcare professionals to ensure comprehensive care and patient education.
6. Documentation: Maintaining accurate and detailed records of the patient's progress, treatment plans, and responses to interventions.
7. Critical Thinking: Applying critical thinking skills to analyze complex situations, make informed decisions, and prioritize patient care.

By honing these fundamental skills, Rehabilitation Registered Nurses can optimize the management of their patients' neurological and complex medical conditions to achieve positive outcomes.

2.2.6.1 Assessing cognition, perception, sensation, apraxia, perseveration, and pain:

Assessing cognition, perception, sensation, apraxia, perseveration, and pain are important aspects of managing a patient's neurological and complex medical conditions in the field of rehabilitation nursing. Cognition refers to mental processes such as memory, attention, and problem-solving, while perception involves the interpretation of sensory information. Sensation assessment evaluates the patient's ability to feel or respond to stimuli. Apraxia assessment focuses on evaluating the patient's ability to perform purposeful movements. Perseveration assessment looks at the patient's tendency to repeat actions or thoughts. Pain assessment is crucial for identifying and managing the patient's discomfort. These assessments aid in understanding the patient's functional health patterns and designing individualized rehabilitation plans. By applying the nursing process, rehabilitation registered nurses can optimize the management of patients' neurological and complex medical conditions, ensuring improved outcomes.

2.2.6.2 Implementing and evaluating strategies for safety (e.g., personal response devices, alarms, helmets, padding):

Implementing and evaluating strategies for safety is a crucial aspect of the rehabilitation nurse's role in optimizing patient management. These strategies may include the use of personal response devices, alarms, helmets, and padding. Personal response devices can enhance patient safety by allowing them to call for help when needed. Alarms can be used to alert healthcare providers when a patient is in distress or attempting to leave a safe environment. Helmets and padding can protect patients from injury during falls or seizures. The nurse must assess the patient's needs, determine the appropriate safety measures to implement, and regularly evaluate their effectiveness. This involves monitoring the patient's response to the safety strategies, ensuring proper use and fit of devices, and making necessary adjustments to enhance safety. By implementing and evaluating these strategies, the rehabilitation nurse can create a safer environment for their patients.

2.2.6.3 Teaching strategies for neurological deficits:

Teaching strategies for neurological deficits are crucial for Rehabilitation Registered Nurses. These strategies aim to optimize patient management by addressing complex medical conditions and functional health patterns. One important aspect is assessing the patient's current deficits and understanding their specific neurological condition. This helps in tailoring individualized teaching plans. Proper communication and collaboration with the patient and their family is essential to ensure understanding and participation. Nurses must use clear and concise language, provide visual aids, and utilize repetition to enhance learning. Breaking down complex tasks into smaller, easy-to-understand steps can facilitate the patient's ability to absorb and apply new information. In addition, incorporating different teaching methods such as demonstrations, role-playing, and hands-on activities can enhance comprehension and retention. Continuous evaluation of the patient's progress is important to modify teaching strategies accordingly. By employing these teaching strategies, Rehabilitation Registered Nurses can help patients with neurological deficits achieve optimal outcomes in their rehabilitation journey.

2.2.6.4 Teaching strategies for pain and comfort management (e.g., pharmacological, nonpharmacological):

Teaching strategies for pain and comfort management are crucial for rehabilitation registered nurses in optimizing the management of patients' neurological and complex medical conditions. These strategies encompass both pharmacological and nonpharmacological approaches.

Pharmacological interventions involve the use of medications to relieve pain and provide comfort. Nurses must have a deep understanding of various pain medications and their side effects. They should educate patients on the appropriate use of these medications, potential adverse effects, and the importance of adhering to prescribed dosages.

Nonpharmacological interventions focus on holistic approaches to pain and comfort management. Nurses can teach patients relaxation techniques, such as deep breathing exercises and guided imagery, to help reduce pain and promote comfort. Additionally, physical therapy, massage, and heat/cold therapy can provide relief.

Patient education plays a vital role in pain and comfort management. Rehabilitation registered nurses must effectively communicate with patients and their families to empower them with knowledge about pain management strategies. By incorporating both pharmacological and nonpharmacological approaches into teaching strategies, nurses can optimize patient outcomes and overall well-being.

2.2.6.5 Using medical equipment and technology (e.g., TENS unit, baclofen pump, LVAD):

Using medical equipment and technology plays a crucial role in optimizing the management of patients' neurological and other complex medical conditions for the Rehabilitation Registered Nurse. One important piece of equipment is the TENS unit, which stands for Transcutaneous Electrical Nerve Stimulation. It helps relieve pain by sending low-voltage electrical currents through electrodes placed on the skin. Another device is the baclofen pump, which delivers the medication directly into the spinal cord to treat spasticity. It is especially useful in patients with conditions such as spinal cord injury or multiple sclerosis. Additionally, the Left Ventricular Assist Device (LVAD) is a mechanical pump implanted in patients with heart failure to support and improve heart function. Understanding how to properly use and monitor these devices is crucial for the Rehabilitation Registered Nurse's role in patient care. By effectively applying the nursing process, the nurse can ensure optimal outcomes for patients with complex medical conditions.

2.2.6.6 Implementing behavioral management strategies (e.g., contracts, positive reinforcement, rule setting):

Implementing behavioral management strategies is an integral aspect of the Rehabilitation Registered Nurse's role in optimizing the management of patients with neurological and other complex medical conditions. These strategies include the use of contracts, positive reinforcement, and rule setting.

Contracts help establish clear expectations and goals between the nurse and the patient, ensuring a collaborative approach to care. Positive reinforcement involves offering rewards or praise to encourage desired behaviors or outcomes, motivating patients to actively participate in their rehabilitation. Rule setting is important in providing structure and boundaries, helping patients understand and adhere to the necessary protocols for their recovery.

By employing these strategies, Rehabilitation Registered Nurses can effectively address behavioral issues, promote patient engagement, and enhance the overall effectiveness of the nursing process. Their implementation allows for a patient-centered approach, empowering individuals to take an active role in their own healing journey while ensuring a safe and conducive environment for their rehabilitation.

2.2.6.7 Teaching the patients and the caregivers about the purpose and caring for central lines, ports, and catheters:

Teaching patients and caregivers about the purpose and care of central lines, ports, and catheters is crucial for their management during rehabilitation. Central lines, ports, and catheters are commonly used in patients with complex medical conditions to deliver medication, fluids, or nutrients directly into the bloodstream. By educating patients and caregivers about these devices, they can better understand their purpose and importance in their overall care. Providing clear instructions on how to properly clean, flush, and care for these devices ensures their optimal functioning and reduces the risk of infection. Additionally, teaching patients and caregivers about the signs and symptoms of complications related to central lines, ports, and catheters enables prompt intervention and improves patient outcomes. Overall, educating patients and caregivers about the purpose and care of these devices empowers them to actively participate in their treatment and promotes safe and effective management during rehabilitation.

2.2.6.8 Task 5: Apply the nursing process to optimize the patient's ability to communicate effectively.:

Task 5: Apply the nursing process to optimize the patient's ability to communicate effectively in rehabilitation settings is a critical aspect of patient care. Effective communication is crucial for understanding the patient's needs, concerns, and goals, and it helps develop a strong nurse-patient relationship.

In order to optimize communication, nurses can follow the nursing process, which consists of assessing, diagnosing, planning, implementing, and evaluating the patient's condition and needs. During the assessment phase, nurses can observe the patient's communication skills, identify any barriers or difficulties, and gather information about their preferred mode of communication.

Based on this assessment, nurses can diagnose any communication issues or deficits that may be affecting the patient's ability to effectively communicate. This involves analyzing the data collected during the assessment phase and identifying relevant nursing diagnoses related to communication.

After the diagnosis, nurses can develop a plan of care to address the identified communication issues. This may include interventions such as providing adaptive communication devices, facilitating communication aids or techniques, or providing education to the patient and their families on effective communication strategies.

The next step is the implementation of the care plan, which involves putting the interventions into action. Nurses can collaborate with other healthcare team members, such as speech therapists or occupational therapists, to provide comprehensive care and support the patient's communication needs.

Lastly, evaluating the effectiveness of the interventions is crucial to determine if the patient's ability to communicate effectively has improved. Nurses can use various assessment tools or techniques to measure the patient's progress and make any necessary adjustments to the care plan.

By applying the nursing process, rehabilitation registered nurses can play a vital role in optimizing the patient's ability to communicate effectively, ultimately enhancing their overall quality of life and facilitating their recovery process.

2.2.7 Knowledge in:

Knowledge of communication is crucial for a Rehabilitation Registered Nurse to effectively optimize the patient's ability to communicate. This includes understanding different communication methods, such as verbal, nonverbal, and alternative communication strategies. The nurse should have knowledge of various functional health patterns related to communication, such as language abilities, hearing impairments, and cognitive impairments. They should also be familiar with assessment tools to evaluate the patient's communication skills and identify any limitations or barriers. Additionally, the nurse should possess knowledge about therapeutic interventions and techniques to promote effective communication, such as active listening, clarification, and the use of visual aids. Understanding cultural and individual differences in communication styles is also essential. By utilizing this knowledge, the Rehabilitation Registered Nurse can create a supportive environment and develop tailored interventions to optimize the patient's ability to communicate effectively during the rehabilitation process.

2.2.7.1 Anatomy and physiology (e.g., cognition, comprehension, sensory deficits):

Anatomy and physiology refers to the study of the structure and function of the human body. In relation to cognition, comprehension, and sensory deficits, it is important for a Rehabilitation Registered Nurse to have a solid understanding of these concepts. Cognition refers to the mental processes involved in acquiring knowledge and understanding, such as thinking, memory, and problem-solving. Comprehension is the ability to understand and interpret information, while sensory deficits relate to impaired or decreased sensory function, such as vision or hearing loss. In order to effectively optimize a patient's ability to communicate, a nurse must be knowledgeable about how these processes and deficits can impact communication. This includes understanding the pathways and structures involved in communication, as well as the impact of sensory deficits on a patient's ability to send and receive messages. Nurses must be able to assess and evaluate these areas to develop appropriate interventions and strategies to support effective communication for their patients.

2.2.7.2 Communication techniques (e.g., active listening, anger management, reflection):

Communication techniques, such as active listening, anger management, and reflection, are crucial for rehabilitation registered nurses to optimize a patient's ability to communicate effectively. Active listening involves giving full attention to what the patient is saying, using non-verbal cues to indicate understanding, and providing feedback to show that their feelings and thoughts are being heard. Anger management techniques help nurses respond calmly and empathetically to patients who may express anger or frustration, ensuring a therapeutic environment. Reflection involves analyzing one's own communication style and identifying areas for improvement in order to enhance patient-centered care. By applying these techniques, nurses can foster trust and rapport with patients, promote effective communication, and ultimately improve patient outcomes in the rehabilitation setting.

2.2.7.3   Cultural diversity:

Cultural diversity refers to the coexistence of various cultures within a society or organization. It encompasses differences in language, beliefs, traditions, values, and behaviors. Understanding cultural diversity is crucial for a Rehabilitation Registered Nurse as it directly impacts patient care and communication. By acknowledging and respecting cultural differences, nurses can optimize a patient's ability to effectively communicate their needs and concerns. They need to be knowledgeable about the cultural norms, customs, and preferences of their patients to provide culturally sensitive care. Nurses should also be aware of the potential barriers that cultural diversity can pose and find ways to overcome them. This includes using interpreters, providing translated materials, utilizing non-verbal communication, and being mindful of body language. By embracing cultural diversity, Rehabilitation Registered Nurses can foster an inclusive and equitable healthcare environment that promotes a patient's overall well-being.

2.2.7.4   Developmental factors:

Developmental factors refer to the age-related changes that occur throughout a person's life and impact their ability to communicate effectively. These factors are important for a Rehabilitation Registered Nurse to consider in order to optimize patient communication. Infants and young children have limited communication skills and may rely on nonverbal cues. They may also have difficulty understanding complex language.
Adolescents are developing their communication skills but may struggle with expressing their emotions and thoughts effectively.
Adults typically have well-developed communication skills but may face challenges due to physical or cognitive impairments.
Elderly individuals may experience age-related changes that affect their communication, such as hearing loss or memory decline.
Understanding these developmental factors allows the Rehabilitation Registered Nurse to tailor communication strategies and techniques to meet the needs of each patient. This ensures effective communication and promotes patient engagement in their rehabilitation process.

2.2.7.5   Linguistic deficits (e.g., aphasia, dysarthria, language barriers):

Linguistic deficits, including aphasia, dysarthria, and language barriers, can significantly impact a patient's ability to communicate effectively. Aphasia is a language disorder often caused by stroke or other brain injuries, leading to difficulty understanding or producing speech. Dysarthria is a condition that affects the muscles used for speech, resulting in slurred or unclear speech. Language barriers can arise when patients and healthcare providers do not share a common language, making it challenging to convey needs or understand medical instructions. As a Rehabilitation Registered Nurse, it is crucial to address these linguistic deficits to optimize patient communication. This includes using alternative communication methods, such as visual aids or technology, working with speech-language pathologists to develop strategies, and collaborating with interpreters or language services to bridge language barriers. Understanding these deficits and implementing appropriate interventions can improve patient outcomes and overall communication in rehabilitation settings.

2.2.7.6   Assistive technology and adaptive equipment:

Assistive technology and adaptive equipment play a crucial role in optimizing a patient's ability to communicate effectively in the field of rehabilitation nursing. These devices are designed to assist individuals with physical disabilities, cognitive impairments, or communication disorders.
Assistive technology includes devices such as speech synthesizers, augmentative and alternative communication tools, or text-to-speech software. These technologies aid patients in expressing themselves and interacting with others.
Adaptive equipment, on the other hand, focuses on modifying the environment to meet an individual's specific needs. This may involve providing wheelchairs, walkers, or home modifications to improve mobility and accessibility.
By utilizing assistive technology and adaptive equipment, rehabilitation registered nurses can enhance the patient's functional health patterns, allowing them to engage in meaningful communication and improve their overall quality of life. These tools not only assist patients in expressing their needs but also facilitate their participation in social interactions and activities.

2.2.8   Skill in:

Skill in effective communication is crucial for a Rehabilitation Registered Nurse. Communication is essential in caring for patients in order to establish rapport, gather important information, and provide appropriate treatments. It involves both verbal and nonverbal skills. Verbal communication includes expressing empathy, actively listening, and using appropriate language and tone. Nonverbal communication involves interpreting body language, facial expressions, and gestures. To optimize patient communication, the nurse must consider cultural and language differences. Additionally, the nurse should be skilled in documenting and conveying patient information accurately to other healthcare professionals. Good communication enhances patient satisfaction, improves outcomes, and promotes teamwork among the healthcare team. Therefore, developing and honing communication skills is essential for a Rehabilitation Registered Nurse.

2.2.8.1   Assessing comprehension and communication (e.g., oral, written, auditory, visual):

Assessing comprehension and communication is a crucial aspect of optimizing a patient's ability to communicate effectively in rehabilitation nursing. This involves evaluating the patient's understanding and expression of information through various means, such as oral, written, auditory, and visual communication.
To assess comprehension, the nurse may ask the patient questions or provide written materials for them to read and interpret. They can also evaluate the patient's ability to follow verbal instructions or comprehend visual aids, like diagrams or charts.
In terms of communication, assessing the patient's ability to express themselves verbally or in writing is important. The nurse may observe their speech patterns, articulation, and vocabulary, as well as their ability to write coherently. They may also assess the patient's use of non-verbal communication, such as gestures or facial expressions.

The nurse should also consider any barriers to communication, like hearing or vision impairments, and tailor their assessment strategies accordingly. By thoroughly assessing comprehension and communication skills, the nurse can develop appropriate interventions and strategies to optimize the patient's ability to effectively communicate during their rehabilitation process.

2.2.8.2   Implementing and evaluating communication interventions:

Implementing and evaluating communication interventions is an essential aspect of a Rehabilitation Registered Nurse's role in optimizing a patient's ability to communicate effectively. In order to effectively implement these interventions, it is crucial to follow the nursing process.

The first step in the process is assessing the patient's communication abilities and needs. This includes identifying any barriers or challenges they may face in expressing themselves. The nurse may also assess the patient's non-verbal cues and understanding of instructions.

Based on the assessment, the nurse will develop a plan of care that includes specific interventions to address the patient's communication needs. These interventions may involve using alternative communication methods such as sign language or picture boards, providing assistive devices, or facilitating communication through technology.

Once the interventions are implemented, the nurse will continuously evaluate their effectiveness. This includes monitoring the patient's progress in communication, addressing any concerns or issues that arise, and making adjustments to the plan of care as needed.

By implementing and evaluating communication interventions, Rehabilitation Registered Nurses play a vital role in improving the overall functional health patterns of their patients.

2.2.8.3   Involving and educating support systems:

Involving and educating support systems is an essential aspect of the rehabilitation process for a Rehabilitation Registered Nurse. It involves engaging and educating the individuals or groups who provide support to the patient, such as family members, friends, and caregivers. By involving support systems, the nurse can ensure that the patient receives holistic care and support. The nurse educates the support systems about the patient's condition, treatment plans, and specific needs. This education empowers support systems to actively participate in the patient's care and rehabilitation journey. The nurse may also provide resources, guidance, and skills training to the support systems, helping them to better understand and meet the patient's needs. By involving and educating support systems, the nurse can enhance communication, promote positive relationships, and improve the patient's overall rehabilitation outcomes.

2.2.8.4   Using assistive technology and adaptive equipment (e.g., Passy Muir):

Using assistive technology and adaptive equipment, such as the Passy Muir valve, is essential for optimizing a patient's ability to communicate effectively. These devices allow individuals with communication impairments, such as those with tracheostomy tubes, to speak and express their needs, facilitating their participation in daily activities and improving their quality of life. The Passy Muir valve is a one-way valve that attaches to the tracheostomy tube, redirecting airflow to the vocal cords. This enables the patient to produce speech. Nurses play a vital role in assessing the patient's communication needs and providing appropriate assistive technology. They should be knowledgeable about the different types of assistive devices available and their usage. Nurses should also educate patients and caregivers on the correct and safe use of these devices. Ongoing support and follow-up are crucial to ensure the patient's successful implementation and continued use of the assistive technology.

2.2.8.5   Using communication techniques:

Using communication techniques is an essential skill for Rehabilitation Registered Nurses when optimizing a patient's ability to communicate effectively. Effective communication techniques play a vital role in the nursing process, ensuring that patients can express their needs and concerns clearly. Nurses can utilize various communication strategies, including active listening, asking open-ended questions, using appropriate body language, and providing empathetic responses. These techniques help build rapport with patients and foster a trusting and therapeutic relationship. Additionally, nurses should be mindful of non-verbal cues and cultural considerations that may impact communication. By refining their communication skills, Rehabilitation Registered Nurses can facilitate effective exchanges with patients, leading to better patient outcomes and enhanced overall care.

2.2.8.6   Teaching self-advocacy skills to patients and caregivers:

Teaching self-advocacy skills to patients and caregivers is an important aspect of the rehabilitation registered nurse's role. By equipping patients and their caregivers with these skills, the nurse helps to optimize their ability to communicate effectively. Self-advocacy involves empowering patients to actively participate in their own care and make informed decisions about their health.

One important aspect of teaching self-advocacy skills is providing information and education to patients and their caregivers. This can include explaining their rights and responsibilities as healthcare consumers, as well as teaching them how to navigate the healthcare system and access the resources and support they need.

Another important aspect is fostering effective communication between patients, caregivers, and healthcare professionals. This involves teaching patients and caregivers how to ask questions, express their concerns, and effectively communicate their needs and preferences to the healthcare team.

Furthermore, the rehabilitation registered nurse can educate patients and caregivers on how to advocate for themselves or their loved ones, ensuring that their voices are heard in decision-making processes. This can involve teaching them how to gather information, explore different options, and collaborate with healthcare providers to make informed choices.

Overall, teaching self-advocacy skills to patients and caregivers is crucial in promoting their autonomy, improving communication, and enhancing their overall rehabilitation experience.

2.2.8.7   Task 6: Apply the nursing process to promote optimal nutrition and hydration.:

Task 6: Apply the nursing process to promote optimal nutrition and hydration in rehabilitation nursing.

In rehabilitation nursing, it is crucial to ensure that patients are receiving adequate nutrition and hydration to support their recovery. To accomplish this, nurses apply the nursing process, which involves assessment, diagnosis, planning, implementation, and evaluation.

During the assessment phase, nurses gather information about the patient's dietary habits, medical history, and any specific dietary restrictions. They may also conduct physical examinations to identify any signs of malnutrition or dehydration.

Based on the assessment findings, nurses make a diagnosis related to nutrition and hydration, such as inadequate oral intake or impaired swallowing.

Once the diagnosis is made, nurses develop a plan of care, which may include consulting with a dietitian to create a personalized meal plan, providing education on healthy eating habits, and monitoring the patient's fluid intake.

The implementation phase entails carrying out the planned interventions, such as assisting with meal preparation, administering medications or supplements, and ensuring adequate hydration.

Lastly, nurses evaluate the effectiveness of the interventions and make adjustments as needed to promote optimal nutrition and hydration.

By applying the nursing process, rehabilitation nurses play a vital role in helping patients achieve their nutritional goals, supporting their overall recovery.

2.2.9   Knowledge of:

As a Rehabilitation Registered Nurse, it is essential to have knowledge of promoting optimal nutrition and hydration by applying the nursing process. This knowledge involves understanding the importance of nutrition and hydration in the rehabilitation process and its impact on overall health. It is crucial to assess patients' nutritional needs by considering factors such as their medical history, dietary preferences, and any specific dietary restrictions they may have. Furthermore, it is important to develop individualized nutrition plans that meet the patients' specific needs and goals. This may involve collaborating with dietitians to ensure that patients receive appropriate nutrients and maintain a balanced diet. Monitoring patients' dietary intake and providing education and support for healthy eating habits are also essential aspects of promoting optimal nutrition and hydration. By having knowledge of these concepts, as a Rehabilitation Registered Nurse, you can contribute to the overall well-being and recovery of your patients.

2.2.9.1   Adaptive equipment and feeding techniques (e.g., modified utensils, scoop plates, positioning):

Adaptive equipment and feeding techniques, such as modified utensils, scoop plates, and positioning, are essential for promoting optimal nutrition and hydration in patients. Modified utensils, like weighted or angled forks and spoons, assist individuals with limited grip strength or coordination to feed themselves more easily. Scoop plates have raised edges and a sloped design, allowing individuals to scoop food onto their utensils with less difficulty. Proper positioning during meals, such as sitting upright or using supportive pillows, ensures the person's safety and comfort while eating.

These adaptive techniques and tools can benefit patients with a range of conditions, including stroke, neurological disorders, arthritis, or physical disabilities. By utilizing these strategies, a rehabilitation registered nurse can enable patients to maintain their independence and dignity while enjoying meals. This promotes adequate nutrition and hydration, which is vital for the overall health and well-being of individuals undergoing rehabilitation. Therefore, knowledge of adaptive equipment and feeding techniques is crucial for a rehabilitation registered nurse to effectively support their patients' nutritional needs.

2.2.9.2   Enteral and parenteral nutrition and hydration:

Enteral and parenteral nutrition and hydration are vital aspects of providing optimal nutrition and hydration to patients. Enteral nutrition involves providing nutrients and fluids directly into the gastrointestinal tract through a feeding tube. This method is commonly used when a patient is unable to eat or swallow normally. On the other hand, parenteral nutrition involves delivering nutrients and fluids intravenously, bypassing the digestive system. This approach is used when the gastrointestinal tract is not functioning properly or when oral or enteral intake is insufficient. It is crucial for rehabilitation registered nurses to assess the patient's nutritional status, including their needs for protein, carbohydrates, fats, vitamins, and minerals. They must also monitor the patient's fluid balance and maintain adequate hydration. Proper nutrition and hydration promote healing, support immune function, and optimize overall health and well-being during the rehabilitation process.

2.2.9.3   Anatomy and physiology related to nutritional and metabolic patterns (e.g., endocrine, obesity, swallowing):

Anatomy and physiology play a crucial role in understanding nutritional and metabolic patterns. The endocrine system, which consists of various glands producing hormones, is closely tied to nutrition. Hormones like insulin, produced by the pancreas, regulate glucose metabolism, while the thyroid hormone affects metabolism overall. Obesity, a complex condition, involves an imbalance between energy intake and expenditure, often influenced by genetic and environmental factors. Understanding the anatomy and physiology behind obesity helps in developing targeted interventions. Swallowing, a vital process, relies on coordination between various anatomical structures like the tongue, larynx, and esophagus. Disruptions in this process can result in dysphagia, impacting nutrition and hydration. Nurses need to apply the nursing process to assess and address these issues in rehabilitation settings, ensuring optimal nutrition and hydration for their patients.

2.2.9.4   Diagnostic testing:

Diagnostic testing is an essential component of the nursing process in promoting optimal nutrition and hydration for the Rehabilitation Registered Nurse. It involves various procedures that aid in identifying the underlying causes of patients' conditions. These tests help determine the nutritional status, hydration levels, and any potential deficiencies or abnormalities that may affect a patient's overall well-being. Diagnostic tests commonly performed include blood tests, urine analysis, imaging studies, and endoscopic procedures. Blood tests provide valuable information about nutrient levels, organ function, and potential deficiencies. Urine analysis helps assess hydration status and kidney function. Imaging studies such as x-rays, CT scans, or MRIs aid in visualizing any structural abnormalities. Endoscopic procedures allow for direct examination of the gastrointestinal tract. Understanding the importance of diagnostic testing enables the Rehabilitation Registered Nurse to formulate appropriate nutrition and hydration interventions tailored to each patient's specific needs.

2.2.9.5   Diet types (e.g., cardiac, diabetic, renal, dysphagia):

A rehabilitation registered nurse must have knowledge of different types of diets, including cardiac, diabetic, renal, and dysphagia diets.

A cardiac diet is designed for patients with heart conditions, focusing on reducing fat, salt, and cholesterol intake. It emphasizes lean proteins, fruits, vegetables, and whole grains.

A diabetic diet is essential for individuals with diabetes, aiming to regulate blood sugar levels. It involves monitoring carbohydrate intake, choosing low glycemic index foods, and spreading meals throughout the day.

A renal diet is customized for patients with kidney disease, requiring controlled protein, sodium, and potassium intake. It aims to lessen the workload on the kidneys and maintain proper electrolyte balance.

A dysphagia diet is prescribed for those with swallowing difficulties. It involves modifying the texture of foods and thickening liquids to prevent choking or aspiration.

Understanding these diet types enables the rehabilitation registered nurse to provide optimal nutrition and hydration to their patients, promoting their overall health and well-being.

2.2.9.6   Fluid and electrolyte balance:

Fluid and electrolyte balance is an important aspect of maintaining optimal nutrition and hydration in rehabilitation nursing. It involves the regulation of fluids and electrolytes in the body to ensure proper functioning of cells, organs, and systems.

Dehydration can occur when fluid intake is insufficient or excessive fluid is lost, leading to imbalances in electrolytes such as sodium, potassium, and calcium. This can result in symptoms like dry mouth, increased thirst, weakness, dizziness, and confusion. On the other hand, overhydration can lead to fluid overload, causing symptoms like swelling, shortness of breath, and increased blood pressure.

As a rehabilitation registered nurse, it is crucial to assess and monitor patients' fluid and electrolyte status, including intake and output, laboratory values, and signs of imbalance. Nursing interventions may include promoting oral fluid intake, administering intravenous fluids or electrolyte replacement, and educating patients on the importance of maintaining proper hydration.

2.2.9.7   Nutritional requirements:

Nutritional requirements play a crucial role in promoting optimal nutrition and hydration for patients in rehabilitation. These requirements vary depending on the individual's age, sex, weight, medical conditions, and activity level. It is important for Rehabilitation Registered Nurses to assess and identify the nutritional needs of their patients accurately. Providing the right amount of calories, macronutrients, micronutrients, and fluids is essential for supporting the recovery process and preventing complications. Additionally, understanding suitable meal planning, special diets for specific conditions, and therapeutic nutrition interventions is essential. Collaborating with dieticians, identifying risks for malnutrition, and monitoring patients' nutritional status are vital aspects of a Rehabilitation Registered Nurse's role. By addressing these nutritional requirements, Rehabilitation Registered Nurses can contribute to their patients' overall well-being and enhance their rehabilitation outcomes.

2.2.9.8   Skin integrity (e.g., Braden scale, pressure ulcer staging):

Skin integrity refers to the condition of the skin and its ability to withstand pressure and prevent damage. It is an important aspect of nursing care, especially in the rehabilitation setting. The Braden scale is a widely used tool to assess and predict the risk of pressure ulcers in patients. It takes into consideration factors such as sensory perception, moisture, activity, mobility, nutrition, and friction/shear. Pressure ulcers, also known as bedsores, are classified into four stages based on the extent of tissue damage. Stage 1 involves non-blanchable erythema, while stage 4 is characterized by full-thickness tissue loss. Prompt identification and staging of pressure ulcers are crucial for appropriate treatment and prevention. Nurses play a vital role in assessing and monitoring skin integrity, implementing preventive measures, and promoting optimal nutrition and hydration to maintain skin health in rehabilitation settings.

2.2.9.9   Pharmacology (e.g., antispasmodics, anticholinergics, antidepressants, analgesics):

Pharmacology is a branch of medicine that focuses on the study of how drugs interact with the body. In the context of nursing, understanding pharmacology is crucial for promoting optimal nutrition and hydration in patients. Several types of medications are commonly used in rehabilitation settings to manage various conditions.

Antispasmodics are medications that help alleviate muscle spasms. They work by relaxing muscle contractions, reducing pain and discomfort. Anticholinergics, on the other hand, block the effects of certain neurotransmitters in the body, helping to control conditions such as overactive bladder or chronic obstructive pulmonary disease.

Antidepressants are commonly prescribed to treat depression and other mental health conditions. They work by affecting the balance of chemicals in the brain, improving mood and overall well-being.

Analgesics, also known as painkillers, are medications used to relieve pain. They can be either prescription or over-the-counter drugs and are available in various forms, such as opioids, nonsteroidal anti-inflammatory drugs (NSAIDs), and acetaminophen.

When administering these medications, nurses need to consider factors such as patient allergies, potential drug interactions, and any contraindications or precautions. They must monitor patients for any adverse effects and educate them on proper medication use to ensure optimal outcomes.

Overall, understanding the different classifications of medications within pharmacology is essential for the rehabilitation registered nurse to provide effective care and promote optimal nutrition and hydration in patients.

2.2.9.10   Safety concerns and interventions (e.g., swallowing, positioning, food textures, fluid consistency):

Safety concerns and interventions related to nutrition and hydration are important considerations for Rehabilitation Registered Nurses. One aspect of safety concerns is swallowing difficulties, which can result from various conditions such as stroke or neurological disorders. Nurses must carefully assess patients' ability to swallow and implement appropriate interventions, such as modified food textures or fluid consistency. Positioning is another crucial aspect to ensure safe swallowing and prevent choking. Nurses should educate patients on proper body positioning during meals and provide necessary support or adaptive devices. Additionally, the texture of food and consistency of fluids should be carefully chosen to accommodate patients' individual needs and abilities. These interventions aim to promote optimal nutrition and hydration while ensuring the safety and well-being of patients during their rehabilitation journey.

2.2.9.11   Cultural and religious practices related to dietary habits:

Cultural and religious practices play a significant role in shaping dietary habits. Different cultures and religions have their own unique food preferences and restrictions based on tradition, belief systems, and values. Understanding and respecting these practices is crucial for a Rehabilitation Registered Nurse in order to provide optimal care and promote proper nutrition and hydration.

Some cultures may have specific dietary rituals, such as offering certain foods during religious ceremonies or fasting during specific times of the year. These practices can impact a patient's nutritional status and require adaptations in their care plan.

Religious restrictions on dietary choices, such as avoiding certain meats or consuming only vegetarian or vegan diets, must also be taken into consideration. These restrictions may be based on religious beliefs or ethical values, and it is important to respect and accommodate these preferences.

Cultural practices can also influence portion sizes, meal timings, and food preparation techniques. Some cultures prioritize communal dining and emphasize the importance of sharing meals, while others may have specific rituals or customs related to food preparation and consumption.

By understanding and incorporating cultural and religious practices into care plans, Rehabilitation Registered Nurses can promote inclusivity, respect cultural diversity, and provide culturally sensitive care to their patients.

2.2.10   Skill in:

As a Rehabilitation Registered Nurse, it is important to possess a range of skills related to promoting optimal nutrition and hydration. These skills include assessing the nutritional needs of patients, identifying any deficiencies, and developing appropriate care plans.

One aspect of this skill set involves conducting comprehensive nutritional assessments to determine the patient's current nutritional status. This may include evaluating dietary intake, reviewing laboratory results, and assessing the patient's overall health.

Another important skill is the ability to identify nutritional deficiencies and develop interventions to address them. This may involve collaborating with a multidisciplinary team of healthcare professionals, implementing dietary modifications, and monitoring the patient's progress.

Additionally, as a Rehabilitation Registered Nurse, it is essential to educate patients and their families about the importance of proper nutrition and hydration. This may include providing information about healthy eating habits, demonstrating meal planning techniques, and offering guidance on the appropriate intake of fluids.

By possessing these skills, a Rehabilitation Registered Nurse can play a crucial role in promoting optimal nutrition and hydration for their patients, ultimately supporting their overall recovery and well-being.

2.2.10.1   Using and managing manual and mechanical devices to provide nutrition and hydration:

Using and managing manual and mechanical devices to provide nutrition and hydration is an essential skill for Rehabilitation Registered Nurses. This topic involves the application of the nursing process to promote optimal nutrition and hydration in patients. The use of manual devices, such as feeding tubes or syringes, and mechanical devices, like enteral pumps, is necessary for patients who are unable to consume food or fluids orally.

The nurse must be knowledgeable about the different types of devices available and how to properly use and manage them. This includes understanding how to calculate and administer the appropriate amount of nutrition and fluids, as well as monitoring the patient's response and making adjustments as needed.

Subtopics that should be covered include the importance of nutrition and hydration in the rehabilitation process, the various types of manual and mechanical devices used, the steps involved in using and managing these devices, and the potential complications or risks associated with their use.

By effectively utilizing manual and mechanical devices, Rehabilitation Registered Nurses can ensure that their patients receive the necessary nutrition and hydration for optimal recovery and rehabilitation.

2.2.10.2   Assessing nutritional and metabolic patterns (e.g., nutritional intake, fluid volume deficits, skin integrity, metabolic functions, feeding and swallowing):

Assessing nutritional and metabolic patterns is a crucial aspect of the nursing process to promote optimal nutrition and hydration in rehabilitation patients. It involves evaluating various factors such as nutritional intake, fluid volume deficits, skin integrity, metabolic functions, and feeding and swallowing abilities.

To assess nutritional intake, the nurse examines the patient's diet history, including food preferences, allergies, and any dietary restrictions. This information helps determine if the patient is receiving adequate nutrients for healing and recovery. Assessing fluid volume deficits involves monitoring the patient's hydration status, urine output, and signs of dehydration. The nurse ensures that the patient's fluid intake matches their needs.

Skin integrity assessment is essential to identify any pressure ulcers or potential risks. The nurse inspects the skin for redness, swelling, or breakdown, and takes appropriate measures to prevent skin damage.

To evaluate metabolic functions, the nurse assesses the patient's weight, body mass index (BMI), and laboratory results, such as blood glucose levels and lipid profiles. These findings help identify any metabolic imbalances or nutritional deficiencies requiring intervention.

Assessing feeding and swallowing abilities involves observing the patient's ability to chew, swallow, and tolerate oral intake. This assessment helps determine the appropriate diet consistency and any need for feeding assistance, such as a soft or pureed diet or a feeding tube.

Overall, a thorough assessment of nutritional and metabolic patterns allows the rehabilitation registered nurse to develop a comprehensive care plan tailored to the individual patient's needs and promote optimal nutrition and hydration during the rehabilitation process.

2.2.10.3   Implementing and evaluating interventions for nutrition:

Implementing and evaluating interventions for nutrition is a crucial aspect of a Rehabilitation Registered Nurse's role. This involves applying the nursing process to promote optimal nutrition and hydration, as well as addressing functional health patterns. To effectively implement these interventions, the nurse must first assess the patient's nutritional status and identify any underlying issues. This could include evaluating their overall health, dietary habits, and any specific dietary restrictions or allergies. Once this assessment is complete, the nurse can develop individualized care plans that focus on improving nutrition and hydration. These plans may involve providing education on proper nutrition, monitoring food and fluid intake, and collaborating with other healthcare professionals to address any underlying medical conditions. It is essential for the nurse to regularly evaluate the effectiveness of these interventions to ensure positive outcomes for the patients. By continuously monitoring and adjusting the care plans as needed, the nurse can help patients achieve optimal nutrition and overall wellness during their rehabilitation journey.

2.2.10.4   Implementing and evaluating interventions for skin integrity (e.g., skin assessment, pressure relief, moisture reduction, nutrition and hydration):

Implementing and evaluating interventions for skin integrity is crucial in promoting optimal nutrition and hydration for rehabilitation registered nurses. They need to have the skills to assess the skin condition, provide pressure relief, reduce moisture, and ensure adequate nutrition and hydration.

Skin assessment is the first step in identifying any areas of concern such as pressure ulcers or wounds. This involves carefully examining the skin for redness, swelling, or signs of breakdown. Pressure relief techniques, such as repositioning patients regularly and using specialized mattresses or cushions, can help alleviate pressure on vulnerable areas. Moisture reduction techniques, like using moisture barriers and regularly changing wet dressings, are also important to maintain skin integrity.

Proper nutrition and hydration are essential to support the healing process and prevent further skin damage. Rehabilitation registered nurses should assess patients' dietary needs and provide appropriate recommendations. They may collaborate with dietitians and encourage patients to consume a balanced diet rich in vitamins, minerals, and protein. Adequate hydration is also crucial for skin health, so nurses should monitor fluid intake and encourage patients to drink enough fluids. By conducting thorough skin assessments, providing pressure relief, reducing moisture, and promoting proper nutrition and hydration, nurses can contribute to optimal patient outcomes.

2.2.10.5   Teaching interventions for swallowing deficits:

Teaching interventions for swallowing deficits are crucial in promoting optimal nutrition and hydration in patients. These interventions aim to address difficulties in swallowing, which can lead to complications such as malnutrition and dehydration.

One important aspect of teaching interventions is educating patients and their caregivers about proper techniques for safe swallowing. They should be taught strategies to improve swallowing function, such as changing body positioning, modifying food consistency and texture, and using swallowing maneuvers.

Another aspect is teaching patients about the importance of maintaining good oral hygiene to prevent infections. Regular dental care and ensuring proper mouth care after meals can contribute to overall swallowing health.

Additionally, rehabilitation registered nurses can assist in coordinating interdisciplinary care with speech-language pathologists and dieticians to develop individualized treatment plans. These plans may include exercises to strengthen swallowing muscles, dietary modifications, and adaptive equipment recommendations.

Overall, teaching interventions for swallowing deficits aim to improve patients' ability to swallow safely, thereby promoting optimal nutrition and hydration.

2.2.10.6   Using adaptive equipment:

Using adaptive equipment is an important skill for a Rehabilitation Registered Nurse, especially when promoting optimal nutrition and hydration. Adaptive equipment refers to devices that help individuals with physical limitations or disabilities to perform daily tasks more independently. In the context of nutrition and hydration, adaptive equipment can be used to assist patients in feeding themselves or drinking fluids.

There are various types of adaptive equipment available, including specialized utensils with larger handles or modified grips to aid patients with limited hand mobility. Other examples include weighted cups and plates, straw holders, angled utensils, and adaptive tableware designed for individuals with swallowing difficulties. These devices promote independence, improve safety, and enhance the overall dining experience for patients.

In addition to facilitating physical tasks, the use of adaptive equipment also involves assessing patients' needs, educating them on proper usage, and monitoring their progress. Rehabilitation Registered Nurses need to stay up-to-date with the latest advancements in adaptive equipment and collaborate with occupational therapists and speech-language pathologists to ensure comprehensive care. Overall, the skill of using adaptive equipment is crucial for Rehabilitation Registered Nurses to support their patients in achieving optimal nutrition and hydration while promoting independence and enhancing their quality of life.

2.3   Task 7: Apply the nursing process to optimize the patient's elimination patterns.

When it comes to optimizing a patient's elimination patterns, the nursing process plays a crucial role. This process consists of five steps: assessment, diagnosis, planning, implementation, and evaluation.

During the assessment phase, the rehabilitation registered nurse gathers relevant information about the patient's elimination patterns. This includes factors such as frequency, consistency, and any associated symptoms or difficulties. The nurse also considers the patient's medical history, medications, and overall health status.

Based on the assessment findings, a diagnosis is formulated. This involves identifying any altered elimination patterns or potential issues that may affect the patient's bowel or bladder function. Common diagnoses in this context include urinary retention, urinary incontinence, constipation, and fecal impaction.

After the diagnosis, a plan is developed to address the patient's specific needs and optimize their elimination patterns. This plan may involve interventions such as implementing a toileting schedule, offering dietary recommendations to promote regular bowel movements, and providing education on proper hydration.

The implementation phase focuses on executing the planned interventions. This may include assisting the patient with toileting, providing support and encouragement, and ensuring the proper use of assistive devices such as bedpans or commodes.

Lastly, the evaluation phase allows the nurse to assess the effectiveness of the interventions and determine if the patient's elimination patterns have improved. Modifications to the plan can be made as needed to ensure optimal outcomes.

Overall, by applying the nursing process, the rehabilitation registered nurse can effectively address and optimize the patient's elimination patterns. This includes conducting a comprehensive assessment, formulating a diagnosis, developing a tailored plan, implementing interventions, and evaluating the outcomes.

2.3.1   Knowledge of:

As a Rehabilitation Registered Nurse, it is crucial to have knowledge of various aspects related to optimizing the patient's elimination patterns. This knowledge includes understanding the normal elimination processes of the body and identifying any deviations from the norm. It also involves knowing how to assess the patient's elimination patterns, which includes evaluating their bowel and bladder function, as well as any issues with sweating or respiratory secretions. Knowledge of the nursing process is vital to effectively address any elimination problems that patients may have. This process includes assessment, diagnosis, planning, implementation, and evaluation. Additionally, knowledge of interventions such as promoting hydration, encouraging regular exercise, providing assistance with toileting, and implementing medication management strategies is essential in optimizing a patient's elimination patterns. Overall, having a comprehensive understanding of the various factors that affect elimination patterns enables Rehabilitation Registered Nurses to provide optimal care to their patients.

2.3.1.1   Anatomy and physiology of altered bowel and bladder function:

The anatomy and physiology of altered bowel and bladder function is an essential consideration for Rehabilitation Registered Nurses in optimizing a patient's elimination patterns. Understanding the structure and function of the gastrointestinal and urinary systems is crucial for providing effective care.

In terms of bowel function, the colon plays a vital role in absorbing water and electrolytes from the intestine, forming stool, and promoting regular bowel movements. Alterations in this process can result in constipation or diarrhea. Factors such as diet, medication, neurological disorders, and surgical interventions can impact bowel function.

Regarding bladder function, the kidneys produce urine, which is stored in the bladder until it is eliminated through urination. The muscles of the bladder and the urethra control the release of urine. Altered bladder function can manifest as urinary retention or incontinence. Various factors, including neurological conditions, pelvic floor dysfunction, and medications, can disrupt normal bladder function.

To optimize a patient's elimination patterns, Rehabilitation Registered Nurses must assess their bowel and bladder function, including frequency, consistency, and any associated symptoms. This assessment helps in identifying any abnormalities or potential issues. Nurses can then collaborate with other healthcare professionals to develop a care plan that may include interventions such as dietary modifications, medication management, bowel and bladder training, and pelvic floor exercises. Continual evaluation and monitoring of the patient's response to interventions are also important to ensure optimal results.

2.3.1.2   Bladder and bowel adaptive equipment and technology (e.g., bladder scan, types of catheters, suppository inserter):

Bladder and bowel adaptive equipment and technology play a crucial role in optimizing a patient's elimination patterns. One important piece of equipment is the bladder scan, which is used to measure the amount of urine in the bladder non-invasively. This information helps healthcare professionals determine the need for bladder emptying interventions.

There are various types of catheters available, such as intermittent catheters, indwelling catheters, and condom catheters. Intermittent catheters are commonly used for patients who require periodic bladder emptying, while indwelling catheters are inserted and remain inside the bladder for a longer duration. Condom catheters are external devices suitable for male patients who can self-manage their urination.

Suppositories are another type of adaptive technology used for bowel management. They are solid medications inserted into the rectum to induce bowel movement. Suppository inserters are devices that assist in the insertion of suppositories accurately and comfortably.

Overall, understanding the use of bladder and bowel adaptive equipment and technology is essential for rehabilitation registered nurses to optimize the patient's elimination patterns effectively.

2.3.1.3   Bladder and bowel training (e.g., scheduled self- catheterization, timed voiding, elimination programs):

Bladder and bowel training refers to various techniques used to optimize a patient's elimination patterns. This includes scheduled self-catheterization, timed voiding, and elimination programs. Scheduled self-catheterization involves teaching patients how to insert and remove their own catheters at regular intervals to empty their bladders. Timed voiding involves establishing a regular schedule for patients to empty their bladders, helping them regain control and avoid accidents. Elimination programs are designed to address issues such as constipation or incontinence by implementing strategies such as diet modifications, exercise, and medication management. These interventions are important for rehabilitation registered nurses as they play a crucial role in helping patients regain independence and improve their quality of life. By implementing bladder and bowel training techniques, nurses can promote optimal elimination patterns and prevent complications associated with urinary and bowel dysfunction.

2.3.1.4   Pharmacologic and non-pharmacological interventions:

Pharmacologic and non-pharmacological interventions are strategies used by rehabilitation registered nurses to optimize a patient's elimination patterns. These interventions aim to improve bowel and bladder function, as well as promote regular and healthy bowel movements and urination.

Pharmacologic interventions involve the administration of medications that help regulate bowel movements or relax the bladder muscles. This may include laxatives, stool softeners, or anticholinergic drugs.

Non-pharmacological interventions, on the other hand, focus on lifestyle modifications and behavioral changes. This may include dietary adjustments, such as increasing fiber intake or managing fluid intake, as well as exercise and physical activity to stimulate bowel function. Nurses may also educate patients about proper toileting techniques and the use of assistive devices, such as commodes or bedpans.

It is crucial for rehabilitation registered nurses to assess the patient's specific needs and tailor interventions accordingly. Patient education and collaboration with other healthcare professionals are also essential in optimizing the patient's elimination patterns.

2.3.2 Skill in:

As a Rehabilitation Registered Nurse, having skill in optimizing the patient's elimination patterns is crucial. This skill involves implementing the nursing process to ensure the patient's elimination functions are functioning properly. Firstly, it requires the nurse to assess and gather data related to the patient's elimination patterns, including frequency, consistency, and any associated symptoms. Then, the nurse must analyze the data to identify any abnormalities or potential issues. This analysis helps in establishing a nursing diagnosis. Afterward, a care plan is developed, which may involve interventions such as promoting fluid intake, dietary modifications, and providing education on bowel and bladder habits. Implementation of the care plan involves providing direct care to the patient, while evaluation helps assess the effectiveness of the interventions and make necessary adjustments. Ultimately, having skill in optimizing elimination patterns helps improve the patient's overall health and well-being.

2.3.2.1 Assessing elimination patterns (e.g., elimination diary, patient's history):

Assessing elimination patterns is an important aspect of optimizing a patient's elimination patterns in rehabilitation nursing. One way to assess elimination patterns is through the use of an elimination diary, where the patient records their bowel movements and urinary patterns. This diary helps the nurse monitor the frequency, consistency, and other characteristics of elimination. Another valuable tool for assessment is the patient's history, which provides insights into any previous elimination issues, surgeries, or medication use that may impact current patterns. When assessing elimination, it is crucial to consider factors such as diet, fluid intake, and physical activity level. By understanding the patient's elimination patterns, the rehabilitation registered nurse can develop appropriate interventions and educate the patient on healthy elimination habits. Effective assessment of elimination patterns contributes to overall patient well-being and helps track progress in rehabilitation.

2.3.2.2 Implementing and evaluating interventions for bladder and bowel management (e.g., nutrition, exercise, pharmacological, adaptive equipment):

Implementing and evaluating interventions for bladder and bowel management is a crucial aspect of optimizing a patient's elimination patterns for Rehabilitation Registered Nurses. There are several important aspects to consider within this topic.

One aspect is nutrition, where nurses must assess the patient's dietary intake and make appropriate recommendations. This may involve increasing dietary fiber and fluid intake to promote regular bowel movements.

Exercise is another important intervention, as physical activity can help stimulate bowel and bladder function. Nurses can assess the patient's mobility and develop a customized exercise plan to improve elimination patterns.

Pharmacological interventions may be necessary in some cases, such as the use of laxatives or antispasmodic medications to manage bowel or bladder dysfunction. Nurses should closely monitor the patient's response to these medications and adjust the treatment plan as needed.

Additionally, adaptive equipment can be utilized to support bladder and bowel management. This may include devices such as commodes, bedpans, or urinary catheters. Nurses should evaluate the patient's needs and provide appropriate training and education on how to use these devices effectively.

Overall, implementing and evaluating interventions for bladder and bowel management requires a comprehensive approach, incorporating nutrition, exercise, pharmacological interventions, and adaptive equipment to optimize a patient's elimination patterns.

2.3.2.3 Teaching interventions to prevent complications (e.g., constipation, urinary tract infections, autonomic dysreflexia):

Teaching interventions are an essential aspect of a Rehabilitation Registered Nurse's role in optimizing a patient's elimination patterns and preventing complications such as constipation, urinary tract infections (UTIs), and autonomic dysreflexia (AD).

To prevent constipation, the nurse can educate the patient on the importance of adequate fluid intake, a high-fiber diet, and regular exercise. They can also teach the patient proper toileting techniques and the use of laxatives or stool softeners if necessary.

For preventing UTIs, the nurse can educate the patient on maintaining proper hygiene, like wiping from front to back, and the importance of emptying the bladder regularly. They can also encourage the patient to drink plenty of fluids and avoid irritants such as caffeine and alcohol.

To prevent autonomic dysreflexia, the nurse can educate patients with spinal cord injuries on the signs and symptoms of AD, such as sudden high blood pressure and severe headache. They can teach them the importance of regular bladder and bowel management, as well as proper skin care to prevent pressure ulcers, which can trigger AD.

Overall, teaching interventions play a crucial role in preventing complications and optimizing the patient's elimination patterns in rehabilitation settings.

2.3.2.4 Providing patient and caregiver education related to bowel and bladder management:

Providing patient and caregiver education related to bowel and bladder management is an integral aspect of optimizing a patient's elimination patterns in rehabilitation nursing. This education aims to enhance the patient's understanding of their bowel and bladder functions, as well as strategies for maintaining optimal management.

The education process involves explaining the importance of regularity and consistency in their bowel and bladder routines, promoting a balanced diet and fluid intake, and encouraging physical activity. It is also crucial to provide information on proper techniques for toileting, including correct positioning, relaxation techniques, and adequate time for voiding.

Moreover, helping patients and caregivers understand the significance of recognizing and reporting any changes or abnormalities in bowel or bladder patterns is essential. Teaching them how to manage potential issues, such as constipation, incontinence, or urinary tract infections, is also a vital component of education.

Through effective patient and caregiver education, a rehabilitation registered nurse can empower individuals to take an active role in their own bowel and bladder management, ultimately improving their overall functional health patterns.

2.3.2.5 Using adaptive equipment and technology:

Using adaptive equipment and technology is essential in optimizing a patient's elimination patterns for Rehabilitation Registered Nurses. This involves identifying the patient's specific needs and implementing the appropriate adaptive equipment and technology to enhance their mobility and independence. This may include providing assistive devices like canes, walkers, and wheelchairs to support the patient's mobility. Additionally, technology such as electric lifts, bed rails, and grab bars can aid with safe transfers and positioning. Use of adaptive technology may also involve implementing communication devices, such as speech recognition software or augmentative and alternative communication (AAC) systems, to help patients with communication impairments. The Rehabilitation Registered Nurse must assess the patient's condition, select appropriate adaptive equipment, provide education and training to the patient on its use, and periodically reevaluate their needs to ensure optimal effectiveness.

2.4   Task 8: Apply the nursing process to optimize the patient's sleep and rest patterns.

As a Rehabilitation Registered Nurse, it is important to prioritize the optimization of a patient's sleep and rest patterns. This can greatly affect their overall health and well-being. To achieve this, the nursing process can be applied.

First, a comprehensive assessment should be conducted to determine the patient's current sleep patterns, any potential disturbances, and factors contributing to their sleep issues. This may include asking about their sleeping habits, medical history, and any medications they are taking.

Once the assessment is complete, a nursing diagnosis can be formulated, identifying specific sleep-related problems and the underlying causes. Common sleep-related diagnoses may include insomnia, sleep apnea, or restless leg syndrome.

Based on the nursing diagnosis, an individualized plan of care should be developed. This plan may involve implementing strategies to promote a conducive sleep environment, such as reducing noise and implementing calming routines before bedtime. It may also include education on sleep hygiene and relaxation techniques.

Throughout the patient's stay in rehabilitation, the nursing interventions should be regularly evaluated and adjusted as needed. Documentation is important to track the effectiveness of interventions and provide continuity of care.

By applying the nursing process to optimize a patient's sleep and rest patterns, Rehabilitation Registered Nurses can contribute to improved patient outcomes and overall well-being.

2.4.1   Knowledge of:

Knowledge of: Sleep and rest patterns is crucial for a Rehabilitation Registered Nurse. Understanding the factors that influence sleep and rest is important in optimizing patient care. This includes knowledge about the physiological and psychological processes involved in sleep, as well as the impact of various conditions and interventions on sleep quality. RNs should be aware of the individual variations in sleep patterns and the importance of tailoring interventions to meet the specific needs of each patient. Additionally, knowledge of sleep disorders and their management is necessary in order to identify and address any issues that may be affecting the patient's sleep. RNs should also be familiar with non-pharmacological interventions that can promote better sleep and rest, such as relaxation techniques and environmental modifications. Overall, possessing a comprehensive understanding of sleep and rest patterns allows Rehabilitation RNs to implement effective strategies for optimizing the patient's sleep and rest.

2.4.1.1   Factors affecting sleep and rest (e.g., diet, sleep habits, alcohol, pain, environment):

Sleep and rest are essential for overall health and well-being. Several factors can affect sleep and rest patterns, including diet, sleep habits, alcohol consumption, pain, and environment.

Diet plays a significant role in sleep quality. Consuming heavy or spicy meals close to bedtime can cause indigestion and discomfort, leading to disrupted sleep. On the other hand, a balanced diet that includes foods rich in tryptophan, magnesium, and melatonin can promote better sleep.

Establishing healthy sleep habits is crucial. Maintaining a consistent sleep schedule, practicing relaxation techniques, and creating a comfortable sleep environment can improve sleep and rest.

Alcohol can negatively impact sleep. While it may help you fall asleep initially, it can disrupt the sleep cycle, reducing the overall quality of sleep.

Chronic pain can interfere with sleep. Managing pain effectively through appropriate medications and therapies can promote better sleep and rest.

Lastly, the sleep environment should be conducive to rest. Factors such as noise, light, temperature, and comfort of the bed can affect sleep quality.

By addressing these factors, rehabilitation registered nurses can optimize their patients' sleep and rest patterns, thereby enhancing their recovery and overall well-being.

2.4.1.2   Pharmacological and non-pharmacological sleep aids:

Pharmacological and non-pharmacological sleep aids are essential for optimizing a patient's sleep and rest patterns in rehabilitation nursing. Pharmacological sleep aids include medications such as sedatives and hypnotics, which can help induce sleep and address underlying sleep disorders. Non-pharmacological sleep aids, on the other hand, focus on lifestyle modifications and behavioral interventions. These may include creating a conducive sleep environment, practicing good sleep hygiene, engaging in relaxation techniques, and incorporating regular exercise into the daily routine. Additionally, cognitive-behavioral therapy for insomnia (CBT-I) is a non-pharmacological approach that helps patients modify their thoughts and behaviors associated with sleep. By combining both pharmacological and non-pharmacological approaches, rehabilitation registered nurses can effectively address sleep disturbances and promote optimal rest for their patients.

2.4.1.3   Physiology of sleep and rest cycles:

The physiology of sleep and rest cycles is an essential aspect of understanding the patient's sleep and rest patterns. Sleep is a complex process influenced by various factors, including circadian rhythms, hormones, and neurotransmitters. The sleep-wake cycle, also known as the circadian rhythm, is controlled by the suprachiasmatic nucleus in the brain. Melatonin, a hormone produced by the pineal gland, plays a crucial role in regulating sleep.

During sleep, the body goes through different stages, including NREM (non-rapid eye movement) and REM (rapid eye movement) sleep. NREM sleep is further divided into four stages, with each stage having distinct characteristics. REM sleep is associated with dreaming and essential for cognitive function and emotional processing.

Optimizing patients' sleep and rest patterns involves assessing their sleep quality and quantity, identifying any sleep disorders, and implementing interventions to promote better sleep hygiene. Nurses can educate patients on good sleep habits, such as maintaining a regular sleep schedule, creating a comfortable sleep environment, and avoiding stimulants before bedtime.

2.4.1.4   Technology:

Technology plays a significant role in today's healthcare industry, including the field of rehabilitation nursing. As a Rehabilitation Registered Nurse, understanding and utilizing technology can optimize a patient's sleep and rest patterns. One aspect of technology that can enhance sleep is the use of smart beds and mattresses. These innovative products can adjust the position of the bed, provide pressure relief, and track patient movements during sleep. Another important technology is wearable devices, such as activity trackers, which can monitor sleep patterns and provide feedback on sleep quality. Additionally, noise-canceling headphones or white noise machines can help create a peaceful sleeping environment for patients. Finally, the use of electronic health records and telemedicine allows healthcare providers to access patient information and provide virtual consultations, reducing the need for physical appointments. Being knowledgeable about these technologies can help Rehabilitation Registered Nurses optimize sleep and rest patterns for their patients.

2.4.2   Skill in:

'Nursing skills related to optimizing the patient's sleep and rest patterns are crucial for a Rehabilitation Registered Nurse. These skills include assessing the patient's sleep and rest patterns, identifying any disruptions or issues, and implementing interventions to enhance sleep quality. The nurse should possess strong observational skills to identify sleep disturbances, such as insomnia or sleep apnea. They should be knowledgeable about various relaxation techniques and assistive devices that can aid in improving sleep and rest. Additionally, the nurse should educate the patient and their family members about the importance of sleep hygiene and provide guidance on creating a conducive sleep environment. They should also collaborate with the interdisciplinary team to develop individualized care plans that promote optimal sleep and rest for the patient. Overall, skill in optimizing sleep and rest patterns is vital for a Rehabilitation Registered Nurse to support patients' recovery and overall well-being.'.

2.4.2.1   Assessing sleep and rest patterns:

Assessing sleep and rest patterns is a crucial component of optimizing a patient's sleep and rest patterns as a Rehabilitation Registered Nurse. By applying the nursing process, an accurate assessment of the patient's sleep and rest patterns can be achieved. This assessment involves gathering data about the patient's sleep and rest routines, duration and quality of sleep, any disturbances or interruptions that may occur, and the patient's perceived level of rest and relaxation. Additionally, it is important to evaluate the patient's environment, including noise levels, lighting, and comfort. By conducting a thorough assessment, the nurse can identify any potential problems or areas for improvement in the patient's sleep and rest patterns. This allows for the development of a personalized care plan that addresses the patient's specific needs. Regular monitoring and reassessment are essential to track the effectiveness of interventions and make necessary adjustments to the care plan. Overall, assessing sleep and rest patterns is vital in promoting optimal rest and recovery for rehabilitation patients.

2.4.2.2   Evaluating effectiveness of sleep and rest interventions:

Evaluating the effectiveness of sleep and rest interventions is an essential task for Rehabilitation Registered Nurses in optimizing the patient's sleep and rest patterns. This process involves assessing various interventions implemented to improve sleep and rest quality in patients. The nurse will collect data on the patient's sleep habits, routines, and any factors that may contribute to sleep disturbances. They will then analyze the effectiveness of interventions such as medication administration, environmental changes, relaxation techniques, and sleep hygiene education. Monitoring the patient's sleep patterns before and after implementing these interventions helps determine their success. The nurse may also collaborate with other healthcare professionals to develop personalized strategies to address specific sleep and rest issues. Regular evaluation allows nurses to modify and adjust interventions as necessary, ensuring the best possible outcomes for their patients' sleep and rest patterns.

2.4.2.3   Teaching interventions and strategies to promote sleep and rest (e.g., energy conversation, environmental modifications):

Teaching interventions and strategies can play a crucial role in optimizing sleep and rest patterns for patients in the rehabilitation setting. Energy conservation techniques can be taught to patients to help them prioritize and allocate their energy throughout the day. This may involve teaching them to plan activities, delegate tasks, or use assistive devices effectively. Environmental modifications, such as adjusting lighting, temperature, and noise levels, can also promote better sleep and rest. Teaching patients relaxation techniques, such as deep breathing or progressive muscle relaxation, can help them manage stress and induce sleep. Additionally, educating patients about sleep hygiene practices, such as maintaining a regular sleep schedule, avoiding caffeine and electronics before bedtime, and creating a comfortable sleep environment, can further support their sleep and rest patterns. By incorporating these teaching interventions and strategies, rehabilitation registered nurses can enhance the quality of their patients' sleep and rest, leading to improved overall well-being and recovery.

2.4.2.4   Using technology (e.g., sleep study, CPAP, BiPAP, relaxation technology):

Using technology in the field of sleep and rest optimization is crucial for Rehabilitation Registered Nurses. One important aspect is sleep studies, which involve monitoring a patient's sleep patterns using various tools and techniques. These studies provide valuable insights into the underlying causes of sleep disorders and help in developing personalized treatment plans. Another important technology is Continuous Positive Airway Pressure (CPAP) and Bi-level Positive Airway Pressure (BiPAP) devices. These devices provide a steady flow of air pressure to keep the airways open during sleep, ensuring proper breathing and preventing conditions like sleep apnea. Additionally, relaxation technology such as calming music, meditation apps, and white noise machines can help patients relax and fall asleep faster. These technological interventions greatly aid Rehabilitation Registered Nurses in improving patients' sleep and rest patterns to enhance overall well-being and optimize rehabilitation outcomes.

3   The Function of the Rehabilitation Team and Transitions of Care:

The function of the rehabilitation team is essential for providing optimal care to patients and ensuring successful transitions of care. When a patient enters the rehabilitation setting, a team of healthcare professionals, including rehabilitation registered nurses, work together to assess the patient's needs, set goals, and develop an individualized care plan. The rehabilitation team consists of various disciplines such as physical therapists, occupational therapists, speech-language pathologists, social workers, and psychologists. Each member of the team plays a specific role in the patient's care and contributes to their overall recovery. The rehabilitation registered nurse coordinates the care provided by the team, monitors the patient's progress, and communicates with other healthcare professionals involved in the patient's care. Transitions of care occur when a patient moves from one level of care to another, such as from the acute care hospital to a rehabilitation facility or back home. The rehabilitation team ensures a smooth transition by collaborating with other healthcare providers, educating the patient and their family on the discharge plan, and providing necessary resources for continued recovery. Overall, the function of the rehabilitation team is vital in promoting positive outcomes and improving the quality of life for patients in need of rehabilitation services.

3.1   Task 1: Collaborate with the interdisciplinary team to achieve patient- centered goals.:

Task 1: Collaborating with the interdisciplinary team is essential for a Rehabilitation Registered Nurse to achieve patient-centered goals. In order to provide holistic care, it is important to work together with professionals from different disciplines such as doctors, therapists, social workers, and case managers. Collaboration improves communication and ensures that all aspects of the patient's care are addressed. By sharing knowledge and expertise, the team can create a comprehensive treatment plan that meets the individual needs of each patient. This collaboration also helps in setting goals that prioritize the patient's preferences and values, ultimately leading to better outcomes. Effective teamwork and coordination contribute to a smoother transition of care between different healthcare settings, improving continuity and ensuring that the patient's needs are met consistently. Overall, collaboration with the interdisciplinary team plays a crucial role in enhancing the quality of care provided by Rehabilitation Registered Nurses.

3.1.1   Knowledge of:

Knowledge of the topic "Knowledge of:" is important for Rehabilitation Registered Nurses who are working in interdisciplinary teams to achieve patient-centered goals. To effectively collaborate with the team, nurses need to have a comprehensive understanding of the various aspects involved in patient care. They need to possess knowledge about the function of the rehabilitation team, including the roles and responsibilities of each team member.

Additionally, nurses should be well-versed in transitions of care, which involve the transfer of patients from one healthcare setting to another. This knowledge enables them to ensure a smooth and seamless transition for patients, minimizing any potential risks or disruptions in their care.

Subtopics that fall under this broad topic include effective communication and collaboration with team members, understanding the goals and objectives of rehabilitation, promoting patient safety and well-being, coordinating care and services, and advocating for the needs of the patient.

Overall, having a strong knowledge base in these areas allows Rehabilitation Registered Nurses to provide holistic and patient-centered care, facilitating successful outcomes for their patients.

3.1.1.1   Goal setting and expected outcomes:

Goal setting and expected outcomes are crucial aspects in achieving patient-centered care in rehabilitation nursing. The interdisciplinary team collaborates to establish specific goals for the patient's rehabilitation journey. These goals should be realistic, measurable, and focused on improving the patient's quality of life. Common goals include restoring physical function, enhancing mobility, reducing pain, and promoting independence in daily activities. The rehabilitation team works together to develop personalized care plans that reflect the patient's individual needs and preferences. These plans consider the patient's medical history, current condition, and long-term goals. Expected outcomes are the expected results of the rehabilitation interventions, such as improved range of motion, increased strength, or decreased reliance on assistive devices. Regular evaluation and reassessment are essential to track progress towards these expected outcomes and make any necessary adjustments to the care plan. Effective goal setting and expected outcomes help guide the rehabilitation process and ensure optimal outcomes for the patient.

3.1.1.2   Models of healthcare teams (e.g., interdisciplinary, multidisciplinary, transdisciplinary):

Models of healthcare teams, such as interdisciplinary, multidisciplinary, and transdisciplinary, are essential for effective patient care and achieving patient-centered goals.

Interdisciplinary teams consist of professionals from various disciplines who collaborate to provide comprehensive care. Each team member contributes their expertise and works together to develop a holistic treatment plan.

Multidisciplinary teams involve professionals from different disciplines who work independently in their specific roles and communicate regularly to ensure coordinated care. While each member focuses on their area of specialization, collaboration is key to avoid fragmented care.

Transdisciplinary teams take collaboration a step further, blurring boundaries between disciplines. They integrate their knowledge, skills, and perspectives to provide seamless and patient-centered care. This approach encourages shared decision-making and promotes a sense of unity among team members.

These models promote effective communication, teamwork, and information sharing, leading to improved patient outcomes and smoother transitions of care.

3.1.1.3   Rehabilitation philosophy and definition:

Rehabilitation philosophy refers to the underlying principles and beliefs that guide the practice of rehabilitation. It is centered around the idea that individuals with disabilities or injuries can improve their quality of life and functional abilities through comprehensive and individualized care. The primary goal of rehabilitation is to restore optimal physical, emotional, cognitive, and social functioning, enabling patients to regain independence and actively participate in their daily lives.

The definition of rehabilitation involves a multidisciplinary approach, with a team of healthcare professionals working collaboratively to deliver patient-centered care. This team typically includes rehabilitation nurses, physical therapists, occupational therapists, speech therapists, psychologists, and social workers, among others. They assess the patient's unique needs, develop a personalized treatment plan, and monitor progress towards achieving goals. Rehabilitation does not solely focus on treating the physical aspects of an injury or disability but also addresses the psychosocial and environmental factors that may affect a patient's recovery. The philosophy of rehabilitation emphasizes empowerment, education, and support to help individuals overcome obstacles and reach their full potential.

3.1.1.4   Role of the rehabilitation nurse and other team members:

The role of the rehabilitation nurse and other team members is crucial in providing patient-centered care and achieving goals in the rehabilitation process. The rehabilitation nurse collaborates with an interdisciplinary team, including physicians, therapists, social workers, and case managers, to develop and implement individualized care plans. They work together to address the physical, psychological, and social needs of the patient and guide them through the various stages of rehabilitation.

The nurse plays a key role in assessing the patient's condition, developing goals, and coordinating care. They provide education and support to patients and their families, helping them to understand and participate in the recovery process. The team members work together to provide a comprehensive approach to rehabilitation, utilizing their expertise and knowledge to maximize the patient's functional abilities and independence. Effective communication and teamwork are essential for ensuring a smooth transition of care between different settings, such as acute care, inpatient rehabilitation, and home care. By working collaboratively, the rehabilitation team can provide holistic care and improve the outcomes for patients.

3.1.1.5   Related theories (e.g., change, leadership, communication, team function, organizational):

Related theories play a crucial role in the success of a rehabilitation registered nurse working within an interdisciplinary team to achieve patient-centered goals. These theories encompass various aspects such as change, leadership, communication, team function, and organizational dynamics.

Change theories help nurses understand the process of implementing and managing changes in the healthcare setting. Leadership theories provide insights into effective leadership styles and strategies that foster collaboration and motivation within the team. Communication theories highlight the importance of clear and effective communication to ensure smooth coordination and information sharing.

Understanding team function theories enables nurses to comprehend the dynamics of working within an interdisciplinary team, emphasizing the importance of roles, responsibilities, and effective collaboration. Organizational theories provide valuable knowledge about the healthcare organization's structure, culture, and policies, which impact the overall functioning of the rehabilitation team.

By incorporating these related theories, rehabilitation registered nurses can optimize their practice, enhance patient outcomes, and contribute to the smooth transition of care for patients.

3.1.2   Skill in:

As a Rehabilitation Registered Nurse, having strong skills in collaboration with interdisciplinary teams is essential to achieve patient-centered goals. Collaboration requires effective communication, active listening, and the ability to work collectively with professionals from various disciplines. By working together, the team can tailor treatment plans to meet the specific needs of each patient.

One important skill is the ability to understand and respect the expertise of other team members, including physicians, physical therapists, occupational therapists, and social workers. This understanding allows for comprehensive care that addresses all aspects of a patient's rehabilitation. Additionally, being able to contribute valuable insights from the nursing perspective is crucial to ensure holistic care.

Another skill in collaboration is the ability to advocate for the patient's goals and wishes within the team. This involves advocating for appropriate resources, interventions, and supports to help patients achieve their desired outcomes. Collaboration also involves effective coordination of care during transitions, such as from the acute care setting to a rehabilitation facility or from inpatient to outpatient care.

3.1.2.1   Applying appropriate theories (e.g., change, leadership, communication, team function, organizational):

Applying appropriate theories is crucial when collaborating with an interdisciplinary team to achieve patient-centered goals in rehabilitation nursing. These theories include change, leadership, communication, team function, and organizational theories.

Change theories help predict and manage the process of change, ensuring a smooth transition within the team and facilitating patient care. Leadership theories equip rehabilitation nurses with the necessary skills to guide and motivate team members towards common goals. Effective communication theories provide strategies to enhance information exchange and understanding among team members, improving collaboration and patient outcomes.

Understanding team function theories allows rehabilitation nurses to utilize the strengths and expertise of each team member, maximizing the overall effectiveness of the team. Lastly, organizational theories assist nurses in navigating the complex organizational structures within healthcare settings, promoting efficient resource allocation and decision-making.

By applying these theories appropriately, rehabilitation nurses can foster a cohesive and effective interdisciplinary team, ultimately achieving patient-centered goals and successful transitions of care.

3.1.2.2   Communicating and collaborating with the interdisciplinary team:

Communicating and collaborating with the interdisciplinary team is crucial for a Rehabilitation Registered Nurse in order to achieve patient-centered goals. This involves working together with professionals from various disciplines, such as physical therapists, occupational therapists, social workers, and physicians. Effective communication is key to ensure seamless coordination and a holistic approach to patient care. It is important for the nurse to actively participate in team meetings, share knowledge and expertise, and provide updates on the patient's progress. Building strong relationships with team members and establishing trust is essential for effective collaboration. The nurse should also be open to input and feedback from the interdisciplinary team, as it contributes to better patient outcomes. In addition, clear and concise documentation of information and care plans is vital for the team's understanding and continuity of care. Overall, effective communication and collaboration with the interdisciplinary team are foundational skills for a Rehabilitation Registered Nurse to provide comprehensive and patient-centered care.

3.1.2.3   Developing and documenting plans of care to attain patient- centered goals:

Developing and documenting plans of care to attain patient-centered goals is a crucial aspect of a Rehabilitation Registered Nurse's role. This task requires collaboration with the interdisciplinary team to ensure that the care provided is centered around the patient's individual needs and goals.

The first step in this process involves gathering relevant information about the patient, such as their medical history, current condition, and personal preferences. This information helps to create a comprehensive plan of care that addresses the specific needs of the patient.

The next step is to establish patient-centered goals that are realistic and attainable, taking into account the patient's abilities and limitations. These goals should be measurable and time-bound, allowing for regular evaluation and adjustment as needed.

Once the goals are established, the Rehabilitation Registered Nurse works closely with other members of the interdisciplinary team, such as physical therapists, occupational therapists, and social workers, to develop a detailed plan of care. This plan outlines specific interventions and strategies that will be implemented to help the patient reach their goals.

Documentation plays a crucial role in this process, as it ensures that the care provided is well-documented and easily accessible to all members of the healthcare team. Accurate and detailed documentation also helps to track the patient's progress and make any necessary adjustments to the plan of care. Through collaboration with the interdisciplinary team, careful goal-setting, and comprehensive documentation, the nurse can enhance the quality of care provided and improve patient outcomes.

3.1.2.4   Appropriate delegation of responsibilities to team members:

One of the skills required for a Rehabilitation Registered Nurse is the ability to appropriately delegate responsibilities to team members. This involves assigning tasks to individuals based on their skills and expertise, while considering the needs of the patient and the goals of the interdisciplinary team. Effective delegation helps distribute the workload and allows team members to contribute their skills to achieve patient-centered goals. It is important to clearly communicate expectations and provide support and resources to aid team members in carrying out their delegated tasks. The Rehabilitation Registered Nurse must also ensure that tasks are delegated in a fair and equitable manner, taking into account each team member's workload and abilities. Successful delegation promotes collaboration, improves efficiency, and enhances the overall quality of patient care within the rehabilitation team.

3.2   Task 2: Apply the nursing process to promote the patient's community reintegration or transition to the next level of care.:

Task 2: Apply the nursing process to promote the patient's community reintegration or transition to the next level of care in the field of rehabilitation nursing involves several important aspects. Firstly, the nursing process includes assessment, where the nurse gathers information about the patient's condition, needs, and goals for community reintegration or transition. This assessment helps in identifying the specific areas that need to be addressed for a successful transition.

Next, the nursing process involves planning, where the nurse collaborates with the patient, family, and interdisciplinary team to develop a comprehensive care plan. This plan includes specific interventions and goals that aim to support the patient's community reintegration or transition to the next level of care.

Following planning, the nursing process moves to implementation, where the nurse carries out the planned interventions and provides care to promote the patient's community reintegration. This may involve coordinating with other healthcare professionals, providing education and support to the patient and family, and facilitating access to resources and services.

Finally, the nursing process includes evaluation, where the nurse assesses the effectiveness of the interventions and the patient's progress towards achieving their goals. This evaluation helps in identifying any necessary modifications to the care plan and ensures that the patient's needs are being met.

Overall, applying the nursing process to promote the patient's community reintegration or transition to the next level of care is a collaborative and holistic approach that focuses on addressing individual needs and goals to support a successful transition.

3.2.1   Knowledge of:

As a Rehabilitation Registered Nurse, it is important to have knowledge of various aspects related to promoting a patient's community reintegration or transition to the next level of care. This includes understanding the nursing process and how it can be applied in these situations. The nursing process involves assessment, diagnosis, planning, implementation, and evaluation of care. When working with a rehabilitation team, collaboration and communication are essential in order to provide holistic care to patients. Effective teamwork ensures a coordinated approach and helps address any barriers to community reintegration or transitions of care. It is also important to have knowledge of different levels of care, such as home-based care, outpatient care, or long-term care facilities, and understand the specific needs and challenges associated with each level. By staying up-to-date with current research and evidence-based practice, rehabilitation nurses can provide the best possible care and support for their patients.

3.2.1.1   Technology and adaptive equipment (e.g., electronic hand- held devices, electrical simulation, service animals, equipment to support activities of daily living):

Technology and adaptive equipment play a crucial role in promoting the community reintegration and transitioning of patients to the next level of care in rehabilitation nursing. These tools, such as electronic handheld devices, electrical simulation, service animals, and equipment for activities of daily living, help individuals with disabilities regain their independence and improve their quality of life. Electronic handheld devices, like smartphones and tablets, provide patients with easy access to information, communication, and entertainment. They can assist individuals in managing their schedules, medications, and therapy exercises. Electrical simulation devices, such as nerve stimulators, help restore motor function and alleviate pain. They are often used in conjunction with physical therapy to enhance muscle strength and coordination.

Service animals, such as guide dogs, hearing dogs, or therapy animals, offer emotional support and assistance with daily tasks. They can help individuals with visual or hearing impairments navigate their environment and perform specific tasks. Additionally, adaptive equipment, like modified utensils, grab bars, and wheelchair ramps, enables patients to independently engage in activities of daily living, such as eating, bathing, and mobility.

As a rehabilitation registered nurse, it is crucial to have knowledge about these technological advancements and adaptive equipment. By understanding how to incorporate and utilize these tools effectively, nurses can assist patients in their community reintegration and transition to the next level of care. This knowledge empowers nurses to provide comprehensive care, support independence, and improve overall patient outcomes.

3.2.1.2 Community resources (e.g., housing, transportation, community support systems, social services, recreation, CPS, APS):

Community resources play a vital role in promoting the community reintegration or transition of patients to the next level of care. These resources include housing options, transportation services, community support systems, social services, recreation facilities, and child or adult protective services (CPS and APS).

Housing resources ensure that patients have a safe and suitable place to live after their rehabilitation. This can include transitional housing, assisted living facilities, or home modifications.

Transportation services help patients access medical appointments, therapy sessions, and community resources. This may involve arranging for accessible vehicles or coordinating with public transportation systems.

Community support systems provide ongoing assistance and guidance to patients as they reintegrate into their communities. This can involve support groups, case management services, and peer mentorship programs.

Social services connect patients with resources such as food banks, financial assistance, and employment opportunities, which are crucial for their well-being and successful community reintegration.

Recreation facilities and programs promote socialization, physical activity, and overall well-being. They can range from community centers to adaptive sports programs.

CPS and APS ensure the safety and welfare of vulnerable individuals, such as children or older adults, who may require protective services. These resources address various aspects of a patient's life, including housing, transportation, support systems, social services, recreation, and protective services.

3.2.1.3 Personal resources (e.g., financial, caregiver support systems, caregivers, spiritual, cultural):

Personal resources play a crucial role in promoting the community reintegration or transition to the next level of care for patients. These resources may include financial support, caregiver support systems, caregivers themselves, spiritual beliefs, and cultural background.

Financial resources are important as they ensure that patients have access to necessary medical equipment, medications, and therapies. This may involve insurance coverage, assistance programs, or personal savings.

Caregiver support systems are essential for patients who require assistance with daily activities or medical care. These support systems may include family members, friends, or professional caregivers who provide physical and emotional support to the patient.

The role of caregivers is invaluable in helping patients fully reintegrate into their community or transition to a new level of care. Caregivers provide assistance with mobility, personal care, medication management, and emotional support. They play a vital role in the patient's overall well-being and recovery.

Spiritual beliefs can also contribute to a patient's recovery process. Spiritual resources, such as prayer, meditation, or religious practices, can provide comfort, hope, and emotional strength.

Cultural background is another important personal resource that must be considered. Understanding a patient's cultural values and traditions helps healthcare professionals provide culturally sensitive care, which promotes better patient outcomes and enhances community reintegration. Healthcare professionals must recognize and utilize these resources to provide holistic and patient-centered care.

3.2.1.4 Professional resources (e.g., psychologist, neurologist, clergy, teacher, case manager, vocational rehabilitation counselor, home health, outpatient therapy):

Professional resources play a vital role in promoting a patient's community reintegration or transition to the next level of care in rehabilitation nursing. The multidisciplinary team consists of professionals such as psychologists, neurologists, clergy, teachers, case managers, vocational rehabilitation counselors, home health professionals, and outpatient therapists.

Psychologists provide mental health support and counseling, helping patients cope with emotional challenges during the transition process. Neurologists assess and treat patients with neurological conditions, addressing any physical limitations or impairments.

Clergy members offer spiritual guidance and support, catering to the patient's individual beliefs and values. Teachers may facilitate educational programs to enhance skill development and adjustment to daily activities.

Case managers coordinate services and resources, ensuring a smooth transition and continuity of care. Vocational rehabilitation counselors assist with vocational assessments, job training, and placement.

Home health professionals deliver healthcare services in the comfort of the patient's home, promoting independence and self-care. Outpatient therapists provide ongoing therapy sessions to optimize the patient's physical and functional abilities.

These professionals collaborate with the rehabilitation registered nurse to develop comprehensive care plans and individualized interventions that promote successful community reintegration or transition to the next level of care.

3.2.1.5 Teaching and learning strategies for self-advocacy:

Teaching and learning strategies for self-advocacy are crucial in promoting patients' community reintegration or transition to the next level of care. As a Rehabilitation Registered Nurse, it is essential to equip patients with the necessary skills and knowledge to advocate for themselves effectively.

One important strategy is providing education about their condition, treatment options, and available resources. Patients need to understand their rights, responsibilities, and how to make informed decisions about their care. This can be achieved through one-on-one teaching sessions, group education classes, or through the use of educational materials.

Another strategy is encouraging patients to actively participate in their care planning and decision-making process. This involves empowering them to voice their needs, preferences, and concerns, ensuring that their perspectives are taken into account.

Additionally, utilizing motivational interviewing techniques can help patients explore their goals, strengths, and resources, enabling them to develop self-advocacy skills.

Overall, teaching and learning strategies for self-advocacy play a vital role in facilitating patients' successful transition back to their community or the next level of care.

3.2.1.6   Different levels of care and care continuum (e.g., acute rehab, home care, assisted living):

The care continuum refers to a range of healthcare services available to patients as they progress through different levels of care. This includes acute rehabilitation, home care, and assisted living. Each level of care provides a specific type and intensity of services based on the patient's needs.

Acute rehabilitation involves providing intensive medical and therapeutic care in a hospital setting. It is typically for patients who have experienced a major illness, injury, or surgery and require specialized rehabilitation interventions. The goal is to improve the patient's functional abilities and maximize their independence.

Home care focuses on providing healthcare services in the patient's own home. This can include nursing care, assistance with activities of daily living, medication management, and therapy services. It allows patients to receive care in a familiar environment and promotes their recovery and overall well-being.

Assisted living provides a supportive living arrangement for individuals who may need assistance with daily activities but do not require the level of care provided in a nursing home. It offers services such as meals, housekeeping, transportation, medication management, and social activities to promote independence and quality of life.

The different levels of care in the care continuum aim to meet the diverse needs of patients as they transition through various stages of their healthcare journey. A comprehensive approach involving healthcare professionals, such as rehabilitation nurses, therapists, and care coordinators, ensures a smooth and effective transition between these different levels of care.

3.2.2   Skill in:

Skill in: The skill set required for a Rehabilitation Registered Nurse in promoting the patient's community reintegration or transition to the next level of care is multifaceted. Firstly, a nurse must possess effective communication skills to establish rapport with patients, their families, and the interdisciplinary rehabilitation team. This allows for clear, comprehensive assessment and goal-setting. Additionally, a nurse must have a strong understanding of the nursing process, which involves assessing the patient's current functional abilities, identifying areas of improvement, implementing evidence-based interventions, and evaluating outcomes. The ability to provide patient education about self-care techniques, medication management, and symptom recognition is crucial. Furthermore, a Rehabilitation Registered Nurse must possess excellent time management and organizational skills to coordinate care and navigate healthcare systems. They should also be proficient in documentation and possess knowledge of local community resources to support the patient's continued progress. Overall, a Rehabilitation Registered Nurse plays a vital role in facilitating the patient's smooth transition back to their community or the next level of care through their diverse skill set.

3.2.2.1   Accessing community resources:

Accessing community resources is an essential aspect of a Rehabilitation Registered Nurse's role in promoting a patient's community reintegration or transition to the next level of care. These resources can provide the necessary support and services to facilitate the patient's successful return to the community.

One important aspect of accessing community resources is identifying and connecting the patient with local support organizations that can provide assistance with various aspects of daily living, such as transportation, housing, or financial support. This can help the patient overcome barriers and challenges they may face upon discharge.

Additionally, accessing community resources involves collaborating with healthcare professionals, social workers, and case managers to ensure a smooth transition and continuity of care for the patient. This includes coordinating appointments, referrals, and follow-up care to ensure the patient receives the necessary medical, therapeutic, and psychosocial support.

Furthermore, Rehabilitation Registered Nurses play a crucial role in educating patients and their families about available community resources and empowering them to actively participate in their own care. This may involve providing information about support groups, educational programs, and recreational opportunities that can enhance the patient's well-being and promote their engagement within the community.

Overall, accessing community resources is a vital component of the Rehabilitation Registered Nurse's role in promoting the patient's successful reintegration into the community and facilitating a seamless transition to the next level of care.

3.2.2.2   Assessing readiness for discharge:

Assessing readiness for discharge is an essential aspect of the rehabilitation process for a Rehabilitation Registered Nurse. This involves evaluating the patient's physical, psychological, and social abilities and determining if they are prepared to leave the healthcare facility and reintegrate into their community or transition to the next level of care. The nurse considers various factors such as the patient's medical condition, functional status, support system, and ability to manage their own healthcare needs. Additionally, the nurse assesses the patient's understanding of their treatment plan, medications, and follow-up care requirements. Subtopics that may be explored during this assessment include the patient's readiness to manage activities of daily living, cognitive abilities, emotional well-being, and financial resources. By conducting a thorough assessment of readiness for discharge, the Rehabilitation Registered Nurse can ensure a smooth transition and promote successful community reintegration.

3.2.2.3   Assessing barriers to community reintegration:

Assessing barriers to community reintegration is an essential aspect of the nursing process for promoting a patient's transition back into the community or to the next level of care. The Rehabilitation Registered Nurse plays a crucial role in identifying and addressing these barriers to ensure a successful reintegration.

One important aspect of assessing barriers is understanding the patient's physical and cognitive abilities. This involves evaluating their functional capacity, mobility, and any limitations they may have. It also includes assessing their mental health, including factors such as depression or anxiety that may affect their ability to reintegrate.

Social support is another key consideration. The nurse must assess the patient's relationships, both within their family and in the community. Identifying any lack of social support or strained relationships can help determine whether additional resources or interventions are necessary to facilitate successful community reintegration.

Financial constraints may also pose barriers to community reintegration. The nurse should assess the patient's financial situation and identify any challenges in accessing essential resources, such as housing or transportation. This evaluation can inform appropriate referrals or assistance programs to overcome these barriers.

Lastly, the Rehabilitation Registered Nurse should assess the patient's level of involvement and motivation to reintegrate into the community. Identifying any ambivalence or resistance can guide the development of strategies to address these issues effectively.

Overall, assessing barriers to community reintegration involves evaluating physical and cognitive abilities, social support, financial constraints, and the patient's motivation. By identifying these barriers, the nurse can develop individualized plans of care to promote successful transitions and maximize the patient's overall well-being.

3.2.2.4 Evaluating outcomes and adjusting goals (e.g., interdisciplinary team and patientcentered):

Evaluating outcomes and adjusting goals are crucial aspects of promoting a patient's community reintegration or transition to the next level of care in rehabilitation nursing. This process involves the collaboration of an interdisciplinary team, consisting of healthcare professionals from various disciplines, working together to optimize patient outcomes. The team may include physicians, therapists, psychologists, social workers, and nurses.

The evaluation of outcomes involves assessing the effectiveness of the interventions and treatments provided to the patient. This assessment is done by analyzing various indicators such as the patient's functional abilities, pain levels, quality of life, and overall satisfaction. The interdisciplinary team plays a pivotal role in this evaluation process, as they bring diverse perspectives and expertise to comprehensively evaluate the patient's progress.

Adjusting goals is a continuous process that ensures that the patient's care plan remains patient-centered and adaptable to changing circumstances. It involves identifying and addressing any barriers or challenges that may hinder the patient's progress. The interdisciplinary team collaborates to modify the goals and interventions accordingly, keeping in mind the patient's unique needs and preferences.

By consistently evaluating outcomes and adjusting goals, rehabilitation registered nurses can optimize the rehabilitation process, facilitate the patient's community reintegration, and ensure a successful transition to the next level of care.

3.2.2.5 Identifying financial barriers and providing appropriate resources:

Identifying financial barriers and providing appropriate resources is a crucial aspect of promoting a patient's community reintegration or transition to the next level of care as a Rehabilitation Registered Nurse. Financial barriers can hinder a patient's ability to access the necessary resources, services, and support for their rehabilitation journey. The first step in addressing financial barriers is to conduct a thorough assessment to identify any financial constraints the patient may face. This assessment involves gathering information about the patient's insurance coverage, income level, available financial resources, and potential sources of support, such as grants or community organizations. Once the financial barriers are identified, the rehabilitation team can work together to develop a plan to mitigate these obstacles. This plan may include exploring alternative funding options, connecting patients with financial counseling services, assisting with insurance navigation, or advocating for necessary services. Additionally, the rehabilitation team can collaborate with social workers, case managers, or financial assistance programs to facilitate access to appropriate resources and financial support. By addressing financial barriers, Rehabilitation Registered Nurses can ensure that patients have the financial means to achieve optimal outcomes in their rehabilitation journey and successfully reintegrate into their community or transition to the next level of care.

3.2.2.6 Facilitating appropriate referrals:

Facilitating appropriate referrals is an important aspect of the rehabilitation registered nurse's role in promoting the patient's community reintegration or transition to the next level of care. This involves identifying the patient's needs and connecting them with appropriate resources and services.

One aspect of facilitating appropriate referrals is conducting a thorough assessment of the patient's physical, psychological, and social needs. This helps the nurse determine what services are necessary for the patient's successful reintegration or transition.

Once the patient's needs are identified, the nurse can then make referrals to various professionals and services, such as physical therapists, occupational therapists, social workers, and support groups. The nurse ensures that these referrals are appropriate and align with the patient's goals and preferences.

Effective communication is crucial in facilitating referrals. The nurse collaborates with the patient, their family, and the healthcare team to ensure that everyone is informed and involved in the referral process. The nurse also follows up with the patient and the referral sources to ensure that the appropriate care is being provided.

Overall, facilitating appropriate referrals requires the nurse to have a comprehensive understanding of the patient's needs and available resources. By connecting the patient with the right professionals and services, the nurse plays a vital role in promoting the patient's successful community reintegration or transition to the next level of care.

3.2.2.7 Participating in team and patient caregiver conferences:

Participating in team and patient caregiver conferences is an important role for a Rehabilitation Registered Nurse. During these conferences, the nurse collaborates with other healthcare professionals, such as physical therapists, occupational therapists, and social workers, to develop and implement a comprehensive plan for the patient's community reintegration or transition to the next level of care. The nurse actively participates in discussions to understand the patient's needs, goals, and progress. They also share their expertise, observations, and recommendations to ensure the best possible outcomes for the patient. Additionally, the Rehabilitation Registered Nurse communicates with the patient's caregiver to provide education, support, and guidance throughout the rehabilitation process. By actively participating in these conferences, the nurse helps facilitate effective teamwork and promotes coordinated care for the patient's successful transition back into the community or to another level of care.

3.2.2.8   Planning discharge (e.g., home visits, caregiver teaching):

Planning discharge is a crucial component of the nursing process to ensure the patient's successful transition to the community or the next level of care. This involves various activities, including home visits and caregiver teaching. Home visits help the rehabilitation registered nurse assess the patient's living environment and determine any modifications or adaptations needed for a safe and supportive homecoming. During these visits, the nurse may also identify potential barriers or challenges the patient might face and provide education on how to manage them. Caregiver teaching is another essential aspect of discharge planning, as it equips the patient's family members or caregivers with the knowledge and skills necessary to provide optimal care at home. This may include training on wound care, medication management, mobility assistance, and disease management strategies. By addressing these areas, the rehabilitation registered nurse ensures a smooth and successful transition for the patient, promoting their community reintegration and overall well-being.

3.2.2.9   Teaching health, wellness, and life skills maintenance:

Teaching health, wellness, and life skills maintenance is a crucial aspect of the rehabilitation process for a Rehabilitation Registered Nurse. This involves educating patients on how to take care of their physical and mental well-being, as well as developing and maintaining essential life skills. The nurse plays a vital role in providing information and guidance to patients on various topics such as healthy eating habits, exercise routines, medication management, stress management, and personal hygiene. Teaching these skills helps patients to maximize their independence and quality of life after they transition to the next level of care or return to their community. By empowering patients with the knowledge and skills to manage their health and wellness, the nurse promotes a successful transition and long-term sustainability of their progress.

3.2.2.10   Using adaptive equipment and technology (e.g., voice activated call systems, computer supported prosthetics):

Using adaptive equipment and technology such as voice activated call systems and computer supported prosthetics is an important aspect of promoting a patient's community reintegration or transition to the next level of care as a Rehabilitation Registered Nurse. Voice activated call systems allow patients with limited mobility or physical impairments to easily communicate their needs and summon assistance. This technology enhances their independence and safety by reducing the need for physical assistance. Additionally, computer supported prosthetics enable patients to regain their ability to perform tasks with greater ease and functionality. These prosthetics can be controlled by the patient's movements or through advanced technology like neural interfaces. By utilizing adaptive equipment and technology, Rehabilitation Registered Nurses can support patients in their transition back into the community or to higher levels of care, empowering them to regain their independence and improve their overall quality of life.

4   Legislative, Economic, Ethical, and Legal Issues:

As a Rehabilitation Registered Nurse, it is essential to have an understanding of legislative, economic, ethical, and legal issues that may arise in the healthcare field.

Legislative issues refer to laws and regulations that govern the practice of nursing and healthcare in general. These laws ensure patient safety, privacy, and informed consent. Nurses must be knowledgeable about their scope of practice, licensing requirements, and documentation standards to comply with legislative mandates.

Economic issues involve the financial aspects of healthcare, such as reimbursement models, insurance coverage, and healthcare costs. Rehabilitation nurses must navigate these economic factors to provide efficient and cost-effective care to their patients.

Ethical considerations encompass moral values and principles that guide nursing practice. Nurses face dilemmas that require ethical decision-making, such as balancing the autonomy of patients with their well-being.

Legal issues pertain to the application of laws and regulations specific to healthcare. Rehabilitation nurses need to be aware of legal obligations, such as reporting incidents, maintaining patient confidentiality, and avoiding negligence or malpractice.

Overall, understanding and addressing legislative, economic, ethical, and legal issues is crucial for Rehabilitation Registered Nurses to provide quality care while upholding professional standards and maintaining patient satisfaction.

4.1   Task 1: Integrate legislation and regulations in the management of care.:

As a Rehabilitation Registered Nurse, it is important to integrate legislation and regulations in the management of care. This means understanding and following the laws and rules that govern healthcare practice. This includes regulations related to patient safety, privacy, documentation, and ethical standards.

One aspect of integrating legislation and regulations in the management of care is staying up-to-date with current laws and regulations that pertain to rehabilitation nursing. This involves regularly reviewing and understanding government and organizational policies and guidelines.

Another aspect is accurately documenting and maintaining patient records, following legal requirements for confidentiality and information security. Rehabilitation nurses must also be aware of ethical considerations, ensuring that the care provided is in the best interest of the patient and within legal boundaries.

Furthermore, collaborating with interdisciplinary teams and involving patients in their care planning helps to ensure compliance with legislation and regulations. This includes respecting patients' rights and autonomy while also meeting legal obligations.

Overall, as a Rehabilitation Registered Nurse, integrating legislation and regulations in the management of care is vital to provide safe, ethical, and effective care to patients.

4.1.1   Knowledge of:

As a Rehabilitation Registered Nurse, having knowledge of legislation and regulations in the management of care is crucial. Understanding the laws and policies that govern healthcare practices is essential for providing safe and effective patient care.

One important aspect of this topic is understanding legislative requirements for documentation and record-keeping. This includes knowing the proper way to document patient assessments, progress notes, and treatment plans. It also involves understanding the legal obligations regarding confidentiality and privacy of patient information.

Additionally, being knowledgeable about economic issues related to healthcare is necessary. This includes understanding insurance policies, reimbursement procedures, and the financial impact of different treatments and interventions.

Ethical considerations are another important aspect of this topic. Rehabilitation nurses must understand the principles of medical ethics and be able to navigate ethical dilemmas that arise in their practice. This includes respecting patient autonomy, promoting beneficence, and avoiding conflicts of interest.

Lastly, being aware of legal issues in healthcare is crucial. This includes understanding laws related to informed consent, advanced directives, and patient rights. Knowledge of legal standards and guidelines helps ensure that rehabilitation nurses provide care within the boundaries of the law.

Overall, having a comprehensive knowledge of legislation, economic factors, ethical considerations, and legal issues in the management of care is essential for Rehabilitation Registered Nurses to provide safe, effective, and ethical patient care.

4.1.1.1 Agencies related to regulatory, disability, and rehabilitation (e.g., CARF, The Joint Commission, APS, CPS, CMS, SSA, OSHA):

The management of care in rehabilitation nursing involves integrating legislation and regulations that govern various agencies related to regulatory, disability, and rehabilitation. These agencies play a crucial role in ensuring quality care and safety for individuals with disabilities.

CARF (Commission on Accreditation of Rehabilitation Facilities) is a nonprofit organization that accredits and certifies rehabilitation programs. The Joint Commission is another accrediting body that evaluates healthcare organizations for compliance with standards. APS (Adult Protective Services) and CPS (Child Protective Services) are agencies that investigate and intervene in cases of abuse or neglect. CMS (Centers for Medicare and Medicaid Services) oversees government healthcare programs. SSA (Social Security Administration) provides disability benefits to eligible individuals. OSHA (Occupational Safety and Health Administration) enforces workplace safety regulations.

As a rehabilitation registered nurse, understanding these agencies and their role in maintaining standards of care is essential. Compliance with regulations and standards ensures the provision of high-quality, ethical, and legal care for patients with disabilities.

4.1.1.2 Specific legislation related to disability and rehabilitation (e.g., Medicare, Medicaid, ADA, rehabilitation acts, HIPAA, Affordable Care Act, workers' compensation, IDEA, Vocational, IMPACT Act):

Specific legislation related to disability and rehabilitation includes various acts and laws that aim to protect the rights and improve the quality of life for individuals with disabilities. Medicare and Medicaid provide health insurance coverage for eligible individuals with disabilities and ensure access to necessary medical services and supports. The Americans with Disabilities Act (ADA) prohibits discrimination against individuals with disabilities in public accommodations, employment, and other areas. Rehabilitation acts, such as the Rehabilitation Act of 1973, provide support and funding for vocational rehabilitation services. The Health Insurance Portability and Accountability Act (HIPAA) protects the privacy and security of patient health information. The Affordable Care Act expands access to healthcare and includes provisions related to disability and rehabilitation. Workers' compensation laws provide benefits to workers who experience work-related injuries or disabilities. The Individuals with Disabilities Education Act (IDEA) guarantees free appropriate public education for children with disabilities. Vocational rehabilitation programs assist individuals with disabilities in gaining employment or maintaining workplace accommodations. Lastly, the IMPACT Act promotes care coordination and improved outcomes for individuals receiving post-acute care. These legislations and acts play a vital role in ensuring equal opportunities, healthcare access, and rights for individuals with disabilities and guide the practice of rehabilitation registered nurses.

4.1.2 Skill in:

As a Rehabilitation Registered Nurse, there are several important skills required in integrating legislation and regulations in the management of care. Firstly, it is crucial to have a thorough understanding of the legislative and regulatory framework pertaining to rehabilitation nursing. This involves staying updated on current laws and guidelines related to patient care, privacy, and safety. Secondly, effective communication and collaboration with interdisciplinary teams is essential. The ability to work together and coordinate care ensures compliance with regulations and promotes patient-centered care. Furthermore, critical thinking skills are necessary to interpret and apply legislation and regulations to specific patient scenarios. This involves understanding ethical principles, such as patient autonomy and confidentiality, and making decisions that align with these principles. Finally, documentation and record-keeping must be accurate and up-to-date to comply with legal requirements.

4.1.2.1 Accessing, interpreting, and applying legal, regulatory, and accreditation information:

Accessing, interpreting, and applying legal, regulatory, and accreditation information is crucial for a Rehabilitation Registered Nurse. By integrating legislation and regulations into the management of care, they ensure compliance with industry standards and ethical guidelines. This involves understanding and accessing various sources of information such as federal and state laws, Medicare and Medicaid requirements, and accreditation standards. The nurse must interpret this information accurately to determine its relevance to their practice. They must then apply these laws and regulations to their daily responsibilities, such as patient care, documentation, and professional conduct. By staying up-to-date with legal and regulatory changes, the nurse ensures the provision of safe and effective care, while also protecting themselves and their healthcare facility from legal liability.

4.1.2.2 Using standardized assessment tools:

Using standardized assessment tools is an essential aspect of a Rehabilitation Registered Nurse's skill set. These tools help evaluate the patient's physical, cognitive, and functional abilities, enabling the nurse to design appropriate care plans. Standardized assessment tools provide objective measurements and allow for consistent evaluation across different healthcare settings. These tools are evidence-based and have been developed and validated to ensure accuracy and reliability.

By using standardized assessment tools, Rehabilitation Registered Nurses can gather comprehensive and consistent data about their patients' strengths, limitations, and overall functional status. This information assists in identifying areas for improvement and determining appropriate interventions. It also helps in tracking patients' progress over time and measuring the effectiveness of different interventions.

Some common subtopics within this topic may include the selection and administration of standardized assessment tools, the interpretation of assessment results, and the integration of assessment findings into the care planning process. Overall, using standardized assessment tools enhances the Rehabilitation Registered Nurse's ability to provide individualized and effective care to their patients.

4.2   Task 2: Use the nursing process to deliver cost effective patient- centered care.:

The nursing process is an essential tool for rehabilitation registered nurses to deliver cost-effective patient-centered care. It involves a systematic approach that includes assessment, diagnosis, planning, implementation, and evaluation.

During the assessment phase, nurses gather information about the patient's condition, needs, and goals. This includes physical, mental, and emotional assessments.

In the diagnosis phase, nurses identify the patient's health problems and potential risks. This helps in developing a plan of care that is patient-centered and cost-effective.

The planning phase involves setting goals and developing interventions to address the patient's needs. This includes coordinating with other healthcare professionals and utilizing resources efficiently.

In the implementation phase, nurses carry out the planned interventions and provide the necessary treatments and therapies. This may involve education, counseling, and coordinating care.

The evaluation phase is crucial in determining the effectiveness of the interventions and making necessary adjustments. This ensures that the patient's progress is monitored and that the care provided is cost-effective.

By utilizing the nursing process, rehabilitation registered nurses can deliver high-quality, patient-centered care while considering the economic aspects. They can effectively manage resources, collaborate with the interdisciplinary team, and promote positive outcomes for their patients.

4.2.1   Knowledge of:

A rehabilitation registered nurse needs to have knowledge of various aspects related to legislative, economic, ethical, and legal issues in order to deliver cost-effective patient-centered care. In terms of legislative issues, the nurse should be familiar with laws and regulations that govern healthcare delivery, such as licensing requirements and patient rights. Understanding economic issues is important to ensure efficient use of resources and minimize costs associated with rehabilitation services. This knowledge can include reimbursement methodologies, budgeting, and cost-benefit analysis. Ethical considerations are crucial for providing ethical and culturally sensitive care, respecting patient autonomy, and upholding professional integrity. Legal issues involve understanding legal responsibilities, including documentation, confidentiality, and informed consent. Additionally, the nurse should be knowledgeable about healthcare policies and guidelines related to rehabilitation practices. Overall, possessing comprehensive knowledge in these areas enables the rehabilitation registered nurse to deliver high-quality and cost-effective care to their patients.

4.2.1.1   Clinical practice guidelines:

Clinical practice guidelines are evidence-based recommendations that guide healthcare professionals in delivering optimal patient care. These guidelines are developed by experts in the field and are derived from the latest research and best practices. They provide a framework for healthcare providers to make informed decisions and ensure that patients receive consistent and high-quality care.

The use of clinical practice guidelines can help rehabilitation registered nurses in several ways. Firstly, they ensure that nurses are up-to-date with the latest evidence and recommendations for providing rehabilitation care. This promotes better patient outcomes and reduces the risk of adverse events.

Guidelines also promote cost-effective care by avoiding unnecessary interventions and promoting the use of evidence-based treatments. By following these guidelines, nurses can make informed decisions about resource allocation and help manage healthcare costs.

Furthermore, clinical practice guidelines contribute to patient-centered care by prioritizing the individual needs and preferences of patients. They help nurses tailor their care plans to meet the unique circumstances of each patient, ensuring that their rehabilitation goals are met. They promote evidence-based and cost-effective patient care while also emphasizing the importance of personalized, patient-centered care.

4.2.1.2   Community and public resources:

Community and public resources play a crucial role in the delivery of patient-centered care by Rehabilitation Registered Nurses. These resources encompass a wide range of services and supports that are available in the community to assist individuals in their rehabilitation journey. They include community health clinics, social service agencies, vocational rehabilitation programs, and support groups.

One subtopic under community resources is healthcare facilities. These facilities provide medical services, such as physical therapy, occupational therapy, and speech therapy, which are essential for patients� recovery and rehabilitation. Another subtopic is social services, which offer assistance with housing, transportation, and financial support. These services help patients regain independence and improve their overall well-being.

Additionally, vocational rehabilitation programs help patients reintegrate into the workforce, leading to increased self-esteem and economic stability. Lastly, support groups provide a sense of community and emotional support for patients and their families, which are vital for the rehabilitation process.

By accessing and utilizing these community and public resources, Rehabilitation Registered Nurses can deliver cost-effective and patient-centered care, ensuring that individuals receive the necessary support to achieve their rehabilitation goals.

4.2.1.3   Insurance and reimbursement (e.g., PPS, workers' compensation):

Insurance and reimbursement play a crucial role in the delivery of cost-effective, patient-centered care for Rehabilitation Registered Nurses. One important aspect of insurance is the Prospective Payment System (PPS). PPS is a reimbursement method where a fixed amount is paid for specific medical services or procedures. Understanding PPS is essential for nurses to effectively manage resources and provide quality care while staying within budget.

Additionally, nurses should be knowledgeable about workers' compensation insurance. This type of coverage compensates employees who suffer work-related injuries or illnesses. Rehabilitation nurses need to understand the process of filing workers' compensation claims and ensuring proper reimbursement for their patients.

Other subtopics to consider when discussing insurance and reimbursement are the ethical and legal issues associated with billing and reimbursement practices. Rehabilitation nurses must adhere to ethical standards, such as accurately documenting patient care and avoiding fraudulent billing practices.

4.2.1.4 Regulatory agency audit processes:

Regulatory agency audit processes involve the evaluation of healthcare facilities to ensure compliance with standards and regulations. These audits are conducted by regulatory agencies, such as the Joint Commission, state health departments, and Medicare/Medicaid. The purpose of these audits is to assess the quality of care provided to patients and identify any deficiencies that need to be addressed. The audit process typically includes a review of documentation, interviews with staff and patients, and on-site inspections. Some subtopics that may be covered in the audit process include infection control, medication management, patient safety, and quality improvement. Rehabilitation registered nurses play a crucial role in this process by providing input and ensuring compliance with regulations. They may also be involved in developing and implementing corrective action plans based on audit findings. Overall, regulatory agency audit processes help to promote patient-centered care, improve outcomes, and maintain accountability in healthcare settings.

4.2.1.5 Staffing patterns and policies:

Staffing patterns and policies are crucial for the delivery of cost-effective, patient-centered care by Rehabilitation Registered Nurses. These policies encompass various aspects such as the allocation of staff, work schedules, and patient-to-nurse ratios. It is essential to establish appropriate staffing patterns to ensure optimal patient outcomes and safety. By analyzing patient needs and acuity levels, the organization can determine the ideal number and types of staff required. Additionally, policies should address the utilization of temporary or agency staff during times of increased demand. Adequate staffing helps prevent burnout among nursing staff and promotes quality care. It is crucial to regularly review and update staffing policies to align with legislative, economic, ethical, and legal requirements. Ultimately, effective staffing patterns contribute to the overall success and satisfaction of both patients and healthcare providers in the rehabilitation setting.

4.2.1.6 Utilization review processes:

Utilization review processes play a crucial role in delivering cost-effective and patient-centered care in rehabilitation nursing. These processes involve the assessment of the medical necessity and appropriateness of healthcare services provided to patients. By conducting utilization reviews, healthcare providers can ensure that resources are used efficiently and effectively.

One important aspect of utilization review processes is the evaluation of the patient's condition and treatment plan. This involves reviewing medical records, conducting interviews, and utilizing evidence-based guidelines to determine the most appropriate course of action. Case managers and utilization review nurses are often involved in this process.

Another aspect is the identification of potential gaps or deviations from established standards of care. By identifying these issues, healthcare professionals can implement strategies to address them and improve patient outcomes. This may involve modifying treatment plans, providing additional education or resources, or promoting alternative care options.

Utilization review processes also include collaboration with payers and insurance companies to ensure that reimbursement is appropriately allocated and that the care provided aligns with established guidelines and policies.

4.2.1.7 Patient-centered care:

Patient-centered care is an essential aspect of nursing practice, particularly for Rehabilitation Registered Nurses. It focuses on providing individualized care that is tailored to meet the specific needs and preferences of each patient. This approach recognizes that patients are experts in their own experiences and empowers them to actively participate in their healthcare decisions. Patient-centered care involves effective communication, shared decision-making, and mutual respect between healthcare providers and patients. It also takes into consideration the physical, emotional, and psychosocial aspects of care. By prioritizing the patient's values, preferences, and goals, Rehabilitation Registered Nurses can ensure that the care they deliver is holistic and meaningful. Implementing patient-centered care requires a collaborative approach among healthcare professionals, patients, and their families, as well as a commitment to continuous improvement.

4.2.2 Skill in:

Skill in rehabilitation nursing requires proficiency in various aspects of patient care. This includes effective communication with patients, their families, and the interdisciplinary team. Rehabilitation nurses must possess the ability to assess patients' needs and develop individualized care plans. They should also be skilled in providing patient-centered care that promotes independence and functional abilities.

In addition, rehabilitation nurses must have a good understanding of legislative, economic, ethical, and legal issues that may impact patient care. They need to comply with healthcare regulations, advocate for patient rights, and provide cost-effective care. These nurses must be knowledgeable about reimbursement systems, insurance coverage, and the availability of community resources.

Furthermore, rehabilitation nurses must adhere to ethical principles, ensuring the privacy and confidentiality of patient information. They must also understand and follow legal protocols regarding informed consent, advance directives, and documentation. By integrating these skills into their practice, rehabilitation registered nurses can deliver effective and comprehensive care to their patients.

4.2.2.1 Analyzing quality and utilization data:

Analyzing quality and utilization data is an essential task for Rehabilitation Registered Nurses. This process helps in delivering cost-effective and patient-centered care. Quality data analysis involves evaluating the overall performance of healthcare services, focusing on indicators such as patient outcomes, safety, and satisfaction. Utilization data analysis, on the other hand, involves examining the patterns of healthcare service use and resource allocation. By analyzing these data, nurses can identify areas for improvement, implement evidence-based practices, and optimize resource utilization. Subtopics within this area may include collecting and evaluating patient outcomes, monitoring healthcare service utilization, identifying cost-saving opportunities, and ensuring compliance with legislative, economic, ethical, and legal requirements. This analysis also contributes to the development of healthcare policies and guidelines, and ultimately, enhances the overall quality and efficiency of rehabilitation nursing care.

4.2.2.2   Collaborating with private, community, and public resources:

Collaborating with private, community, and public resources is essential for a Rehabilitation Registered Nurse to deliver cost-effective, patient-centered care. By working together with these different resources, nurses can ensure that patients receive the support and services they need to achieve optimal rehabilitation outcomes.

Private resources, such as private healthcare providers and insurance companies, can offer specialized services, therapies, and funding options for patients. Community resources, such as local support groups, non-profit organizations, and community centers, can provide additional support and resources for patients during their rehabilitation journey. Public resources, such as government programs and agencies, can provide funding, assistance, and regulations to support rehabilitation efforts.

In order to effectively collaborate with these different resources, Rehabilitation Registered Nurses need to have strong communication and networking skills. They must also be knowledgeable about the various resources available in their community and how to access them for their patients. By leveraging these resources, nurses can enhance their ability to deliver holistic, comprehensive care to their patients, improving their overall well-being and quality of life.

4.2.2.3   Incorporating clinical practice guidelines:

Incorporating clinical practice guidelines is a vital aspect of delivering cost-effective patient-centered care as a Rehabilitation Registered Nurse. These guidelines provide evidence-based recommendations for clinical decision-making and help to standardize practices across the healthcare system. By following clinical practice guidelines, nurses can ensure that their interventions are based on the best available evidence, resulting in improved patient outcomes and reduced healthcare costs.

One important aspect of incorporating these guidelines is understanding the legislative, economic, ethical, and legal issues surrounding their implementation. Nurses must be aware of any laws or regulations that govern the use of clinical practice guidelines in their practice setting. They must also consider the economic implications, such as the cost-effectiveness of implementing these guidelines and any potential financial incentives or penalties associated with their use.

Ethical considerations are another important aspect to consider. Rehabilitation Registered Nurses must ensure that the guidelines align with their professional values and ethical obligations towards their patients. They must also consider the legal implications, such as any potential liability associated with deviating from or not following these guidelines.

To effectively incorporate clinical practice guidelines, Rehabilitation Registered Nurses should stay updated on the latest evidence-based practices. They should also collaborate with interdisciplinary healthcare teams to ensure that these guidelines are implemented consistently across all levels of care. This collaboration can help to address any challenges or barriers that may arise in incorporating the guidelines into daily practice. By adhering to these guidelines, nurses can improve patient outcomes, reduce healthcare costs, and ensure ethical and legal compliance in their practice.

4.2.2.4   Managing current and projected resources in a cost-effective manner:

Managing current and projected resources in a cost-effective manner is an essential skill for Rehabilitation Registered Nurses. It involves optimizing the use of available resources to deliver high-quality patient-centered care while minimizing costs. This includes efficiently allocating staff, supplies, equipment, and facilities based on the projected needs of the patients. Nurses must have a comprehensive understanding of the nursing process to effectively manage resources. They must assess the needs of each patient, plan and implement appropriate interventions, and evaluate the outcomes. Additionally, Rehabilitation Registered Nurses must stay updated on legislative, economic, ethical, and legal issues that impact resource management. This includes understanding healthcare policies, reimbursement systems, ethical guidelines, and legal regulations. By effectively managing resources, Rehabilitation Registered Nurses can ensure optimal patient outcomes and provide cost-effective care.

4.2.2.5   Documentation to support regulatory requirements:

Documentation to support regulatory requirements is a crucial aspect of delivering patient-centered care as a Rehabilitation Registered Nurse. It involves the creation and maintenance of accurate and comprehensive records that comply with legislative, economic, ethical, and legal regulations. This documentation serves as evidence of the care provided and ensures accountability and transparency. Key aspects of documentation for regulatory purposes include patient assessments, care plans, medication administration records, progress notes, and discharge summaries. Adhering to regulatory requirements helps protect patient rights, ensures accurate billing and reimbursement, promotes quality improvement, and aids in legal defense if necessary. Regular audits and reviews are also important to ensure documentation accuracy and completeness. Proper training and knowledge of regulatory requirements are essential for Rehabilitation Registered Nurses to effectively document patient care and maintain compliance.

4.3   Task 3: Incorporate ethical considerations and legal obligations that affect nursing practice.:

Task 3: Incorporate ethical considerations and legal obligations that affect nursing practice in the field of Rehabilitation Registered Nursing involves addressing important aspects related to ethics and laws. As a Rehabilitation Registered Nurse, it is essential to consider ethical principles such as autonomy, beneficence, and confidentiality when providing care to patients. Respecting patients' choices, promoting their well-being, and safeguarding their privacy are crucial ethical considerations in nursing practice.

In addition to ethical concerns, legal obligations play a significant role in nursing practice. Nurses are bound by the law to provide care within their scope of practice, ensuring patient safety and protecting their rights. Understanding legal frameworks, such as informed consent, documentation, and reporting requirements, is vital for Rehabilitation Registered Nurses.

Subtopics to consider may include the duty to report any suspected abuse or neglect, ensuring patient privacy in the era of electronic health records, and adhering to legal requirements when administering medications or performing procedures.

By incorporating ethical considerations and meeting legal obligations, Rehabilitation Registered Nurses can provide high-quality care while upholding patient rights and professional standards.

4.3.1   Knowledge of:

As a Rehabilitation Registered Nurse, having knowledge of legislative, economic, ethical, and legal issues is crucial for effective nursing practice. Understanding legislation related to healthcare, such as the Health Insurance Portability and Accountability Act (HIPAA), ensures patient privacy and confidentiality. Being aware of economic factors, such as reimbursement policies, allows healthcare providers to deliver cost-effective care. Ethical considerations involve respecting patient autonomy, informed consent, and maintaining professional boundaries. Legal obligations entail following the standards of nursing practice, reporting any concerns related to patient safety, and safeguarding patient rights. Knowledge of these topics is essential for providing safe and ethical care to patients in a rehabilitation setting. Subtopics may include specific legislation, healthcare economics, ethical principles, and legal issues in nursing practice.

4.3.1.1   Ethical theories and resources (e.g., deontology, ombudsperson, ethics committee):

Ethical theories and resources play a crucial role in nursing practice, including rehabilitation nursing. These theories provide a framework for guiding ethical decision-making in patient care. Deontology, for example, emphasizes duty and moral obligations, focusing on actions rather than consequences. This theory helps nurses determine their ethical responsibilities and make decisions based on principles such as autonomy, beneficence, and nonmaleficence.

In addition to ethical theories, resources like ombudsperson and ethics committee are valuable in supporting ethical practice. An ombudsperson acts as an impartial advocate who helps resolve conflicts and concerns within healthcare settings. They serve as a resource for nurses to seek guidance and advice on ethical dilemmas. On the other hand, an ethics committee comprises interdisciplinary professionals who provide consultation and recommendations on ethical issues in patient care. They review complex cases, mediate conflicts, and ensure that ethical standards are met.

Overall, incorporating ethical theories and utilizing resources such as deontology, ombudspersons, and ethics committees can enhance the ethical decision-making process for rehabilitation registered nurses, ensuring that patients receive the highest quality of care while upholding ethical standards in practice.

4.3.1.2   Legal implications of healthcare related policies and documents (e.g., HIPAA, advance directives, powers of attorney, POLST/MOLST, informed consent):

As a Rehabilitation Registered Nurse, it is essential to have a comprehensive understanding of the legal implications surrounding healthcare-related policies and documents. These policies and documents, such as HIPAA, advance directives, powers of attorney, POLST/MOLST, and informed consent, play a crucial role in patient care and protection.

HIPAA (Health Insurance Portability and Accountability Act) ensures patient confidentiality and privacy by regulating the use and disclosure of patient health information. As a nurse, you must understand how to handle and protect patients' sensitive information in accordance with HIPAA regulations.

Advance directives empower patients to communicate their treatment preferences, even when they are unable to do so. This legal document provides guidance to healthcare providers and family members regarding end-of-life decisions, ensuring that patients' wishes are respected.

Powers of attorney grant a designated individual the authority to make healthcare decisions on behalf of patients who are unable to do so. Nurses must acknowledge and respect the decisions made by the designated caregiver.

POLST (Physician Orders for Life-Sustaining Treatment) or MOLST (Medical Orders for Life-Sustaining Treatment) forms are crucial in providing patients with appropriate end-of-life care. These documents contain specific medical orders that healthcare professionals must follow.

Informed consent is an ethical and legal requirement for any medical treatment or procedure. As a nurse, it is your responsibility to ensure that patients fully understand the risks, benefits, and alternatives before obtaining their consent.

By having a thorough understanding of these healthcare-related policies and documents, Rehabilitation Registered Nurses can uphold legal obligations and ethical considerations in their practice, ensuring patient safety and satisfaction.

4.3.2   Skill in:

A Rehabilitation Registered Nurse possesses a range of skills necessary for ethical and legal nursing practice. One important skill is the ability to communicate effectively with patients, families, and interdisciplinary teams. This involves being empathetic, respectful, and providing clear information. Another important skill is critical thinking, which enables nurses to assess, analyze, and make decisions based on ethical principles and legal obligations. Rehabilitation nurses should also possess excellent assessment skills to identify potential ethical dilemmas or legal issues. They must be knowledgeable about legislation related to nursing practice and ensure they uphold the standards set by regulatory bodies. In addition, a Rehabilitation Registered Nurse must maintain confidentiality and protect patient rights, respecting their autonomy and informed consent. By staying updated on legislative changes and ethical guidelines, these nurses ensure the provision of safe and ethical care for their patients.

4.3.2.1   Advocating for the patient:

Advocating for the patient is an essential aspect of nursing practice, particularly for Rehabilitation Registered Nurses. It involves speaking up on behalf of patients, ensuring their needs and rights are met. Firstly, advocating for the patient includes actively listening to their concerns and collaborating with them to make informed decisions about their care. Secondly, it entails advocating for appropriate resources, such as therapies and equipment, to optimize patients' rehabilitation outcomes. Advocacy also involves addressing ethical considerations, such as informed consent and respecting patients' autonomy. Furthermore, Rehabilitation Registered Nurses may advocate for patients by navigating complex healthcare systems, ensuring access to necessary services. They may also advocate for policy changes to improve the overall delivery of rehabilitation services.

4.3.2.2 Documenting services provided:

Documenting services provided is an essential aspect of nursing practice, especially for Rehabilitation Registered Nurses. It involves recording all the services, treatments, and interventions provided to patients in a clear and concise manner. This documentation serves as a legal and professional record of the care given, ensuring accountability and continuity of care.

Important aspects of documenting services provided include accurate and timely recording of assessments, interventions, medications, and patient responses. This documentation should be objective, reflecting the patient's condition accurately and avoiding personal opinions or biases. It should also adhere to ethical considerations, such as maintaining confidentiality and privacy.

Subtopics to consider in this context include the use of standardized documentation forms, electronic health records, and the importance of collaboration and communication with other healthcare professionals. Rehabilitation Registered Nurses must also consider legal obligations, such as ensuring their documentation meets the requirements of regulatory and accreditation bodies.

4.3.2.3 Identifying appropriate resources to assist with legal documents:

Identifying appropriate resources to assist with legal documents is an essential skill for Rehabilitation Registered Nurses. This topic falls under the broader category of incorporating ethical considerations and legal obligations that affect nursing practice.

When dealing with legal documents, nurses must be aware of the legislative, economic, ethical, and legal issues that impact their work. They need to stay updated on the latest laws, regulations, and guidelines related to healthcare and rehabilitation.

There are various resources available to assist nurses in navigating legal documents efficiently. These resources include professional associations, government websites, legal databases, and trusted legal advisors or consultants. Nurses can also rely on colleagues and mentors who have experience in dealing with legal matters.

By identifying and utilizing appropriate resources, Rehabilitation Registered Nurses can ensure that they are following proper procedures, complying with legal requirements, and providing the best possible care to their patients. This knowledge helps them maintain ethical standards, protect patient rights, and avoid legal complications.

4.3.2.4 Implementing strategies to resolve ethical dilemmas:

Implementing strategies to resolve ethical dilemmas is an essential skill for Rehabilitation Registered Nurses. These dilemmas often arise when there is a conflict between the nurse's personal values, professional obligations, and legal requirements. To address such situations, nurses need to adopt a systematic approach. The first step is to identify the ethical dilemma and gather all the relevant information. Nurses should then consider the potential alternatives and their consequences. Consultation with colleagues, supervisors, or ethics committees can provide valuable insight and guidance. Once a decision is made, it should be implemented and evaluated for its effectiveness. Ethical dilemmas can range from issues such as patient privacy, informed consent, resource allocation, to end-of-life decisions. By utilizing appropriate strategies, Rehabilitation Registered Nurses can navigate these challenges while upholding their ethical responsibilities and providing optimal care to their patients.

4.3.2.5 Applying ethics in the delivery of care:

Applying ethics in the delivery of care is crucial for rehabilitation registered nurses. Ethical considerations guide their actions and decisions, ensuring quality and patient-centered care. These considerations include respect for autonomy, beneficence, nonmaleficence, and justice. Respect for autonomy means honoring patients' choices and decisions regarding their care. Beneficence involves providing benefits and promoting well-being for patients. Nonmaleficence means refraining from causing harm and avoiding actions that may have a negative impact on patients. Justice refers to the fair allocation of resources and equal treatment of all patients. Rehabilitation registered nurses must assess ethical dilemmas in the delivery of care, seek guidance from ethics committees or consultants, and follow professional ethical codes and frameworks. They must also consider legal obligations such as patient confidentiality and informed consent. By integrating ethics into their practice, rehabilitation registered nurses ensure safe and effective care for their patients.

4.3.2.6 Task 4: Promote a safe environment of care for patients and staff to minimize risk.:

Task 4: Promote a safe environment of care for patients and staff to minimize risk is a crucial aspect of the rehabilitation registered nurse's role. A safe environment is essential to ensure the well-being and recovery of patients.

In order to promote a safe environment, nurses must adhere to various legislative, economic, ethical, and legal guidelines. Legislative requirements include following health and safety regulations, infection control protocols, and privacy laws. Nurses must also consider economic factors, such as managing resources effectively to ensure the availability of necessary equipment and supplies.

Ethical considerations involve respecting patient autonomy and confidentiality, as well as promoting an inclusive and non-discriminatory environment. Legal issues encompass the duty of care, ensuring accurate documentation, and reporting any incidents or breaches.

To minimize the risk of harm, nurses should implement various strategies. This includes conducting risk assessments, identifying potential hazards, and implementing appropriate preventive measures. Safeguarding patients and staff involves promoting effective communication, providing adequate training, and fostering a culture of safety.

Overall, the rehabilitation registered nurse plays a vital role in creating and maintaining a safe environment of care for patients and staff. By adhering to legislative, economic, ethical, and legal principles, they can effectively minimize risk and ensure optimal outcomes for all involved.

4.3.3 Knowledge of:

As a Rehabilitation Registered Nurse, it is vital to have knowledge of various legislative, economic, ethical, and legal issues in order to promote a safe environment of care for patients and staff while minimizing risk.

Legislative issues include understanding and adhering to laws and regulations that govern healthcare practices, such as patient privacy and protection against discrimination.

Economic considerations involve being aware of financial constraints within the healthcare system and ensuring access to necessary resources and services for patients.

Ethical issues encompass maintaining professional integrity, respecting patient autonomy, and making ethically sound decisions regarding patient care.

Legal issues entail understanding healthcare-related laws and legal obligations, such as informed consent and documentation practices.

Having knowledge of these aspects allows the Rehabilitation Registered Nurse to navigate the complexities of the healthcare system and ensure a safe environment of care for all involved.

4.3.3.1   Safe patient handling practices:

Safe patient handling practices are crucial to promoting a safe environment of care for both patients and staff in rehabilitation settings. These practices aim to minimize the risk of injury during patient transfers, repositioning, and mobility activities. By implementing safe patient handling techniques, healthcare providers can prevent musculoskeletal injuries, falls, and pressure ulcers among patients, while also protecting themselves from healthcare-related injuries.

Key aspects of safe patient handling practices include the use of assistive devices such as ceiling lifts, hoists, and transfer belts to aid in patient movement. Staff should also receive proper training on the correct techniques for lifting, transferring, and repositioning patients. This includes proper body mechanics, utilizing teamwork, and communicating effectively during the handling process.

Legislative, economic, ethical, and legal issues play a significant role in promoting safe patient handling practices. Legislative measures in some jurisdictions mandate the implementation of safe patient handling programs in healthcare facilities. From an economic perspective, investing in safe patient handling equipment and training can lead to cost savings in terms of reduced worker compensation claims and improved patient outcomes. Ethically, ensuring the safety and well-being of patients and staff is a fundamental principle of healthcare. Moreover, healthcare organizations have a legal obligation to provide a safe environment for their employees. Implementation of these practices requires appropriate training, the use of assistive devices, and consideration of legislative, economic, ethical, and legal factors.

4.3.3.2   Safety measures (e.g., safe medication practices, restraint and alternatives, fall prevention):

As a Rehabilitation Registered Nurse, it is crucial to promote a safe environment of care for patients and staff to minimize risk. One important aspect of this is implementing safety measures such as safe medication practices, restraint and alternatives, and fall prevention.

Safe medication practices involve following proper protocols for medication administration, including double-checking dosages, verifying patient allergies, and ensuring accurate documentation. This helps prevent medication errors and adverse reactions.

Restraint and alternatives is another aspect to consider. While restraints may be necessary in some cases to ensure patient safety, it is important to explore non-restraint alternatives first. This can include the use of assistive devices or modifying the environment to prevent falls or injuries.

Fall prevention is a critical component of patient safety. This can involve implementing measures such as keeping walkways clear, using bed alarms, providing proper mobility aids, and educating patients and staff about fall risks and prevention strategies.

By addressing these safety measures, Rehabilitation Registered Nurses can create a secure environment that protects both patients and staff from potential harm.

4.3.3.3   Risk factors and mitigation strategies:

Risk factors and mitigation strategies are important aspects of promoting a safe environment of care for patients and staff in rehabilitation settings. Some risk factors include falls, medication errors, infections, and patient aggression. To mitigate these risks, nurses can implement preventive measures such as assessing patients for fall risk, ensuring proper medication administration protocols, maintaining strict infection control practices, and implementing de-escalation techniques in dealing with aggressive patients. Other mitigation strategies include regular staff education and training on safety protocols, maintaining a clean and organized environment, and promoting effective communication among interdisciplinary team members. These strategies help minimize the occurrence of adverse events, enhance patient safety, and create a conducive working environment for staff. Rehabilitation registered nurses play a crucial role in identifying and addressing risk factors to ensure the safety and well-being of patients and staff in rehabilitation settings.

4.3.3.4   Infection control practices:

Infection control practices are essential for a Rehabilitation Registered Nurse to promote a safe environment of care for patients and staff and minimize the risk of infections. These practices involve the implementation of measures to prevent and control the spread of infections in healthcare settings. This includes proper hand hygiene, the use of personal protective equipment, regular cleaning and disinfection of surfaces, and adherence to specific infection control protocols. Additionally, education and training for both healthcare providers and patients are important in preventing the transmission of infections. Nurses should stay updated on the latest guidelines and best practices related to infection control. By following these practices, Rehabilitation Registered Nurses can help protect patients and staff from infections and maintain a safe healthcare environment.

4.3.3.5   Behavioral management techniques:

Behavioral management techniques are important in promoting a safe environment of care for patients and staff in rehabilitation settings. These techniques aim to minimize risk and maintain a peaceful and supportive atmosphere. One key aspect of behavioral management is effective communication, which involves active listening, providing clear instructions, and maintaining a respectful tone. Another technique is positive reinforcement, which involves rewarding desired behaviors to encourage their repetition. Additionally, setting clear boundaries and expectations can help ensure a safe environment. In situations where challenging behaviors arise, the use of de-escalation techniques can be effective in diffusing tense situations. It is also important for rehabilitation registered nurses to collaborate with multidisciplinary teams, including psychiatrists and psychologists, to develop individualized behavior management plans for patients. By implementing these techniques, rehabilitation registered nurses can enhance the overall quality of care provided.

4.3.4   Skill in:

As a Rehabilitation Registered Nurse, having skill in promoting a safe environment of care for patients and staff to minimize risk is crucial. This skill involves understanding and implementing legislative, economic, ethical, and legal issues.

Legislative issues encompass following and adhering to laws and regulations designed to ensure patient and staff safety. This includes guidelines for infection control, medication administration, and patient rights.

Economic issues involve managing resources efficiently to provide a safe environment. This includes budgeting for essential safety equipment, such as hand hygiene supplies and personal protective equipment.

Ethical issues require making decisions that prioritize patient safety and well-being. This involves maintaining confidentiality, respecting patient autonomy, and advocating for the best interest of patients.

Legal issues entail understanding and complying with laws and regulations related to patient care and safety. This includes documentation, informed consent, and reporting of adverse events.

Overall, the skill in promoting a safe environment of care for patients and staff involves understanding and implementing legislative, economic, ethical, and legal issues to minimize risk and ensure the well-being of all involved.

4.3.4.1   Assessing safety risks:

Assessing safety risks is a critical aspect of promoting a safe environment of care for patients and staff in the field of rehabilitation nursing. This process involves identifying potential hazards and implementing measures to minimize risks. A rehabilitation registered nurse must be skilled in evaluating the physical environment and identifying potential dangers such as slippery floors or equipment malfunctions. They also need to be aware of patient-related safety risks, including fall prevention strategies and medication error prevention. Additionally, assessing safety risks involves considering legislative, economic, ethical, and legal issues that affect the safety of patients and staff. This includes adhering to healthcare regulations, ensuring cost-effective safety measures, and ethically managing risks to promote the well-being of all individuals involved. Overall, a comprehensive assessment of safety risks is essential for a rehabilitation registered nurse to ensure a secure and protected healthcare environment.

4.3.4.2   Minimizing safety risk factors:

Minimizing safety risk factors is crucial in promoting a safe environment for patients and staff in rehabilitation settings. As a Rehabilitation Registered Nurse, it is your responsibility to identify and address potential risks that may jeopardize the safety of individuals under your care.

Some key aspects to consider when minimizing safety risk factors include legislative, economic, ethical, and legal issues. This involves complying with relevant laws and regulations, such as those related to patient safety and infection control. Allocating resources effectively is also important, ensuring that necessary equipment and staffing levels are maintained to mitigate potential risks.

Ethical considerations should guide decision-making, ensuring that the rights and well-being of patients and staff are prioritized. This includes maintaining confidentiality and respecting autonomy. Additionally, being aware of legal issues surrounding documentation, consent, and incident reporting is essential in minimizing safety risks.

By proactively addressing safety risk factors, Rehabilitation Registered Nurses can create an environment that promotes the well-being and recovery of patients, while also protecting the staff members involved in their care.

4.3.4.3   Implementing safety prevention measures:

Implementing safety prevention measures is a crucial aspect of promoting a safe environment of care for patients and staff in rehabilitation settings. These measures aim to minimize risks and ensure the well-being of all individuals involved.

One important aspect is ensuring legislative compliance, which involves adhering to laws and regulations related to safety standards. This may include implementing protocols for infection control, fire safety, and patient safety.

Economic factors also play a role, as healthcare facilities need to allocate resources effectively to provide a safe environment. This may involve investing in safety equipment, conducting regular maintenance checks, and providing staff with appropriate training.

Ethical considerations are also important, as individuals have a right to receive care in a safe environment. This may involve respecting patient privacy, maintaining confidentiality, and promoting a culture of mutual respect.

Finally, legal issues come into play, such as liability and negligence. Rehabilitation registered nurses must be knowledgeable about legal guidelines and take appropriate actions to prevent accidents or injuries. By addressing legislative, economic, ethical, and legal issues, rehabilitation registered nurses can minimize risks and ensure the well-being of all individuals involved.

4.3.4.4   Applying behavior management techniques (e.g., de- escalation techniques):

To promote a safe environment of care for both patients and staff, rehabilitation registered nurses must possess the skill of applying behavior management techniques, such as de-escalation techniques. These techniques are crucial in minimizing the risk of violent or disruptive behavior in a healthcare setting.

De-escalation techniques involve effective communication and active listening to defuse potentially volatile situations. The nurse should remain calm, use a respectful tone, and project an empathetic attitude. Non-threatening body language and gestures can help to put the individual at ease.

Subtopics within this topic may include recognizing signs of aggression or agitation, assessing the situation for potential triggers, and implementing appropriate strategies to reduce tension. It is important for rehabilitation registered nurses to receive proper training and education on these techniques to ensure the safety and well-being of patients and staff.

By utilizing behavior management techniques, rehabilitation registered nurses can create a peaceful and secure environment that promotes healing and minimizes the risk of harm.

4.3.4.5   Using appropriate safety devices (e.g., restraints and alternatives, alarms):

The use of appropriate safety devices is crucial in promoting a safe environment of care for both patients and staff in rehabilitation settings. These safety devices include restraints, alternatives to restraints, and alarms.

Restraints are physical devices used to restrict a patient's movement. They are typically used when a patient poses a risk to themselves or others. However, it is important to use restraints as a last resort and for the shortest duration possible. Restraints should be periodically evaluated and discontinued if appropriate.

Alternatives to restraints focus on creating a safe environment without physically restraining the patient. This can include modifying the environment, using visual or auditory cues, and providing adequate supervision and support. These alternatives help promote the autonomy and dignity of the patient.

Alarms are another safety device that can be used to alert healthcare providers to potential risks. They can be used to monitor patient movement, falls, or other safety-related concerns. Alarms should be appropriately calibrated to minimize false alarms and ensure that they are effective in preventing adverse events.

Overall, using appropriate safety devices such as restraints, alternatives, and alarms is vital in minimizing risks and ensuring a safe environment for patients and staff in rehabilitation settings. It is important for rehabilitation registered nurses to be knowledgeable about these devices and to use them judiciously, considering the individual needs and preferences of the patients they care for.

4.3.4.6   Task 5: Integrate quality improvement processes into nursing practice.:

Task 5: Integrate quality improvement processes into nursing practice is an important aspect of the Rehabilitation Registered Nurse's role. Quality improvement processes involve systematically assessing and improving the quality of patient care.

One subtopic is the identification of areas for improvement. Rehabilitation Registered Nurses must be able to identify areas in their practice that need improvement. This can include assessing patient outcomes, patient satisfaction, and adherence to established protocols and guidelines.

Another subtopic is the development and implementation of improvement strategies. Once areas for improvement have been identified, Rehabilitation Registered Nurses must work collaboratively with the healthcare team to develop and implement strategies to address these areas. This may involve changes to workflows, staff education, or the use of evidence-based practices.

Monitoring and evaluating the effectiveness of improvement strategies is also crucial. Rehabilitation Registered Nurses should regularly assess the impact of the implemented improvement strategies on patient outcomes and overall quality of care.

Integrating quality improvement processes into nursing practice requires the Rehabilitation Registered Nurse to be proactive, engaged, and committed to continuously improving patient care. By making quality improvement an integral part of their nursing practice, Rehabilitation Registered Nurses can contribute to providing optimal care and improving patient outcomes.

4.3.5   Knowledge of:

As a Rehabilitation Registered Nurse, it is important to have a strong understanding of legislative, economic, ethical, and legal issues related to quality improvement processes. Firstly, legislative knowledge involves being aware of the laws and regulations that govern healthcare practices, such as those pertaining to patient safety and privacy. Understanding these laws enables the nurse to provide care within legal boundaries. Secondly, economic knowledge is crucial as it involves understanding the healthcare system's financial aspects, such as reimbursement processes and cost-effective interventions. This knowledge helps guide decision-making to provide quality care while considering limited resources. Ethical knowledge is essential in handling ethical dilemmas and maintaining patient autonomy, dignity, and confidentiality. Lastly, legal knowledge encompassing standards of care, the Nurse Practice Act, and informed consent is necessary to protect both patients and healthcare professionals. Developing a comprehensive understanding of these topics ensures that Rehabilitation Registered Nurses can effectively integrate quality improvement processes into their practice.

4.3.5.1   Quality measurement and performance improvement processes (e.g., Agency for Healthcare Research and Quality, Institute of Medicine, National Database of Nursing Quality Indicators):

Quality measurement and performance improvement processes are essential in healthcare, including the field of rehabilitation nursing. These processes aim to assess and enhance the quality of care provided to patients. Several organizations, such as the Agency for Healthcare Research and Quality (AHRQ), the Institute of Medicine (IOM), and the National Database of Nursing Quality Indicators (NDNQI), play significant roles in this area.

The AHRQ is a federal agency that supports research to improve healthcare quality. They develop and provide tools and resources for measuring and monitoring quality indicators. The IOM is an independent organization that provides guidance on healthcare quality improvement. They publish reports highlighting best practices and recommendations for enhancing patient outcomes.

The NDNQI is a database established by the American Nurses Association to measure and benchmark nursing quality indicators. It collects data on various nursing-sensitive measures, such as falls, pressure ulcers, and infections, allowing healthcare facilities to compare their performance and identify areas for improvement.

Integrating quality improvement processes into nursing practice involves utilizing these resources and implementing evidence-based practices. Rehabilitation nurses can utilize these tools and databases to measure and track their performance, identify areas for improvement, and implement interventions to enhance patient outcomes. By continuously monitoring and improving the quality of care, rehabilitation nurses can ensure that they are providing the best possible care to their patients.

4.3.5.2   Models and tools used in process improvement (e.g., Plan, Do, Check, Act; Six Sigma; Lean approach):

Models and tools used in process improvement are valuable in the field of nursing, specifically for Rehabilitation Registered Nurses. One of the widely used models is the Plan, Do, Check, Act (PDCA) cycle, also known as the Deming Cycle. This model involves planning the process, implementing it, checking for any issues or deviations, and acting upon them to improve the process. Six Sigma is another popular model that focuses on reducing defects and variability in processes. It uses statistical analysis to identify and eliminate errors. Lean approach is a philosophy that aims to eliminate waste and increase efficiency by streamlining processes. It emphasizes continuous improvement and customer value. These models and tools provide structured approaches to analyze and improve processes in healthcare settings. They help identify areas for improvement, reduce errors, enhance patient safety, and optimize overall quality of care. Rehabilitation Registered Nurses can benefit from utilizing these models and tools to enhance their practice and deliver better outcomes for their patients.

4.3.5.3   Federal quality measurement efforts:

Federal quality measurement efforts in healthcare aim to assess and improve the quality of care provided to patients. These efforts involve collecting data, analyzing performance, and implementing strategies to enhance the overall patient experience. Under the broad topic of 'Knowledge of: Task 5: Integrate quality improvement processes into nursing practice, Legislative, Economic, Ethical, and Legal Issues,' rehabilitation registered nurses need to be aware of the various federal initiatives promoting quality measurement. One important aspect is the Hospital Compare program, which provides public access to information regarding the quality of care delivered by hospitals. This program enables patients to make informed decisions about their healthcare providers. Another significant effort is the Hospital Consumer Assessment of Healthcare Providers and Systems (HCAHPS) survey, which measures patient satisfaction and evaluates the effectiveness of care.

Rehabilitation registered nurses should also be familiar with the Centers for Medicare and Medicaid Services (CMS) Quality Payment Program, which aims to improve the quality of care for Medicare beneficiaries through value-based incentive programs. These programs reward healthcare providers for delivering high-quality care and penalize those with subpar performance.

Furthermore, understanding the Hospital Readmissions Reduction Program is crucial. This program encourages hospitals to reduce avoidable readmissions by imposing financial penalties on facilities that have higher-than-expected readmission rates.

Overall, rehabilitation registered nurses should stay informed about federal quality measurement efforts to enhance the quality of care they provide and contribute to positive patient outcomes.

4.3.5.4 Reporting requirements (e.g., infection rates, healthcare- acquired pressure injury, sentinel events, discharge to community, readmission rates):

As a Rehabilitation Registered Nurse, it is essential to have knowledge of reporting requirements related to various aspects of healthcare, such as infection rates, healthcare-acquired pressure injuries, sentinel events, discharge to the community, and readmission rates. These reporting requirements are crucial for quality improvement processes in nursing practice.

Infection rates are reported to identify and prevent the spread of infections within healthcare facilities. This information helps healthcare professionals implement effective strategies for infection control and improve patient outcomes. Healthcare-acquired pressure injuries also require reporting to monitor and address the occurrence of these preventable conditions. By tracking and analyzing these incidents, nurses can develop preventive measures and enhance patient care.

Sentinel events, which are severe patient safety events, are reported to ensure appropriate investigations and prevent similar incidents in the future. This reporting helps healthcare providers identify system failures and implement necessary changes to prevent harm to patients.

Discharge to the community and readmission rates are reported to examine the effectiveness of transitional care and to identify areas for improvement. By monitoring these rates, nurses can assess the success of discharge planning and post-acute care interventions, ultimately promoting better patient outcomes. These reports provide essential data for quality improvement processes and enable nurses to enhance patient safety and care.

4.3.6 Skill in:

As a Rehabilitation Registered Nurse, one must possess a variety of skills to effectively integrate quality improvement processes into nursing practice. One important skill is communication, which involves effectively conveying information to patients, their families, and other healthcare professionals. Another crucial skill is critical thinking, which allows nurses to analyze complex situations and make informed decisions. Additionally, problem-solving skills are vital for identifying and resolving issues that may arise during the rehabilitation process. Being knowledgeable about legislative, economic, ethical, and legal issues is also essential to ensure compliance with regulations and provide ethical and patient-centered care. Lastly, being proficient in technology and data management is beneficial for tracking patient progress and monitoring outcomes.

4.3.6.1 Using standardized assessment tools:

Using standardized assessment tools is an important aspect of the Rehabilitation Registered Nurse's role. These tools provide a structured framework for evaluating patients' health conditions, functional abilities, and progress in rehabilitation. By using standardized assessments, nurses can gather objective data to inform their nursing practice and ensure that appropriate interventions are implemented.

One key benefit of using standardized assessment tools is the ability to compare patient outcomes across different settings, ensuring continuity of care. These tools also contribute to quality improvement processes, enabling nurses to identify areas of improvement and address them effectively. Furthermore, standardized assessments assist in documenting and communicating patient status to other healthcare professionals and stakeholders.

Examples of standardized assessment tools commonly used by Rehabilitation Registered Nurses include the Functional Independence Measure (FIM), the Barthel Index, and the Montreal Cognitive Assessment (MoCA). These tools cover various aspects of a patient's health and functioning, including mobility, activities of daily living, cognition, and mood.

Overall, using standardized assessment tools is an essential skill for Rehabilitation Registered Nurses, enabling them to provide evidence-based care, track patient progress, and contribute to quality improvement processes in their practice.

4.3.6.2 Incorporating standards of professional performance:

Incorporating standards of professional performance is crucial for Rehabilitation Registered Nurses in their daily practice. These standards provide guidelines for nurses to ensure they deliver high-quality care and adhere to ethical, legal, and legislative requirements.

One important aspect of incorporating standards of professional performance is integrating quality improvement processes into nursing practice. This involves constantly assessing and improving the care provided to patients. By implementing evidence-based practices, following protocols, and participating in quality improvement initiatives, nurses can enhance patient outcomes.

Furthermore, Rehabilitation Registered Nurses must also stay updated on legislative, economic, ethical, and legal issues that impact their practice. This includes understanding healthcare laws and regulations, maintaining patient confidentiality, advocating for patient rights, and navigating healthcare systems.

By adhering to these standards, Rehabilitation Registered Nurses can provide safe, effective, and compassionate care, while also promoting continuous professional development and upholding the integrity of the nursing profession.

4.3.6.3 Applying quality measurement tools in practice:

Applying quality measurement tools in practice is an essential aspect of integrating quality improvement processes into nursing practice for Rehabilitation Registered Nurses. These tools help in evaluating the effectiveness and efficiency of care provided to patients. They enable nurses to identify areas that require improvement and measure the impact of interventions. Quality measurement tools encompass various parameters such as patient satisfaction, clinical outcomes, and adherence to evidence-based practices. They facilitate the identification of best practices and enable benchmarking against national standards. Nurses can utilize these tools to assess their performance, identify any gaps, and implement strategies to enhance patient care. By measuring the quality of care delivered, nurses can improve patient outcomes and patient safety, as well as effectively utilize healthcare resources. The utilization of quality measurement tools supports legislative requirements, ethical practice, and maintains standards of care. It is crucial for Rehabilitation Registered Nurses to understand these tools and integrate them into their everyday practice to provide optimal care for their patients.

4.3.6.4   Using quality improvement model to improve patient care:

Using a quality improvement model is essential for rehabilitation registered nurses to improve patient care. This model helps nurses to assess current practices and identify areas for improvement in patient care. These models involve several steps, including data collection, analysis, and implementation of changes to improve outcomes. By using quality improvement models, nurses can identify common issues and implement evidence-based interventions to address them. Additionally, these models allow for ongoing monitoring and evaluation of patient care to ensure that improvements are sustained over time. Overall, integrating quality improvement processes into nursing practice is crucial for rehabilitation registered nurses to enhance patient care and outcomes.

CRRN
Practice
Questions

<u>SET 1</u>

Question 1: Which medication is commonly used as an anticholinergic agent to treat muscle spasm and excessive sweating in rehabilitation patients?
A) Amitriptyline
B) Morphine
C) Diazepam
D) Oxybutynin

Question 2: Which nursing model focuses on understanding and addressing the patient's personal values, beliefs, and goals to guide the rehabilitation nursing practice?
A) Orem's Self-Care Deficit Theory
B) Roy's Adaptation Model
C) Neuman's Systems Model
D) Watson's Human Caring Theory

Question 3: Mrs. Johnson, a 70-year-old patient, has recently been admitted to a rehabilitation facility following a stroke. She is experiencing difficulty with mobility and requires assistance with activities of daily living. As a rehabilitation registered nurse, what is the most important aspect of providing patient-centered care for Mrs. Johnson?
A) Ensuring medication administration is timely
B) Promoting independence in activities of daily living
C) Monitoring vital signs every hour
D) Administering pain medication as needed

Question 4: You are working as a Certified Rehabilitation Registered Nurse (CRRN) in a rehabilitation center. The interdisciplinary team is working together to develop a discharge plan for a patient named Rachel, who had a stroke and requires ongoing rehabilitation. As a part of the team, you are responsible for applying appropriate theories in the collaborative process. Which theory would be most suitable to facilitate effective communication and collaboration within the interdisciplinary team during the transition of care for Rachel?
A) Transformational leadership theory
B) Situational leadership theory
C) Systems theory
D) Social exchange theory

Question 5: Which of the following vitamins is required for the absorption of calcium in the gastrointestinal tract?
A) Vitamin C
B) Vitamin D
C) Vitamin K
D) Vitamin A

Question 6: Maria is a registered nurse working in a rehabilitation facility. She is caring for a patient, Mr. Johnson, who recently had a stroke and has limited mobility and difficulty with speech. Mr. Johnson's wife is also experiencing emotional distress and feeling overwhelmed by the new challenges they are facing. Maria believes that connecting both Mr. Johnson and his wife with community resources can help them cope with their situation. Which community resource may provide face-to-face support groups for stroke survivors and their caregivers?
A) Local library
B) Internet search engines
C) Respite care facility
D) Stroke support group

Question 7: Mrs. Adams is a 65-year-old patient who had a stroke and is currently undergoing rehabilitative care at a rehabilitation center. The healthcare team follows a nursing model that emphasizes the integration of physical, social, and psychological aspects of patient care. They believe in providing patient-centered care that addresses the unique needs and goals of each patient. Which nursing model are they most likely following?
A) Roy Adaptation Model
B) Orem's Self-Care Deficit Theory
C) Neuman Systems Model
D) The Rehabilitation Nursing Model

Question 8: Mrs. Thompson, a 70-year-old patient, is admitted to the rehabilitation unit after a total hip replacement surgery. She has a history of hypertension and diabetes. The nurse is assessing Mrs. Thompson's fluid and electrolyte balance. Which finding should the nurse consider as a potential risk for fluid imbalance in this patient?
A) Bradycardia
B) Weight gain of 2 pounds in 24 hours
C) Sodium level of 142 mEq/L
D) Urine output of 50 ml/hour

Question 9: According to the staffing patterns and policies in rehabilitation nursing, which model describes a nursing care delivery system where each team member has a specific role and responsibilities, and each patient is assigned a primary nurse responsible for coordinating the patient's care?
A) Team nursing model
B) Primary nursing model
C) Functional nursing model
D) Case management nursing model

Question 10: Mr. Johnson, a 45-year-old patient with a history of spinal cord injury, has been admitted to a rehabilitation facility. In his care plan, the healthcare team has recommended the use of physical restraints to prevent him from accidentally harming himself during transfers. As the rehabilitation nurse, what is your ethical obligation in this situation?
A) Express your concerns about the use of physical restraints and suggest alternative interventions.
B) Follow the care plan provided by the healthcare team and apply the physical restraints as recommended.
C) Refuse to apply the physical restraints, as they might infringe on the patient's rights and autonomy.
D) Consult with the patient and his family to get their input and consent regarding the use of physical restraints.

Question 11: A rehabilitation nurse is documenting the patient's care in the medical record. Which of the following statements represents accurate documentation to support regulatory requirements?
A) "The patient appears to be in pain."
B) "Administered pain medication at 2:00 pm."
C) "The patient is unable to walk without assistance."
D) "Patient's blood pressure is high."

Question 12: As a Certified Rehabilitation Registered Nurse (CRRN), you are responsible for integrating legislation and regulations in the management of care for your patients. Mr. Johnson is a 40-year-old patient with a traumatic brain injury. He has been receiving inpatient rehabilitation services for the past few weeks. Today, Mr. Johnson's wife informs you that they have received a

medical bill from the hospital and they are unable to afford it. She asks if there are any options for financial assistance or if they can negotiate a lower payment. What would be your best course of action in this situation?
A) Inform Mr. Johnson and his wife that they have to pay the bill in full, as per hospital policy.
B) Advise Mr. Johnson and his wife to contact their insurance company to explore coverage options.
C) Provide Mr. Johnson and his wife with information about financial assistance programs available at the hospital.
D) Suggest Mr. Johnson and his wife to speak with a lawyer for legal advice on negotiating the bill.

Question 13: Maria, a 57-year-old Hispanic female, is admitted to the rehabilitation unit following a stroke. She speaks very limited English and usually relies on her family members to communicate with healthcare providers. As the Certified Rehabilitation Registered Nurse (CRRN), which action should you take to optimize the patient's ability to communicate effectively?
A) Avoid using nonverbal gestures as they may confuse the patient.
B) Speak loudly and repetitively to ensure the patient understands you.
C) Use a professional medical interpreter to facilitate communication.
D) Use complex medical jargon to educate the patient about her condition.

Question 14: Which of the following statements regarding the use of Passy Muir valve is correct?
A) The Passy Muir valve is a device used for urinary incontinence management.
B) The Passy Muir valve is used to facilitate swallowing in patients with dysphagia.
C) The Passy Muir valve is designed to assist with respiratory support and speech rehabilitation.
D) The Passy Muir valve is used for continence management in patients with fecal incontinence.

Question 15: Which quality measurement tool is most commonly used in healthcare settings to assess patient outcomes and identify areas for improvement?
A) Six Sigma
B) Total Quality Management (TQM)
C) Lean methodology
D) National Database of Nursing Quality Indicators (NDNQI)

Question 16: A patient with a spinal cord injury is at risk for developing pressure ulcers due to impaired sensation and mobility. The nurse is implementing measures to prevent pressure ulcers. Which intervention is appropriate for the nursing staff to carry out?
A) Providing a high-protein diet to the patient
B) Applying a heating pad to the patient's skin
C) Bathing the patient with hot water
D) Massaging the patient's bony prominences

Question 17: Which ethical principle advocates for respect for autonomy and the right of individuals to make their own decisions regarding their healthcare?
A) Beneficence
B) Nonmaleficence
C) Autonomy
D) Veracity

Question 18: Mrs. Smith, a 65-year-old patient with a history of dementia, has been admitted to the rehabilitation unit after sustaining a hip fracture. During her stay, she has shown aggressive behavior towards the staff, hitting and scratching them. The nurse is implementing behavioral management techniques to address her aggression. Which of the following strategies would be most appropriate to manage Mrs. Smith's behavior?
A) Restraint Mrs. Smith to prevent physical harm to herself and others.
B) Implement diversion techniques, such as providing her with activities or objects to redirect her attention.
C) Administer sedative medications to calm Mrs. Smith and reduce her aggression.
D) Isolate Mrs. Smith in a secluded area until her aggressive behavior subsides.

Question 19: Which communication technique involves listening carefully to the patient, providing feedback, and demonstrating empathy and understanding?
A) Active listening
B) Anger management
C) Reflection
D) Clarification

Question 20: What teaching intervention is appropriate for a patient with swallowing deficits?
A) Providing a soft diet only
B) Using thickened liquids
C) Encouraging rapid eating
D) Allowing the patient to eat unassisted

Question 21: Which of the following statements accurately describes the concept of acute pain?
A) Acute pain is a persistently uncomfortable sensation that lasts for more than 6 months.
B) Acute pain can be classified into two types: nociceptive and neuropathic pain.
C) Acute pain is characterized by the activation of specialized sensory receptors called nociceptors.
D) Acute pain is generally not responsive to analgesic medications.

Question 22: Which of the following is an appropriate nursing intervention when assessing a patient's functional health patterns?
A) Administering pain medication to manage discomfort
B) Collaborating with the patient's family to create a care plan
C) Encouraging the patient to remain sedentary for enhanced rest
D) Limiting the patient's involvement in decision-making processes

Question 23: Which of the following is an example of a task that falls within the scope of practice for a Certified Rehabilitation Registered Nurse (CRRN)?
A) Prescribing medication for pain management
B) Performing spinal surgeries
C) Developing an individualized rehabilitation plan for a patient with a spinal cord injury
D) Administering anesthesia during surgical procedures

Question 24: What is the purpose of assessing a patient's elimination patterns by using an elimination diary and obtaining their history?
A) To monitor changes in the patient's bowel movements and urinary patterns
B) To track the patient's dietary habits and fluid intake
C) To identify potential triggers for bowel and bladder dysfunction
D) To educate the patient about proper elimination techniques and hygiene

Question 25: A 55-year-old male patient with a history of stroke is admitted to a rehabilitation center. Upon assessment, the patient reports difficulty with balance and coordination, as well as weakness in the left arm and leg. The patient's medical record reveals that he has impaired proprioception on the left side. Which nursing intervention is most appropriate for this patient?
A) Encourage the patient to perform active range of motion exercises on the left side.
B) Assist the patient with transferring and ambulation using a gait belt and appropriate assistive devices.
C) Teach the patient relaxation techniques to reduce muscle tension and promote relaxation.
D) Provide the patient with a cognitive retraining program to improve memory and problem-solving skills.

Question 26: Maggie, a 65-year-old patient, has been admitted to a rehabilitation unit following a hip replacement surgery. The nurse is conducting a fall risk assessment for Maggie. During the assessment, the nurse identifies that Maggie has a history of falls in the past six months, uses a cane for mobility, and has poor balance. What is the most appropriate risk mitigation strategy for Maggie?
A) Placing a bed alarm to alert the staff when Maggie attempts to get out of bed.
B) Assigning a sitter to provide constant supervision for Maggie.
C) Implementing a daily exercise routine to improve her strength and balance.
D) Applying nonslip socks to improve traction and reduce the risk of falls.

Question 27: Which diagnostic test is used to assess blood glucose levels over a period of time?
A) Fasting blood sugar (FBS)
B) Oral glucose tolerance test (OGTT)
C) Glycosylated hemoglobin (HbA1c)
D) Random blood sugar (RBS)

Question 28: In managing current and projected resources in a cost-effective manner, which of the following strategies would be most effective?
A) Reducing staffing levels to minimize labor costs
B) Implementing evidence-based practice to improve patient outcomes
C) Increasing the use of expensive equipment and technology
D) Decreasing the amount of time spent on patient education

Question 29: Which nursing model focuses on the individual's ability to adapt to their environment and emphasizes the importance of self-care?
A) Roy's Adaptation Model
B) Neuman Systems Model
C) Orem's Self-Care Deficit Model
D) Levine's Conservation Model

Question 30: Which professional can provide emotional and psychological support to patients and caregivers?
A) Physician
B) Pharmacist
C) Psychologist
D) Physical therapist

Question 31: Which assessment finding indicates a fluid volume deficit in a patient?
A) Decreased urine output
B) Increased urine output
C) Skin rash

D) Headache

Question 32: Which intervention is most appropriate for a Certified Rehabilitation Registered Nurse (CRRN) to implement to promote optimal nutrition and hydration for a client with dysphagia?
A) Encourage the client to consume foods and fluids with thickened consistency
B) Provide the client with a regular diet, avoiding any modifications
C) Administer a nasogastric tube for feeding purposes
D) Instruct the client to consume small, frequent meals without any restrictions

Question 33: Which teaching intervention is most effective in preventing complications of immobility such as skin integrity and deep vein thrombosis (DVT)?
A) Encouraging regular range of motion exercises
B) Promoting intake of a high-protein diet
C) Applying pressure-relieving devices to bony prominences
D) Administering anticoagulant medications

Question 34: Which of the following is a skill required for rehabilitation nursing practice?
A) Medical coding and billing.
B) Pharmacology knowledge.
C) Physical therapy techniques.
D) Psychological counseling.

Question 35: Ms. Green, a 45-year-old patient, has been admitted to the rehabilitation unit following a traumatic brain injury. She has limited movement and requires assistance for all activities of daily living. The rehabilitation nurse identifies the need to prevent musculoskeletal complications and promote joint mobility in Ms. Green. Which intervention is most appropriate for achieving this goal?
A) Administering medications for pain relief
B) Encouraging active range of motion exercises
C) Applying ice packs to the affected joints
D) Providing complete bed rest

Question 36: A patient with a history of substance abuse has recently been admitted to a rehabilitation unit following a car accident. The patient is displaying signs of anger, frustration, and social withdrawal. The nurse recognizes that these behaviors are most likely related to:
A) Unresolved grief and loss.
B) Lack of personal motivation.
C) Effects of the car accident.
D) Relapse into substance abuse.

Question 37: Which of the following is an example of integrating quality improvement processes into nursing practice?
A) Attending a seminar on evidence-based practice
B) Advocating for patient rights and privacy
C) Participating in a peer review process
D) Documenting patient assessments accurately

Question 38: Ms. Johnson, a Certified Rehabilitation Registered Nurse (CRRN), is responsible for implementing quality improvement processes in a rehabilitation facility. She is reviewing the documentation practices of the nursing staff to ensure compliance with legal and ethical standards. Which of the following actions performed by the nursing staff would be a violation of legal and ethical standards?

A) Documenting medication administration immediately after giving the medication.
B) Falsifying a patient's medical record to cover up a medication error.
C) Documenting the patient's vital signs every 4 hours, as per facility policy.
D) Updating the patient's care plan with the most current goals and interventions.

Question 39: Which stage of grief and loss is characterized by feelings of anger, resentment, and frustration?
A) Denial
B) Bargaining
C) Anger
D) Acceptance

Question 40: When using technology in rehabilitation nursing, it is important for the nurse to:
A) Monitor the patient's vital signs manually
B) Disregard any technological errors and use other methods
C) Ensure proper functioning and calibration of the technology
D) Avoid using any technology to minimize patient dependency

Question 41: Which of the following statements is correct regarding the purpose and caring for central lines, ports, and catheters?
A) Central lines are commonly used for long-term medication administration.
B) Ports are usually inserted into the arm.
C) Catheters are only used for urine collection.
D) Ports are primarily used for short-term medication administration.

Question 42: You are a Certified Rehabilitation Registered Nurse (CRRN) working in a rehabilitation facility. You are part of an interdisciplinary team that focuses on helping patients achieve their goals and facilitating their transition from the acute care setting to rehabilitation. Today, you receive a referral for a new patient named Sarah who recently suffered a stroke and requires rehabilitation services. Question: What is the primary goal of the interdisciplinary team in the rehabilitation process?
A) To provide palliative care to Sarah and manage her symptoms.
B) To collaborate and coordinate care to achieve optimal patient outcomes.
C) To prescribe medications and monitor their efficacy for Sarah's condition.
D) To discharge Sarah from the rehabilitation facility as soon as possible.

Question 43: Which professional resource is instrumental in assisting rehabilitation patients with emotional and psychological support during their recovery process?
A) Neurologist
B) Psychologist
C) Teacher
D) Home health

Question 44: Which part of the nervous system is responsible for controlling bladder function?
A) Sympathetic nervous system
B) Parasympathetic nervous system
C) Central nervous system
D) Somatic nervous system

Question 45: Which nursing theory focuses on the interpersonal processes between nurses and patients as they work towards mutual goal attainment in the rehabilitation setting?
A) King's Theory of Goal Attainment
B) Rogers' Science of Unitary Human Beings
C) Neuman's Systems Model
D) Orem's Self-Care Deficit Theory

Question 46: Mrs. Johnson is a 67-year-old patient admitted to the rehabilitation unit with a diagnosis of stroke. As the nurse, you are responsible for optimizing her sleep and rest patterns. Which intervention would be most appropriate to promote sleep in Mrs. Johnson?
A) Administering a sedative medication at bedtime
B) Providing a quiet and dark sleep environment
C) Encouraging Mrs. Johnson to watch television before bedtime
D) Waking Mrs. Johnson every hour to assess her neurologic status

Question 47: When teaching health, wellness, and life skills maintenance to a patient with a spinal cord injury, which intervention should the Certified Rehabilitation Registered Nurse (CRRN) prioritize?
A) Providing information on proper bowel and bladder management techniques.
B) Conducting a group session on stress management and coping strategies.
C) Teaching techniques for improving upper body strength and mobility.
D) Demonstrating proper skin care and the prevention of pressure ulcers.

Question 48: A rehabilitation nurse is caring for a patient who sustained a brain injury in a motor vehicle accident. The patient's family expresses concerns about the rising medical expenses and asks the nurse for guidance on potential financial assistance programs. Which legislation provides healthcare benefits to individuals with low income and limited resources?
A) Americans with Disabilities Act (ADA)
B) Occupational Safety and Health Act (OSHA)
C) Affordable Care Act (ACA)
D) Emergency Medical Treatment and Active Labor Act (EMTALA)

Question 49: Mr. Smith, a patient with dysphagia, requires enteral feeding. The healthcare provider has prescribed a nasogastric tube for feeding. Which action should the nurse take when providing nutrition using a nasogastric tube?
A) Insert the tube into the patient's mouth.
B) Verify the placement of the tube by listening for air sounds.
C) Administer bolus feeding continuously throughout the day.
D) Flush the tube with water before and after medication administration.

Question 50: Which coping strategy is characterized by the use of physical activity as a means to manage stress and anxiety?
A) Meditation
B) Distraction
C) Exercise
D) Deep breathing

Question 51: Mrs. Johnson, a 45-year-old patient, has been admitted to the rehabilitation unit following a traumatic brain injury. As the Certified Rehabilitation Registered Nurse (CRRN), you are responsible for

providing comprehensive care to Mrs. Johnson. Which skill is essential for the CRRN to apply in optimizing management of Mrs. Johnson's neurological condition?
A) Cardiac assessment
B) Wound care
C) Neurologic assessment
D) Psychosocial assessment

Question 52: Mr. Johnson, a 65-year-old patient with a history of epilepsy, has been admitted to the rehabilitation unit following a recent seizure. Which safety precaution should the nurse prioritize when providing care for Mr. Johnson?
A) Implementing fall precautions
B) Administering antiepileptic medications
C) Assessing for impaired judgment
D) Maintaining seizure precautions

Question 53: A 65-year-old patient with a history of dysphagia following a stroke is being evaluated for the use of an adaptive equipment device called the Passy Muir valve. The nurse wants to assess the patient's understanding of the device. Which of the following statements made by the patient would indicate a correct understanding of the Passy Muir valve?
A) "The Passy Muir valve will help me speak more clearly."
B) "The Passy Muir valve will help improve my balance."
C) "The Passy Muir valve will assist me with my memory."
D) "The Passy Muir valve will help me walk independently."

Question 54: Which of the following behavioral management techniques is based on the concept of positive reinforcement?
A) Time-out
B) Restraints
C) Token economy
D) Seclusion

Question 55: Mrs. Taylor, a 68-year-old patient, has suffered a stroke that has left her with expressive aphasia, an inability to speak fluently. As a Certified Rehabilitation Registered Nurse (CRRN), which communication technique would be most effective in helping Mrs. Taylor express her needs and concerns?
A) Using complex medical terminology to better assess her condition.
B) Using non-verbal communication such as gestures and facial expressions.
C) Ignoring her attempts to communicate until speech therapy can address her aphasia.
D) Encouraging her to give up on speaking and relying solely on writing.

Question 56: Mrs. Johnson, a 40-year-old patient hospitalized after an acute spinal cord injury, expresses feelings of anxiety and frustration related to her condition and future life adjustments. The nurse is assessing Mrs. Johnson's ability to cope and manage stress. Which of the following statements made by Mrs. Johnson reflects an unhealthy coping mechanism?
A) "I have been attending support groups for individuals with spinal cord injuries to find inspiration and learn from their experiences."
B) "I find solace in painting and engaging in other activities that help distract me from my worries."
C) "Whenever I feel overwhelmed, I take deep breaths and practice relaxation techniques to calm myself down."
D) "I frequently isolate myself from family and friends because I don't want them to see me struggling."

Question 57: Emma is a 32-year-old female who sustained a spinal cord injury at the T10 level resulting in paraplegia. As part of her rehabilitation process, the Certified Rehabilitation Registered Nurse (CRRN) assesses her for alterations in sexual function and reproduction. During the assessment, Emma expresses concerns about her ability to have children in the future. Which of the following statements by the nurse is most appropriate?
A) "You will not be able to conceive naturally due to your spinal cord injury."
B) "You may experience difficulty conceiving, but there are assisted reproductive options available to you if you wish to have children."
C) "Your spinal cord injury should not affect your ability to conceive or carry a pregnancy."
D) "Infertility is a common consequence of spinal cord injuries, but miracles do happen, so you never know."

Question 58: Which phase of the nursing process involves analyzing data to determine the client's health needs and formulating a nursing diagnosis?
A) Assessment
B) Diagnosis
C) Outcomes Identification
D) Planning

Question 59: Mr. Johnson, a 68-year-old male, has been admitted to the rehabilitation unit following a stroke. He experiences difficulty with comprehension and communication due to his cognitive deficits. Which area of the brain is most likely affected in Mr. Johnson's case?
A) Frontal lobe
B) Temporal lobe
C) Occipital lobe
D) Parietal lobe

Question 60: Mr. Thompson, a 65-year-old male, has been admitted to a rehabilitation center following a stroke that resulted in mild left-sided weakness. The nurse is discussing the use of assistive devices and technology to improve his mobility and independence. Mr. Thompson expressed concerns about maintaining balance while walking. Which assistive device would be most appropriate for Mr. Thompson to improve his balance during walking?
A) Quad cane
B) Wheelchair
C) Walker
D) Crutches

Question 61: A 45-year-old male patient with a spinal cord injury is experiencing difficulties falling asleep and staying asleep. The rehabilitation nurse is assessing the patient's sleep and rest patterns to identify any contributing factors. Which of the following factors may be affecting the patient's sleep?
A) Consuming caffeine-rich beverages before bedtime.
B) Following a consistent sleep routine.
C) Engaging in regular physical exercise.
D) Having a quiet and dark environment in the bedroom.

Question 62: Mrs. Johnson, a 70-year-old patient with a previous history of stroke, has been admitted to a rehabilitation unit. She has been experiencing weakness and difficulties in walking. What is the most appropriate initial step for the rehabilitation nurse in the assessment phase of the nursing process?
A) Developing a plan of care.
B) Administering medications for pain management.

C) Assessing Mrs. Johnson's cognitive function.
D) Assessing Mrs. Johnson's ability to perform activities of daily living (ADLs).

Question 63: A patient with chronic fatigue syndrome is experiencing limited activity tolerance. Which intervention would be most appropriate for the patient to conserve energy?
A) Encouraging the patient to engage in deep breathing exercises
B) Advising the patient to perform high-intensity aerobic exercises daily
C) Instructing the patient to prioritize tasks and take frequent rest breaks
D) Recommending the patient to engage in rigorous physical therapy sessions

Question 64: A patient admitted to the rehabilitation unit for a spinal cord injury has been experiencing constipation. The nurse understands it is important to promote optimal elimination patterns for the patient's overall health and comfort. Which intervention is appropriate for the nurse to implement?
A) Encouraging the patient to increase fiber intake and drink plenty of fluids
B) Administering a laxative without consulting the healthcare provider
C) Limiting the patient's fluid intake to avoid bladder distention
D) Prescribing a high-protein diet to improve muscle strength

Question 65: Mr. Johnson, a 70-year-old patient with a history of chronic obstructive pulmonary disease (COPD) and heart failure, is admitted to a rehabilitation facility for pulmonary rehabilitation following a recent exacerbation. During his admission, his daughter approaches the nurse and requests access to her father's medical records. Which of the following actions should the nurse take in response to this request?
A) Provide the daughter with immediate access to her father's medical records.
B) Inform the daughter that she must first obtain a court order to access her father's medical records.
C) Direct the daughter to the facility's medical records department to complete the appropriate paperwork for access.
D) Explain to the daughter that access to her father's medical records can only be granted if the patient verbally grants permission.

Question 66: What is the purpose of assistive technology and adaptive equipment in rehabilitation nursing?
A) To improve communication skills
B) To enhance functional abilities and independence
C) To provide emotional support
D) To assist with medication administration

Question 67: You are a Certified Rehabilitation Registered Nurse (CRRN) working in a rehabilitation center. Your patient, Mr. Johnson, is a 68-year-old male who recently suffered a stroke and is experiencing left-sided weakness and difficulty with balance. You are developing a plan of care to help Mr. Johnson attain his patient-centered goals. Which of the following actions would be most appropriate for you to include in the plan?
A) Encourage the patient to participate in physical therapy sessions three times a week.
B) Initiate a home exercise program for the patient to follow independently.

C) Provide education for the patient and family on safety measures, such as installing grab bars in the bathroom.
D) Request a consultation with a psychologist to address the patient's emotional well-being.

Question 68: Which statement best describes patient-centered care in rehabilitation nursing?
A) Patient preferences are disregarded in the decision-making process.
B) The healthcare provider makes all decisions for the patient.
C) The patient and healthcare provider collaborate in decision-making based on the patient's values and goals.
D) The patient's family makes all decisions on behalf of the patient.

Question 69: Ms. Johnson, a 55-year-old patient, has been admitted to the rehabilitation unit after a stroke. She is experiencing difficulty with her communication skills, has limited mobility on her right side, and has been feeling sad and hopeless since the incident. The nurse provides emotional support and encourages her to express her feelings and concerns. Which theory is the nurse applying in this scenario?
A) Developmental theory
B) Coping theory
C) Stress theory
D) Self-esteem theory

Question 70: Which non-pharmacological intervention can be used to optimize a patient's elimination patterns?
A) Adequate fluid intake
B) Administration of laxatives
C) Physical restraints
D) Sedative medications

Question 71: Which reimbursement system is used by Medicare for inpatient rehabilitation facilities (IRFs)?
A) Prospective Payment System (PPS)
B) Fee-for-Service (FFS)
C) Diagnosis-Related Group (DRG)
D) Capitation

Question 72: Which intervention is most appropriate for a patient with incomplete bladder emptying due to a neurogenic bladder?
A) Encouraging the patient to wait for the urge to void before attempting to empty the bladder.
B) Administering an anticholinergic medication to increase bladder capacity.
C) Implementing intermittent self-catheterization to ensure complete bladder emptying.
D) Initiating timed voiding to establish a regular voiding schedule.

Question 73: Which skill is essential for a Certified Rehabilitation Registered Nurse (CRRN) in relation to legislative, economic, ethical, and legal issues?
A) Analyzing financial data and budgeting
B) Advocating for patient rights and informed consent
C) Implementing evidence-based practice guidelines
D) Assessing and managing risks in healthcare

Question 74: Jane, a 68-year-old patient, has been receiving rehabilitation services after a hip replacement surgery. She has made significant progress and is ready for discharge. As the rehabilitation nurse, which of the following would be the most appropriate action for you to take before Jane's discharge?
A) Provide comprehensive written discharge instructions to the patient and her caregiver.

B) Assess the patient's ability to perform activities of daily living (ADLs) independently.
C) Consult with a physical therapist to determine if the patient is capable of using mobility aids.
D) Arrange for a follow-up appointment with the orthopedic surgeon to monitor post-operative progress.

Question 75: Ms. Smith, a 45-year-old patient with a recent diagnosis of multiple sclerosis (MS), is experiencing visual disturbances due to optic neuritis. As a rehabilitation nurse, which teaching strategy would be most effective to help Ms. Smith manage her neurological deficit?
A) Provide written material on the importance of regular eye examinations.
B) Demonstrate techniques for compensatory head movements to improve visual field.
C) Discuss the benefits of proper nutrition and hydration for overall visual health.
D) Encourage participation in support groups to share experiences and coping strategies.

Question 76: Which traditional modality focuses on using healing touch to promote relaxation and pain relief in patients?
A) Botanicals
B) Medications
C) Spiritual practices
D) Mindfulness

Question 77: A 65-year-old patient with a history of chronic back pain is admitted for rehabilitation following a spinal surgery. The patient is currently taking an anticholinergic medication for another condition. The healthcare provider prescribes an antispasmodic medication to alleviate the patient's postoperative muscle spasms. Which of the following statements is true regarding the combination of antispasmodics and anticholinergic medications for this patient?
A) The combination of antispasmodics and anticholinergics can lead to increased sedation and confusion.
B) The combination of antispasmodics and anticholinergics can enhance the analgesic effect of the antispasmodic medication.
C) The combination of antispasmodics and anticholinergics can increase the risk of bleeding in the postoperative period.
D) The combination of antispasmodics and anticholinergics can improve the patient's mobility and functional ability.

Question 78: Under 'Legislative, Economic, Ethical, and Legal Issues', which of the following is essential for a Certified Rehabilitation Registered Nurse (CRRN)?
A) Understanding the ethical principles and standards that guide nursing practice.
B) Applying economic principles to manage healthcare resources efficiently.
C) Advocating for legislative changes to improve the quality of rehabilitation nursing care.
D) Managing legal obligations related to patient confidentiality and privacy.

Question 79: Katherine, a 45-year-old female patient with a spinal cord injury, is admitted to the rehabilitation unit. The nursing team is responsible for promoting optimal nutrition and hydration. Which intervention would be most appropriate for the nurse to implement?
A) Provide Katherine with a high-calorie, high-protein diet
B) Encourage Katherine to drink at least 2 liters of water daily
C) Assist Katherine to eat her meals while lying in a supine position

D) Offer Katherine small, frequent meals throughout the day

Question 80: Mrs. Johnson, a 65-year-old patient, has recently been admitted to the rehabilitation unit following a stroke. As part of her care, the nurse is teaching Mrs. Johnson and her family about self-advocacy skills. Which of the following statements made by Mrs. Johnson's daughter indicates a need for further teaching?
A) "I will make sure to communicate my mother's preferences and concerns to the healthcare team."
B) "I will encourage my mother to ask questions and express her opinions about her care."
C) "I will handle all the decision-making for my mother to reduce her stress."
D) "I will help my mother practice assertiveness and confidence in speaking up for herself."

Question 81: When utilizing standardized assessment tools in rehabilitation nursing practice, which of the following is true?
A) Standardized assessment tools provide subjective information about the patient's condition.
B) Standardized assessment tools are not useful in promoting interprofessional collaboration.
C) Standardized assessment tools are only valid for specific populations and settings.
D) Standardized assessment tools improve the accuracy and consistency of data collection for effective patient care planning.

Question 82: Sarah, a Certified Rehabilitation Registered Nurse (CRRN), is part of an interdisciplinary team caring for Mr. Roberts, a 68-year-old patient who suffered a stroke and is undergoing rehabilitation. The team includes a physical therapist, occupational therapist, speech therapist, social worker, and physician. The team has established patient-centered goals that include increasing Mr. Roberts' mobility, improving his swallowing abilities, and enhancing his ability to communicate effectively. Sarah's role is to coordinate and collaborate with the team to achieve these goals. Which of the following actions by Sarah demonstrates effective collaboration with the interdisciplinary team to achieve patient-centered goals?
A) Sarah schedules therapy sessions without considering Mr. Roberts' preferences or limitations.
B) Sarah shares Mr. Roberts' progress and updates with the team during weekly team meetings.
C) Sarah makes decisions about Mr. Roberts' care without consulting the other team members.
D) Sarah avoids communication with the other team members and focuses solely on her nursing responsibilities.

Question 83: A patient with spinal cord injury has been admitted to the rehabilitation unit. The nurse is implementing infection control practices to prevent the transmission of infections. Which action by the nurse would be the most effective in minimizing the risk of infection?
A) Isolating the patient in a private room.
B) Administering prophylactic antibiotics.
C) Encouraging the patient to perform regular hand hygiene.
D) Wearing a mask and gloves when interacting with the patient.

Question 84: Mrs. Johnson, a 68-year-old patient, was recently discharged from acute rehabilitation following a stroke. She has made significant progress in regaining her functional abilities and is now preparing for the next level of care. As a CRRN, you are responsible for

discussing the options with Mrs. Johnson and her family. Which option represents the most suitable level of care for Mrs. Johnson at this stage?
A) Assisted living facility
B) Home healthcare services
C) Skilled nursing facility
D) Outpatient rehabilitation

Question 85: Which legislation ensures equal access to employment opportunities for individuals with disabilities?
A) Medicare
B) Medicaid
C) Rehabilitation Acts
D) HIPAA

Question 86: Mr. Johnson, a 62-year-old patient, is admitted to the rehabilitation unit following a stroke. As a Certified Rehabilitation Registered Nurse (CRRN), you are responsible for using standardized assessment tools to evaluate his functional abilities. Which assessment tool would be appropriate to assess his mobility and ability to perform activities of daily living (ADLs)?
A) Mini-Mental State Examination (MMSE)
B) Berg Balance Scale
C) Confusion Assessment Method (CAM)
D) Glasgow Coma Scale (GCS)

Question 87: Ms. Anderson, a 48-year-old patient, has recently suffered a spinal cord injury and is struggling with feelings of low self-esteem and dependency. The nurse is working with her to promote self-efficacy and self-concept. Which intervention would be most appropriate in supporting Ms. Anderson's self-efficacy and self-concept?
A) Encouraging Ms. Anderson to set achievable goals for her rehabilitation process.
B) Encouraging Ms. Anderson to rely on others for all activities of daily living.
C) Discouraging Ms. Anderson from expressing her feelings of frustration or sadness.
D) Discouraging Ms. Anderson from participating in activities that challenge her abilities.

Question 88: As a Certified Rehabilitation Registered Nurse (CRRN), you are caring for a patient named Sarah, who recently immigrated from a different country. Sarah speaks limited English and is struggling to communicate her needs effectively. Which action by the nurse best demonstrates cultural competence and fosters effective communication?
A) Providing an interpreter to assist in communicating with Sarah.
B) Relying on non-verbal communication to understand Sarah's needs.
C) Asking Sarah to bring a family member who can translate for her.
D) Assuming Sarah can understand English and continuing to communicate without any assistance.

Question 89: Rachel is a 45-year-old patient who recently suffered a spinal cord injury and is currently undergoing rehabilitation. She is interested in using smart devices to assist her in daily activities. As a CRRN, which of the following options would be the most appropriate device to recommend to Rachel to address her needs?
A) A smart home system
B) A wearable fitness tracker
C) A personal response device

D) A telehealth monitoring system

Question 90: You are caring for a patient admitted for acute stroke rehabilitation. The patient has right-sided weakness and limited range of motion in the upper and lower extremities. The patient's rehabilitation plan includes passive range of motion exercises to prevent contractures. Which statement by the patient indicates a need for further education?
A) "I will ask my family to help me with passive range of motion exercises."
B) "I will make sure to do the exercises at least three times a day."
C) "I will stop the exercises if I feel any pain or discomfort."
D) "I will try to move the unaffected side of my body as well during the exercises."

Question 91: When should a Certified Rehabilitation Registered Nurse (CRRN) facilitate a referral to a mental health professional for a patient?
A) When the patient appears to be experiencing depression or anxiety
B) When the patient is not demonstrating effective coping skills
C) When the patient's psychosocial needs are not being addressed adequately
D) When the patient expresses a desire to seek counseling

Question 92: Sarah, a 45-year-old female, has been diagnosed with multiple sclerosis (MS). She is experiencing muscle spasms and tightness, leading to significant discomfort and limited mobility. As part of her treatment, the healthcare provider prescribes an antispasmodic medication. Which of the following antispasmodic medications is commonly used in the management of muscle spasms associated with MS?
A) Amantadine
B) Gabapentin
C) Baclofen
D) Sertraline

Question 93: Which skill is important for a Certified Rehabilitation Registered Nurse (CRRN) in optimizing the patient's elimination patterns?
A) Administering medications
B) Performing wound care
C) Providing patient education on nutrition
D) Assessing urinary and bowel functions

Question 94: Ms. Anderson is a 35-year-old patient who has recently undergone a knee replacement surgery. She Is currently in the rehabilitation phase and is concerned about managing her pain effectively at home. As a Certified Rehabilitation Registered Nurse (CRRN), which teaching intervention would you prioritize to help Ms. Anderson manage her health and wellness?
A) Encourage her to take excessive amounts of painkillers to ensure maximum pain relief.
B) Teach her relaxation techniques such as deep breathing and guided imagery.
C) Advise her to avoid any form of physical activity until her pain subsides completely.
D) Recommend she engage in high-intensity exercises to improve joint mobility.

Question 95: A 45-year-old patient, Mr. Anderson, is admitted to the rehabilitation unit following a traumatic brain injury. During the assessment, the nurse identifies that Mr. Anderson has been expressing feelings of hopelessness and states, "I don't see the point in living

anymore." What action should the nurse take based on this assessment finding?
A) Document the assessment finding and proceed with the admission process.
B) Recognize the severity of the statement and initiate suicide precautions.
C) Inform the patient that it is natural to feel this way after such an injury.
D) Provide the patient with contact information for a support group after discharge.

Question 96: When advocating for a patient's rights, the nurse should prioritize which of the following actions?
A) Prioritizing the patient's autonomy and self-determination.
B) Focusing on the nurse's personal beliefs and values.
C) Following the recommendations of the healthcare team without question.
D) Ignoring the patient's concerns and preferences.

Question 97: Nurse Jane is providing care to a patient who recently suffered a stroke. The patient has been admitted to the rehabilitation unit and is receiving physical therapy to regain mobility. Nurse Jane is familiar with the clinical practice guidelines for stroke rehabilitation and wants to incorporate them into the patient's care plan. Which of the following actions by Nurse Jane demonstrates the correct use of clinical practice guidelines?
A) Nursing Jane consults the patient's family before implementing any interventions.
B) Nurse Jane ignores the clinical practice guidelines and follows her own experience and expertise.
C) Nurse Jane reviews the clinical practice guidelines and adapts them to fit the patient's unique needs.
D) Nurse Jane uses the clinical practice guidelines as a strict protocol without individualizing the care plan.

Question 98: Mr. Johnson, a 45-year-old patient, has been admitted to the rehabilitation unit after a spinal cord injury. The nurse is assessing his sleep patterns. Which factor is likely to affect Mr. Johnson's sleep and rest the most?
A) Diet
B) Sleep habits
C) Alcohol
D) Pain
.

Question 99: Mrs. Thompson, a 65-year-old female, was recently diagnosed with multiple sclerosis (MS) and has been admitted to the rehabilitation unit. The nurse is developing a plan of care for Mrs. Thompson and wants to include her and her husband in the decision-making process. Which of the following interventions would be most appropriate for the nurse to implement in order to include the patient and caregiver in the plan of care?
A) Provide written educational materials about MS to Mrs. Thompson and her husband.
B) Assign a nursing assistant to take care of Mrs. Thompson's daily needs.
C) Conduct a family meeting to discuss the goals and expectations of the rehabilitation process.
D) Restrict visitation hours to ensure Mrs. Thompson gets enough rest.

Question 100: When resolving ethical dilemmas, which strategy involves collaborating with the interprofessional team and considering their perspectives?
A) Utilizing the ethical decision-making framework

B) Seeking guidance from a supervisor or manager
C) Seeking legal advice from an attorney
D) Seeking input from the patient's family

Question 101: Which of the following theories focuses on the cognitive development of individuals?
A) Psychosocial theory
B) Behavioral theory
C) Cognitive theory
D) Moral theory

Question 102: Which of the following is a safety concern regarding harm to self and others in patients with psychosocial disorders?
A) Aggressive behavior
B) Decreased appetite
C) Excessive sleepiness
D) Hypertension

Question 103: Mrs. Johnson, a 65-year-old patient with a history of stroke and mobility impairments, is currently receiving physical and occupational therapy in a rehabilitation facility. The healthcare team has implemented various sleep and rest interventions to optimize her sleep patterns. Which of the following evaluation methods would be most appropriate to assess the effectiveness of these interventions?
A) Administering a self-report sleep diary
B) Monitoring her vital signs during sleep
C) Conducting a subjective interview about sleep quality
D) Observing her sleep behavior through video surveillance

Question 104: Which of the following brain waves is predominant during NREM sleep?
A) Alpha waves
B) Beta waves
C) Theta waves
D) Gamma waves

Question 105: When it comes to promoting a safe environment of care for patients and staff to minimize risk, which skill is most important for a Certified Rehabilitation Registered Nurse (CRRN)?
A) Ability to navigate and comply with legislative requirements
B) Understanding economic factors that impact healthcare delivery
C) Ethical decision-making in patient care situations
D) Knowledge of legal issues related to patient rights

Question 106: Mr. Johnson, a 60-year-old patient who recently underwent spinal surgery, is having difficulty moving around. He requires assistance with bed mobility and transferring to a wheelchair. In order to prevent potential injuries during these activities, which of the following equipment should the nurse prioritize?
A) Gait belt
B) Transfer board
C) Hoyer lift
D) Knee immobilizer

Question 107: Sarah, a 45-year-old patient, was admitted to a rehabilitation center following a severe spinal cord injury. As the rehabilitation nurse, you are responsible for incorporating nursing models and theories into Sarah's care. Which nursing model or theory is most applicable in this case?
A) The Neuman Systems Model
B) The Self-Care Deficit Theory
C) The Health Belief Model
D) The Transcultural Nursing Model

Question 108: Which of the following is an essential component of quality improvement processes in nursing practice?
A) Continuous assessment and evaluation of outcomes
B) Assigning blame to individuals for errors
C) Ignoring feedback from patients and colleagues
D) Following outdated evidence-based guidelines

Question 109: Which of the following statements best describes the concept of coping in relation to stress management?
A) Coping refers to the process of completely eliminating stress from one's life.
B) Coping involves using adaptive strategies to effectively deal with stressors.
C) Coping refers to the ability to avoid all stressful situations.
D) Coping involves ignoring or denying the presence of stress.

Question 110: Mr. Anderson is a 62-year-old patient who recently had a stroke and is currently receiving rehabilitation therapy in a skilled nursing facility. The nurse is assessing Mr. Anderson's ability to perform self-care activities. Which of the following tasks would be considered an instrumental activity of daily living (IADL)?
A) Dressing himself
B) Bathing himself
C) Managing his medication
D) Feeding himself

Question 111: Maria, a 35-year-old patient, is admitted to the rehabilitation unit following a traumatic brain injury. As part of the assessment, the nurse is using the Rancho Los Amigos Scale to determine the patient's level of cognitive function. Which of the following statements accurately describes the Rancho Los Amigos Scale?
A) The Rancho Los Amigos Scale assesses the patient's level of consciousness and cognitive function.
B) The Rancho Los Amigos Scale measures the patient's level of physical disability and mobility.
C) The Rancho Los Amigos Scale evaluates the patient's pain intensity and location.
D) The Rancho Los Amigos Scale determines the patient's ability to perform activities of daily living.

Question 112: Which of the following statements best describes the philosophy of rehabilitation?
A) Rehabilitation focuses on curing the underlying medical condition.
B) Rehabilitation emphasizes the achievement of optimal physical functioning.
C) Rehabilitation prioritizes the use of pharmacological interventions.
D) Rehabilitation is solely focused on the elimination of pain.

Question 113: Which of the following organizations is responsible for accrediting rehabilitation facilities?
A) The American Nurses Association (ANA)
B) The Centers for Medicare and Medicaid Services (CMS)
C) The National Council of State Boards of Nursing (NCSBN)
D) The Commission on Accreditation of Rehabilitation Facilities (CARF)

Question 114: Which of the following is a symptom commonly associated with substance abuse?
A) Increased appetite
B) Decreased energy
C) Hyperactivity
D) Increased attention span

Question 115: A 65-year-old patient is admitted to the rehabilitation unit following a cerebrovascular accident (CVA). The patient is experiencing difficulties with coordination, balance, and voluntary movement on the left side of the body. The patient's cognition, judgment, sensation, and perception are intact. Which area of the brain is most likely affected?
A) Medulla oblongata
B) Pons
C) Cerebellum
D) Frontal lobe

Question 116: When assessing safety risks for patients, which of the following factors should the certified rehabilitation registered nurse prioritize?
A) Patient's socioeconomic background
B) Patient's religious beliefs
C) Patient's cultural practices
D) Patient's physical limitations

Question 117: Maria is a 35-year-old patient admitted to the rehabilitation unit following a traumatic brain injury. As the Certified Rehabilitation Registered Nurse (CRRN), you are responsible for providing patient-centered care based on relevant nursing models and theories. Which nursing model or theory can guide your practice in this situation?
A) Maslow's Hierarchy of Needs
B) Health Belief Model
C) Orem's Self-Care Deficit Theory
D) Swanson's Theory of Caring

Question 118: Which adaptive equipment would be most appropriate for a patient with limited upper body mobility to perform self-care tasks?
A) A reacher
B) A walker
C) A weighted pen
D) A shower chair

Question 119: Samantha, a 65-year-old patient, was admitted to the rehabilitation unit after a stroke. She has dysphagia and is currently on a pureed diet. Which of the following anatomical structures is responsible for pushing food into the esophagus during swallowing?
A) Epiglottis
B) Uvula
C) Esophagus
D) Pharynx

Question 120: Mr. Smith, a 45-year-old patient, was involved in a severe motor vehicle accident that left him paralyzed from the waist down. He is currently undergoing rehabilitation in the spinal cord injury unit. Which of the following stressors is Mr. Smith most likely experiencing?
A) Physical stressor
B) Psychological stressor
C) Emotional stressor
D) Social stressor

Question 121: Which member of the rehabilitation team is responsible for coordinating the patient's care and ensuring that all interventions are implemented effectively?
A) Physical therapist
B) Speech-language pathologist
C) Occupational therapist
D) Rehabilitation nurse

Question 122: Which of the following is an example of patient-centered goal adjustment in the rehabilitation process?
A) The interdisciplinary team decides to change the patient's goals without consulting the patient.
B) The patient's family decides to modify the goals without the input of the interdisciplinary team.
C) The patient and the interdisciplinary team collaborate to modify the goals based on the patient's progress and preferences.
D) The rehabilitation nurse independently changes the patient's goals without involving the interdisciplinary team.

Question 123: What is the purpose of utilization review processes in rehabilitation nursing?
A) To evaluate the quality and appropriateness of patient care
B) To maximize the revenue of the healthcare facility
C) To expedite the discharge process
D) To increase patient satisfaction

Question 124: According to the SMART goal-setting framework, which of the following is a characteristic of an effective goal?
A) Broad and general
B) Time-limited
C) Vague and immeasurable
D) Subject to change

Question 125: When incorporating cultural awareness and spiritual values in the plan of care, the nurse should:
A) Disregard the patient's cultural and spiritual beliefs as they may interfere with evidence-based practice.
B) Prioritize the nurse's own cultural and spiritual beliefs over those of the patient.
C) Assess and respect the patient's cultural and spiritual beliefs, integrating them into the plan of care.
D) Avoid discussing cultural and spiritual beliefs with the patient to prevent any potential conflicts.

Question 126: You are a Certified Rehabilitation Registered Nurse (CRRN) working in a rehabilitation facility. You receive a report from the night shift nurse on a patient named John, who has been admitted with a traumatic brain injury. The nurse informs you that John's family has expressed concerns about his treatment, and they have requested a meeting with the ombudsperson to discuss their grievances. As the responsible nurse, you need to understand the role of the ombudsperson in resolving ethical conflicts between patients and healthcare providers. Question: Which of the following best describes the role of an ombudsperson in healthcare settings?
A) An ombudsperson is a legal representative who advocates for the rights of the healthcare organization.
B) An ombudsperson acts as a mediator to resolve conflicts between patients and healthcare providers.
C) An ombudsperson ensures that healthcare providers uphold ethical standards and principles.
D) An ombudsperson provides financial assistance to patients in need.

Question 127: Which of the following statements accurately describes the nursing process in relation to optimizing a patient's elimination patterns?
A) The nursing process involves assessing the patient's elimination needs, providing appropriate interventions, and evaluating the outcomes.
B) The nursing process focuses solely on administering medications to regulate the patient's elimination patterns.

C) The nursing process does not play a significant role in optimizing a patient's elimination patterns.
D) The nursing process is not applicable to patients with impaired elimination patterns.

Question 128: You are a Certified Rehabilitation Registered Nurse (CRRN) working in a rehabilitation facility. One of your responsibilities is to promote a safe environment of care for patients and staff to minimize risk. Today, you are conducting an assessment of the facility's safety measures. As you inspect the patient rooms, you notice that one of the rooms has cluttered pathways and the emergency call bell is not within reach of the patient. What is the best action to address this safety concern and minimize risk for the patient?
A) Inform the patient's family about the safety concern and request their assistance in maintaining a clutter-free environment.
B) Immediately remove the clutter and ensure that the emergency call bell is within reach of the patient.
C) Document the safety concern in the patient's medical record and report it to your supervisor.
D) Ignore the safety concern as it is the responsibility of housekeeping staff to ensure a safe environment.

Question 129: Mr. Johnson, a 68-year-old patient with a history of stroke, is receiving rehabilitation services in the inpatient setting. The nurse is assessing Mr. Johnson's functional health patterns. Which of the following statements indicates the nurse's understanding of the Knowledge of: functional health patterns?
A) The nurse assesses Mr. Johnson's cardiovascular system functioning by monitoring his blood pressure and heart rate.
B) The nurse evaluates Mr. Johnson's cognitive abilities by conducting a Mini-Mental State Examination.
C) The nurse observes Mr. Johnson's mobility and balance during his therapy sessions.
D) The nurse asks Mr. Johnson about his social support system and sources of stress.

Question 130: Which intervention should be implemented to optimize bladder and bowel management in a patient receiving rehabilitation care?
A) Providing a balanced diet rich in fiber and fluids
B) Administering laxatives on a daily basis
C) Restricting fluid intake to minimize the need for frequent toileting
D) Encouraging the patient to suppress the urge to void or defecate

Question 131: You are a Certified Rehabilitation Registered Nurse (CRRN) working in a rehabilitation facility. Your facility is implementing quality improvement processes to enhance patient care outcomes. As part of this process, you are reviewing the National Database of Nursing Quality Indicators (NDNQI) to identify areas for improvement. Which of the following statements accurately describes the NDNQI?
A) The NDNQI is a database that collects and analyzes data related to nursing-sensitive quality indicators.
B) The NDNQI is a federal agency that sets standards for healthcare quality improvement.
C) The NDNQI is a research organization focused on rehabilitating patients with chronic conditions.
D) The NDNQI is a professional organization advocating for the rights of rehabilitation nurses.

Question 132: Mrs. Adams, a 65-year-old female patient, is admitted to the rehabilitation unit following a

stroke. She has a history of urinary incontinence and is currently using absorbent pads. The rehabilitation nurse is developing a care plan to address Mrs. Adams' elimination patterns. Which intervention should be included in the plan to promote continence?
A) Limiting fluid intake throughout the day.
B) Encouraging Mrs. Adams to empty her bladder every 4 hours.
C) Administering a diuretic to increase urine output.
D) Providing Mrs. Adams with a bedside commode for easy access.

Question 133: According to the nursing process, what is the first step in promoting optimal psychosocial patterns and coping and stress management skills of the patients and caregivers?
A) Evaluation
B) Assessment
C) Diagnosis
D) Planning

Question 134: Mrs. Johnson is a Certified Rehabilitation Registered Nurse (CRRN) working in a rehabilitation facility. She is responsible for accessing, interpreting, and applying legal, regulatory, and accreditation information to ensure compliance and quality care. While reviewing a patient's medical records, Mrs. Johnson notices that the physician has ordered the use of physical restraints on the patient, Mr. Wilson, without obtaining proper consent from the patient or family members. What action should Mrs. Johnson take to address this situation?
A) Ignore the issue as physical restraints are commonly used in rehabilitation facilities.
B) Consult the facility's legal team for guidance on the situation.
C) Inform the physician and request proper consent from the patient or family members.
D) Remove the physical restraints without informing anyone.

Question 135: Which of the following technologies can be used to optimize the patient's sleep and rest patterns?
A) Virtual reality headsets
B) Robotic assistance devices for mobility
C) Bluetooth-enabled devices for monitoring sleep quality
D) 3D printers for producing personalized sleep masks

Question 136: Laura, a Certified Rehabilitation Registered Nurse (CRRN), is reviewing the medical records of a patient admitted to the rehabilitation unit. The patient, Mr. Johnson, has been receiving physical therapy and occupational therapy to regain his mobility and independence after a stroke. Laura notices that the patient's length of stay is longer than expected for similar cases. She decides to initiate a utilization review to determine the appropriateness of the continued stay. Which of the following statements best describes the utilization review processes in healthcare?
A) Utilization review focuses on ensuring the accuracy of medical coding and billing.
B) Utilization review serves as a quality assurance measure to improve patient outcomes.
C) Utilization review is a process to identify hospital-acquired infections.
D) Utilization review involves monitoring the medical necessity and efficiency of healthcare services.

Question 137: Which tool can be used to evaluate the effectiveness of sleep and rest interventions in patients?
A) Pain Assessment Tool

B) Braden Scale for Predicting Pressure Sore Risk
C) Epworth Sleepiness Scale
D) Johns Hopkins Fall Risk Assessment Tool

Question 138: Mrs. Thompson, a 68-year-old patient, is admitted to a rehabilitation facility after a stroke. She complains of pain in her left arm and shoulder. The nurse is educating Mrs. Thompson about pain management strategies. Which teaching point should the nurse prioritize?
A) Explaining the benefits of nonpharmacological pain management techniques
B) Discussing the potential side effects of opioid pain medication
C) Demonstrating the correct technique for administering IV pain medication
D) Encouraging the use of over-the-counter pain relievers as needed

Question 139: Sarah, a 55-year-old patient, has been admitted to the rehabilitation unit after a stroke. As the nurse, you are responsible for assessing her physical, psychological, and social needs. Which step of the nursing process is this?
A) Diagnosis
B) Planning
C) Implementation
D) Assessment

Question 140: Mark, a 60-year-old male patient, recently experienced a stroke that resulted in right-sided weakness. As part of Mark's rehabilitation plan, the nurse is responsible for implementing and evaluating strategies for safety. Which of the following strategies would be most appropriate for the nurse to implement in order to prevent falls?
A) Providing Mark with a personal response device
B) Placing alarms in strategic areas around Mark's environment
C) Encouraging Mark to wear a helmet whenever he is up and moving
D) Adding padding to the furniture in Mark's room

Question 141: Jennifer is a 60-year-old patient who recently suffered a stroke and has been admitted to the rehabilitation unit. She is experiencing difficulty with her balance and coordination, making mobility challenging. As the rehabilitation nurse, you are implementing the nursing model that focuses on the patient's ability to adapt and maintain independence in their daily activities. Which nursing model is being utilized in Jennifer's care?
A) Roy's Adaptation Model
B) Orem's Self-Care Deficit Model
C) Neuman's Systems Model
D) Leininger's Culture Care Diversity and Universality Theory

Question 142: Which of the following strategies can be utilized to promote coping with role and relationship changes in patients and caregivers?
A) Providing counseling services to patients only
B) Encouraging peer support groups for patients only
C) Educating patients and caregivers about coping techniques
D) Providing caregiver counseling services only

Question 143: Which nursing model emphasizes the importance of the nurse-patient relationship and focuses on meeting the patient's basic physiological, safety, love/belonging, esteem, and self-actualization needs?
A) Orem's Self-Care Deficit Theory

B) Roy's Adaptation Model
C) Neuman's Systems Model
D) Maslow's Hierarchy of Needs

Question 144: What is the purpose of a bladder scan in the assessment of a patient's elimination patterns?
A) To measure the size and shape of the bladder
B) To determine the amount of residual urine in the bladder
C) To assess the type and severity of urinary incontinence
D) To evaluate the effectiveness of bladder training exercises

Question 145: Mr. Smith, a 75-year-old patient, has a history of falls and is at risk for injury. The rehabilitation nurse is implementing fall prevention measures. Which statement by the nurse demonstrates correct knowledge about fall prevention?
A) "I will place the fall risk sign on the door of Mr. Smith's room."
B) "I will encourage Mr. Smith to sleep with the lights on to prevent falls at night."
C) "I will keep the call bell out of Mr. Smith's reach to prevent unnecessary calls for assistance."
D) "I will provide Mr. Smith with non-slip socks to wear to minimize the risk of falls."

Question 146: Mr. Johnson, a 65-year-old patient with a history of stroke and hemiparesis, has been admitted to a rehabilitation facility. The nursing staff has noticed that there are inconsistencies in documentation and communication between team members, leading to potential errors in patient care. The rehabilitation nurse identifies the need to address this issue and improve quality processes. What is the best strategy for the nurse to integrate quality improvement processes into nursing practice?
A) Develop an interdisciplinary communication tool to enhance collaboration.
B) Implement standardized protocols for medication administration.
C) Increase the frequency of team meetings to discuss patient care.
D) Conduct annual performance evaluations for nursing staff.

Question 147: Mr. Smith, a 65-year-old male, was recently admitted to a rehabilitation facility following a cerebrovascular accident (CVA). He is experiencing weakness on the left side of his body and has difficulty with balance and coordination. The rehabilitation team is planning his discharge and is discussing the appropriate setting for his continued care. Which of the following settings would be the most suitable for Mr. Smith's ongoing rehabilitation needs?
A) Assisted living facility
B) Skilled nursing facility
C) Home health care
D) Adult day care center

Question 148: Which federal agency is responsible for overseeing the quality measurement efforts in healthcare?
A) Centers for Medicare and Medicaid Services (CMS)
B) Food and Drug Administration (FDA)
C) National Institutes of Health (NIH)
D) Department of Health and Human Services (HHS)

Question 149: Which safety device is an alternative to physical restraints?
A) Bed alarms
B) Side rails
C) Posey vests
D) Lap belts

Question 150: Which of the following is a priority assessment in assessing potential for harm to self and others?
A) Physical health status
B) Support systems availability
C) Educational background
D) Occupation

ANSWERS WITH DETAILED EXPLANATION (SET 1)

Question 1: Correct Answer: D) Oxybutynin
Rationale: Oxybutynin is an anticholinergic medication commonly used to relieve muscle spasms in patients undergoing rehabilitation. It works by inhibiting the action of acetylcholine, a neurotransmitter responsible for muscle contraction. Oxybutynin helps reduce muscle spasms and excessive sweating by relaxing the smooth muscles. Amitriptyline (option A) is a tricyclic antidepressant commonly used to treat depression but not specifically indicated for antispasmodic effects. Morphine (option B) is an opioid analgesic mainly used for pain relief and is not an anticholinergic agent. Diazepam (option C) is a benzodiazepine primarily used for its sedative and anxiolytic effects and does not possess anticholinergic properties. Hence, the correct answer is option D.
Question 2: Correct Answer: D) Watson's Human Caring Theory

Rationale: Watson's Human Caring Theory emphasizes the importance of establishing a caring relationship between the nurse and patient. It focuses on understanding and valuing the patient's subjective experiences, personal values, beliefs, and goals. As a framework for rehabilitation nursing practice, this model guides nurses to provide holistic care that addresses the physical, emotional, spiritual, and social needs of the patient. By incorporating the patient's personal values, beliefs, and goals into their care, rehabilitation nurses can promote healing, growth, and a sense of well-being in the patient.
Question 3: Correct Answer: B) Promoting independence in activities of daily living
Rationale: Patient-centered care emphasizes the importance of involving the patient in their care and promoting their independence. For Mrs. Johnson, who is experiencing difficulty with mobility, promoting independence in activities of daily living would be of utmost importance. This can include

encouraging her to participate in therapeutic exercises, providing adaptive equipment, and implementing strategies to improve her functional abilities. A) Ensuring medication administration is timely is important but may not be the most important aspect in Mrs. Johnson's case. C) Monitoring vital signs every hour may not be necessary unless there is a specific clinical indication. D) Administering pain medication as needed is important, but promoting independence takes precedence in this scenario.

Question 4: Correct Answer: A) Transformational leadership theory

Rationale: Transformational leadership theory focuses on inspiring and motivating team members to achieve common goals, fostering effective communication, and promoting collaborative teamwork. In the process of transitioning care for Rachel, a transformational leader can inspire team members to provide person-centered care, encourage open communication, and establish a shared vision for optimal patient outcomes. By utilizing transformational leadership theory, the interdisciplinary team can work collaboratively, utilizing their diverse expertise and perspectives to ensure coordinated transitions and seamless continuity of care for Rachel. This theory emphasizes the importance of empowering team members and fostering open communication to achieve patient-centered goals.

Question 5: Correct Answer: B) Vitamin D

Rationale: Vitamin D is essential for the absorption of calcium in the gastrointestinal tract. It helps in the regulation of calcium and phosphate levels in the body, which are important for maintaining healthy bones and teeth. Without sufficient vitamin D, calcium absorption is compromised, leading to conditions like rickets in children and osteoporosis in adults. Vitamin C is important for collagen synthesis and is not directly involved in calcium absorption. Vitamin K plays a role in blood clotting, while vitamin A is important for vision and immune function. Therefore, the correct answer is option B) Vitamin D.

Question 6: Correct Answer: D) Stroke support group

Rationale: Stroke support groups are community resources that provide face-to-face support and information for stroke survivors and their caregivers. These groups often consist of individuals who have experienced similar challenges and can provide a sense of camaraderie, emotional support, and practical guidance. Attending a stroke support group can help Mr. Johnson and his wife connect with others who understand their experiences, learn coping strategies, and access valuable resources. While options A, B, and C may offer other types of services or information, they do not specifically provide face-to-face stroke support groups like option D.

Question 7: Correct Answer: D) The Rehabilitation Nursing Model

Rationale: The Rehabilitation Nursing Model is a patient-centered approach that focuses on integrating physical, social, and psychological aspects of care to help patients achieve their individual goals. It emphasizes the collaborative effort of the healthcare team and the patient in developing a comprehensive rehabilitation plan. The Roy Adaptation Model focuses on the adaptation of individuals to their environment, Orem's Self-Care Deficit Theory emphasizes the importance of meeting patients' self-care needs, and the Neuman Systems Model focuses on the patient's response to stress and the prevention of stressors. None of these models fully capture the holistic and patient-centered approach of the Rehabilitation Nursing Model.

Question 8: Correct Answer: B) Weight gain of 2 pounds in 24 hours

Rationale: An excessive weight gain of 2 pounds in 24 hours indicates possible fluid retention, which can disrupt fluid and electrolyte balance. It is important to monitor weight closely to detect any fluid shifts in patients, especially those with comorbidities like hypertension and diabetes. Bradycardia (Option A) is not directly indicative of fluid imbalance. A sodium level of 142 mEq/L (Option C) falls within the normal range, so it is not a potential risk for fluid imbalance. A urine output of 50 ml/hour (Option D) is slightly low but does not necessarily indicate fluid imbalance on its own. Weight gain is a more reliable indicator in this scenario.

Question 9: Correct Answer: B) Primary nursing model

Rationale: The primary nursing model is a care delivery system in which each patient is assigned a primary nurse who is responsible for coordinating the patient's care. This model promotes continuity of care and ensures that the patient's needs are met by a consistent caregiver. The primary nurse works collaboratively with other members of the healthcare team but maintains overall responsibility for the patient's care. The team nursing model involves a team of healthcare professionals providing care to a group of patients, with each team member having specific roles and responsibilities. The functional nursing model involves dividing responsibilities with different nurses focusing on specific tasks. The case management nursing model focuses on coordinating care across different healthcare settings.

Question 10: Correct Answer: A) Express your concerns about the use of physical restraints and suggest alternative interventions.

Rationale: As a rehabilitation nurse, it is essential to advocate for patients' rights and autonomy. While physical restraints may seem like a viable solution to prevent harm, they should only be used as a last resort. By expressing concerns about the use of physical restraints, the nurse can initiate a discussion with the healthcare team and suggest alternative interventions that promote the patient's safety and well-being. This approach aligns with the ethical principle of beneficence, demonstrating a commitment to the patient's best interests and overall rehabilitation outcome.

Question 11: Correct Answer: B) "Administered pain medication at 2:00 pm."

Rationale: Accurate documentation is essential to support regulatory requirements, ensure continuity of care, and provide evidence for reimbursement. In this scenario, option B is the correct answer as it provides specific information regarding the action taken by the nurse (administering pain medication) at a specific time (2:00 pm). This type of documentation supports accountability, safe medication administration, and adherence to regulatory standards. Options A, C, and D are vague and lack specific details necessary for accurate and comprehensive documentation.

Question 12: Correct Answer: C) Provide Mr. Johnson and his wife with information about financial assistance programs available at the hospital.

Rationale: As a CRRN, it is important to be knowledgeable about financial assistance programs available to patients. Hospitals often have programs in place to assist patients who are unable to afford their medical bills. By providing Mr. Johnson and his wife with information about these programs, you are demonstrating an understanding of the legislative and economic aspects of healthcare management. This approach aligns with the ethical responsibility of advocating for patient's rights and ensuring equitable access to healthcare services. Option A is not the best course of action as it does not consider the financial constraints of the patient. Option B may be a good step, but providing information about financial assistance programs directly aligns with the role of a CRRN. Option D is not necessary at this point as legal advice is not required in this situation.

Question 13: Correct Answer: C) Use a professional medical interpreter to facilitate communication.

Rationale: To optimize communication with culturally diverse patients, it is essential to use qualified interpreters to ensure accurate and effective communication. In this scenario,

Maria's limited English proficiency indicates that using a professional medical interpreter is necessary. Relying on family members may not guarantee accurate translation and may violate patient confidentiality. Using nonverbal gestures or speaking loudly may further confuse or disorient the patient. Additionally, using complex medical jargon may hinder the patient's understanding of her condition. Therefore, option C is the most appropriate action for the CRRN to take in this situation.

Question 14: Correct Answer: C) The Passy Muir valve is designed to assist with respiratory support and speech rehabilitation.

Rationale: The Passy Muir valve is a one-way valve that is used to assist with respiratory support and speech rehabilitation in patients with tracheostomies. It allows for the redirection of airflow through the vocal cords, facilitating the production of speech and improving communication for patients. This valve is not used for urinary or fecal incontinence management or swallowing difficulties. Therefore, option C is the correct answer.

Question 15: Correct Answer: D) National Database of Nursing Quality Indicators (NDNQI)

Rationale: The National Database of Nursing Quality Indicators (NDNQI) is a widely used quality measurement tool in healthcare settings. It allows nurses and healthcare organizations to track and analyze various indicators of patient outcomes, such as falls, pressure ulcers, infections, and staffing levels. By comparing their data to national benchmarks, healthcare providers can identify areas for improvement and develop targeted quality improvement initiatives. NDNQI provides valuable information for evidence-based practice and helps in driving positive changes in nursing care. While Six Sigma, Total Quality Management (TQM), and Lean methodology are also commonly used quality improvement tools, they are more focused on process improvement and may not specifically address patient outcomes and nursing quality indicators like the NDNQI.

Question 16: D) Massaging the patient's bony prominences Correct Answer: A) Providing a high-protein diet to the patient

Rationale: Providing a high-protein diet is an appropriate intervention to prevent pressure ulcers in a patient with a spinal cord injury. A high-protein diet promotes tissue repair and wound healing. Protein is essential for maintaining skin integrity and preventing breakdown. Applying a heating pad, bathing with hot water, and massaging bony prominences can increase the risk of pressure ulcers by causing tissue damage and compromising blood flow. It is important to remember that pressure ulcers are multifactorial, and interventions should focus on reducing pressure, improving nutrition, maintaining skin hygiene, and providing adequate moisture control.

Question 17: Correct Answer: C) Autonomy

Rationale: Autonomy is an ethical principle that emphasizes respect for the individual's right to make decisions regarding their own healthcare. It involves informed consent, shared decision-making, and respecting the choices and values of the individual. Beneficence, on the other hand, refers to the duty to do good and provide benefits to the patient. Nonmaleficence focuses on the duty to do no harm. Veracity pertains to the duty of telling the truth and being honest with patients. While all these principles are important in nursing practice, autonomy specifically addresses the individual's right to make decisions for their own care.

Question 18: Correct Answer: B) Implement diversion techniques, such as providing her with activities or objects to redirect her attention.

Rationale: It is important to implement person-centered care for individuals with dementia like Mrs. Smith, focusing on non-pharmacological approaches. Implementing diversion techniques, such as providing activities or objects that can capture her attention, can redirect her aggression and promote a safer environment for both the staff and the patient. Restraint should only be used as a last resort and only when there is an immediate threat to the patient or others. The use of sedative medication should be minimized due to potentially harmful side effects. Isolating the patient may increase feelings of confusion and distress, potentially worsening her behavior.

Question 19: Correct Answer: A) Active listening

Rationale: Active listening is a valuable communication technique that involves fully concentrating on the speaker, acknowledging their message, and providing verbal and non-verbal feedback. This technique promotes a therapeutic relationship, as it shows genuine interest, empathy, and understanding towards the patient. By actively listening, the nurse can gain a deeper understanding of the patient's concerns, emotions, and needs, thus enhancing the overall quality of communication and collaborative decision-making. Anger management refers to strategies used to control and express anger appropriately, while reflection involves restating and paraphrasing the patient's thoughts and feelings. Clarification is a technique used to ensure understanding by seeking further information. However, active listening encompasses all these aspects and plays a pivotal role in effective communication between the nurse and the patient.

Question 20: Correct Answer: B) Using thickened liquids

Rationale: When a patient has swallowing deficits, using thickened liquids is an appropriate teaching intervention. Thickened liquids help to slow down the rate of fluid intake, making it easier for the patient to swallow safely. Providing a soft diet only may not address the specific swallowing difficulties, and encouraging rapid eating can further exacerbate the problem. It is important to supervise and assist the patient during meals to ensure safe swallowing and prevent aspiration. Therefore, option B is the correct teaching intervention for a patient with swallowing deficits.

Question 21: Correct Answer: C) Acute pain is characterized by the activation of specialized sensory receptors called nociceptors.

Rationale: Acute pain refers to a transient, time-limited uncomfortable sensation that arises suddenly in response to tissue damage or potential harm. It is usually caused by the activation of specialized sensory receptors called nociceptors, which are responsible for detecting noxious stimuli. Acute pain serves as a protective mechanism, alerting the individual to potential or actual tissue damage. It is typically responsive to analgesic medications, such as nonsteroidal anti-inflammatory drugs (NSAIDs) or opioids. Chronic pain, on the other hand, persists for more than 6 months and can have different underlying mechanisms.

Question 22: Correct Answer: B) Collaborating with the patient's family to create a care plan

Rationale: When assessing a patient's functional health patterns, collaborating with the patient's family to create a care plan is an important nursing intervention. The family plays a vital role in the patient's rehabilitation process, and their input can provide valuable insight into the patient's needs and preferences. By involving the family in the care plan, the nurse ensures a holistic approach that promotes the patient's functional ability. Administering pain medication may be necessary, but it is not directly related to the assessment of functional health patterns. Encouraging the patient to remain sedentary may hinder their mobility and functional ability. Limiting the patient's involvement in decision-making processes goes against promoting patient-centered care.

Question 23: Correct Answer: C) Developing an individualized rehabilitation plan for a patient with a spinal cord injury

Rationale: As a rehabilitation nurse, the CRRN has the knowledge and skills to assess the patient's condition, identify their rehabilitation needs, and develop a comprehensive individualized plan to help them achieve their goals. This involves collaborating with the patient, their family, and the interdisciplinary team to create a plan that addresses physical, emotional, and psychosocial aspects of care. Prescribing medication, performing surgeries, and administering anesthesia are tasks typically performed by other healthcare professionals within their respective scopes of practice.

Question 24: Correct Answer: A) To monitor changes in the patient's bowel movements and urinary patterns

Rationale: Assessing a patient's elimination patterns through an elimination diary and history helps to monitor any changes in their bowel movements and urinary patterns. This information is essential in detecting potential issues such as constipation, urinary incontinence, or urinary retention. By closely monitoring and documenting these patterns, healthcare professionals can identify trends or abnormalities, allowing for timely intervention and appropriate treatment. This assessment also assists in identifying potential triggers for bowel and bladder dysfunction, aiding in the development of individualized care plans to optimize the patient's elimination patterns.

Question 25: Correct Answer: B) Assist the patient with transferring and ambulation using a gait belt and appropriate assistive devices.

Rationale: Assisting the patient with transferring and ambulation using a gait belt and appropriate assistive devices is the most appropriate nursing intervention for a patient with impaired proprioception. Impaired proprioception can lead to difficulties with balance and coordination, as well as decreased body awareness. Using a gait belt and assistive devices can provide the patient with the necessary support and stability during transfers and ambulation, reducing the risk of falls and promoting safety. Active range of motion exercises may be more appropriate for patients with limited joint mobility, while relaxation techniques and cognitive retraining programs are not directly related to the patient's impaired proprioception and physical mobility issues.

Question 26: Correct Answer: C) Implementing a daily exercise routine to improve her strength and balance.

Rationale: Implementing a daily exercise routine to improve Maggie's strength and balance is the most appropriate risk mitigation strategy in this scenario. Falls are common among older adults, especially those with poor balance and a history of falls. By implementing a daily exercise routine, Maggie can improve her muscle strength and balance, reducing the risk of falls. Placing a bed alarm or assigning a sitter may be excessive, considering that Maggie is not at a constant risk of falling. Applying nonslip socks alone may not address the underlying risk factors for falls.

Question 27: Correct Answer: C) Glycosylated hemoglobin (HbA1c)

Rationale: The glycosylated hemoglobin (HbA1c) test is used to assess blood glucose levels over a period of time, typically the past 2-3 months. It measures the percentage of hemoglobin that is coated with sugar, providing an average blood sugar level. This test is useful in monitoring long-term blood sugar control in patients with diabetes mellitus. Fasting blood sugar (FBS) measures the glucose level after an overnight fast. Oral glucose tolerance test (OGTT) measures glucose levels after the ingestion of a glucose solution. Random blood sugar (RBS) measures glucose levels at any time, regardless of when the patient last ate.

Question 28: Correct Answer: B) Implementing evidence-based practice to improve patient outcomes

Rationale: Implementing evidence-based practice is a cost-effective strategy as it utilizes research and proven methods to improve patient outcomes. By following evidence-based guidelines, healthcare professionals can ensure the most

effective and efficient use of resources, reducing unnecessary expenses and providing high-quality care. Reducing staffing levels (option A) may result in compromised patient care and increase the risk of adverse events. Increasing the use of expensive equipment and technology (option C) may lead to unnecessary costs without improving patient outcomes. Decreasing the amount of time spent on patient education (option D) can hinder patient understanding, compliance, and overall outcomes. Therefore, option B is the most effective strategy in managing resources cost-effectively.

Question 29: Correct Answer: C) Orem's Self-Care Deficit Model

Rationale: Orem's Self-Care Deficit Model is based on the belief that individuals have the ability to care for themselves but may require assistance in certain circumstances. It emphasizes the importance of self-care and identifies three levels of nursing care required: wholly compensatory, partly compensatory, and supportive-educative. Roy's Adaptation Model focuses on the individual's response to stimuli, Neuman Systems Model looks at the individual's response to stressors, and Levine's Conservation Model focuses on maintaining the individual's integrity and energy. Therefore, the correct answer is C) Orem's Self-Care Deficit Model.

Question 30: Correct Answer: C) Psychologist

Rationale: A psychologist is a healthcare professional who specializes in providing therapy and support for individuals dealing with emotional and psychological issues. They play a crucial role in helping patients and caregivers cope with the emotional challenges that arise during rehabilitation. Psychologists can offer various therapeutic techniques to address anxiety, depression, and other psychological issues and help individuals develop effective coping and stress management skills. Physicians primarily focus on medical treatment, pharmacists are responsible for dispensing medications, and physical therapists focus on physical rehabilitation rather than providing emotional and psychological support. Therefore, the correct option is C) Psychologist.

Question 31: Correct Answer: A) Decreased urine output

Rationale: Decreased urine output is a significant finding that indicates a fluid volume deficit in a patient. This can occur due to inadequate fluid intake, excessive fluid loss (such as through vomiting, diarrhea, or excessive sweating), or fluid shift from the intravascular space to the interstitial space. Decreased urine output is an important assessment finding that should be reported promptly to the healthcare provider as it may indicate dehydration or fluid imbalance. Increased urine output is not consistent with fluid volume deficit. Skin rash and headache may be unrelated to fluid volume status and should be assessed separately.

Question 32: Correct Answer: A) Encourage the client to consume foods and fluids with thickened consistency

Rationale: Dysphagia is a swallowing disorder that may increase the risk of aspiration and malnutrition. The most appropriate intervention for a client with dysphagia is to encourage the client to consume foods and fluids with a thickened consistency. Thickening the consistency of the diet helps control the flow of food and beverages, reducing the risk of aspiration. Providing a regular diet (Option B) or instructing the client to consume small, frequent meals without any restrictions (Option D) may increase the risk of aspiration. Administering a nasogastric tube (Option C) should be considered only when other measures have failed or as a temporary measure while dysphagia management is being planned.

Question 33: Correct Answer: C) Applying pressure-relieving devices to bony prominences

Rationale: Applying pressure-relieving devices to bony prominences is an effective teaching intervention to prevent complications of immobility. Immobility can lead to pressure ulcers due to prolonged pressure on bony areas. By using pressure-relieving devices such as foam padding or cushions, the pressure is redistributed, reducing the risk of skin breakdown. Range of motion exercises, while important for maintaining joint mobility, may not directly address skin integrity or DVT prevention. Although promoting a high-protein diet is essential for overall healing and prevention of complications, it does not directly prevent complications of immobility. Anticoagulant medications are used primarily for DVT prophylaxis in high-risk individuals but do not address skin integrity.

Question 34: Correct Answer: C) Physical therapy techniques.

Rationale: Rehabilitation nursing practice involves providing comprehensive care to patients with physical disabilities and impairments. As part of this role, nurses must possess skills in various areas, including physical therapy techniques. This involves understanding and implementing therapeutic exercises, mobility aids, and positioning techniques to promote functional independence and optimal health outcomes for patients. While knowledge of medical coding and billing, pharmacology, and psychological counseling may be beneficial in certain aspects of rehabilitation nursing, physical therapy techniques are specifically focused on the rehabilitation process and are central to the nurse's role in facilitating patient recovery and rehabilitation.

Question 35: Correct Answer: B) Encouraging active range of motion exercises

Rationale: Encouraging active range of motion exercises is the most appropriate intervention to prevent musculoskeletal complications and promote joint mobility in a patient with limited movement. These exercises help maintain the range of motion, prevent contractures, and preserve muscle strength. Administering medications for pain relief may control pain temporarily but does not address the need for joint mobility. Applying ice packs may provide temporary relief for swelling or acute pain but does not promote joint mobility. Providing complete bed rest can lead to muscle weakness, joint stiffness, and decreased mobility, exacerbating musculoskeletal complications.

Question 36: Correct Answer: D) Relapse into substance abuse.

Rationale: Given the patient's history of substance abuse and the recent car accident, the nurse should consider relapse into substance abuse as the most likely cause for the patient's current behaviors. Anger, frustration, and social withdrawal are common signs of relapse and indicate that the patient may be struggling with their recovery. It is important for the nurse to assess the patient's substance abuse history, provide support and education, and collaborate with the interdisciplinary team to develop a comprehensive care plan that addresses the patient's physical and psychosocial needs.

Question 37:

Correct Answer: C) Participating in a peer review process

Rationale: Participating in a peer review process is an example of integrating quality improvement processes into nursing practice. Peer review involves the evaluation of a nurse's practice by colleagues to ensure the provision of safe and high-quality care. It helps identify areas for improvement, promotes professional development, and contributes to maintaining standards of nursing practice. Attending a seminar on evidence-based practice is important for staying updated with the latest research, but it does not directly involve quality improvement processes. Advocating for patient rights and privacy and documenting patient assessments accurately are essential aspects of nursing practice but not specifically related to integrating quality improvement processes.

Question 38: Correct Answer: B) Falsifying a patient's medical record to cover up a medication error.

Rationale: Falsifying a patient's medical record to cover up a medication error is a serious violation of legal and ethical standards. Nurses are legally and ethically bound to document accurately and honestly. Falsifying medical records can compromise patient safety, undermine trust between the healthcare team and the patient, and lead to legal consequences for the nurse involved. The other options (A, C, and D) are appropriate and align with legal and ethical standards. Documenting medication administration immediately, following facility policies for vital signs, and updating the care plan with current goals and interventions are examples of good documentation practices that reflect professional standards of care.

Question 39: Correct Answer: C) Anger

Rationale: During the stage of anger in the grief and loss process, individuals may experience intense emotions, such as anger, resentment, and frustration. They may direct their anger towards themselves, others, or even the situation itself. This emotional response can be a healthy part of the grieving process, as it allows individuals to express their feelings and work through their pain. It is important for rehabilitation registered nurses to acknowledge and validate these emotions, while providing a supportive and empathetic environment for patients and their families.

Question 40: Correct Answer: C) Ensure proper functioning and calibration of the technology

Rationale: When utilizing technology in rehabilitation nursing, ensuring the proper functioning and calibration of the technology is crucial. This ensures accurate data collection and reliable information for decision-making. Monitoring the patient's vital signs manually (option A) could be time-consuming and may not provide continuous real-time data. Disregarding any technological errors and using other methods (option B) can compromise patient safety and overlook important information. Avoiding the use of technology to minimize patient dependency (option D) overlooks the benefits technology can provide in enhancing patient care and rehabilitation outcomes. Therefore, the correct answer is option C.

Question 41: Correct Answer: A) Central lines are commonly used for long-term medication administration.

Rationale: Central lines are inserted into large veins and are commonly used for long-term medication administration, such as chemotherapy or long-term antibiotic therapy. Ports, on the other hand, are typically surgically implanted under the skin and can be accessed with a needle for medication administration. Catheters, though commonly associated with urine collection, can also be used for other purposes like intravenous fluid administration or drainage of fluids from specific body cavities. It is essential for rehabilitation registered nurses to educate patients and caregivers on the purpose and proper care of these devices to ensure safe and effective use while avoiding complications like infections or dislodgement.

Question 42: Correct Answer: B) To collaborate and coordinate care to achieve optimal patient outcomes.

Rationale: In the rehabilitation process, the primary goal of the interdisciplinary team is to collaborate and coordinate care to achieve optimal patient outcomes. This involves working together with professionals from different disciplines, such as physical therapists, occupational therapists, psychologists, and social workers, to ensure the comprehensive and holistic care of the patient. The team's focus is on maximizing the patient's functional abilities, independence, and overall well-being. Providing palliative care, prescribing medications, or aiming for early discharge may be part of the care plan, but they are not the primary goals of the interdisciplinary team in the rehabilitation process.

Question 43: Correct Answer: B) Psychologist

Rationale: A psychologist is a professional resource that plays a crucial role in assisting rehabilitation patients with emotional and psychological support during their recovery process. They are trained to provide counseling, therapy, and mental health interventions, helping patients cope with the emotional challenges that arise due to their condition or disability. Psychologists work closely with the rehabilitation team to address the psychological aspects of recovery and facilitate the patient's community reintegration or transition to the next level of care. Their expertise is crucial in promoting the patient's overall well-being and mental health during the rehabilitation process. Therefore, option B is the correct answer.

Question 44: Correct Answer: B) Parasympathetic nervous system

Rationale: The parasympathetic nervous system controls the bladder function. It promotes bladder filling by relaxing the detrusor muscle and contracting the internal sphincter to keep the bladder closed. When it's time to empty the bladder, the parasympathetic nervous system stimulates bladder contraction and relaxes the external sphincter to allow urine flow. The sympathetic nervous system plays a role in urinary continence by contracting the internal sphincter, while the central nervous system is involved in coordinating bladder function. The somatic nervous system controls voluntary control over the external sphincter.

Question 45: Correct Answer: A) King's Theory of Goal Attainment

Rationale: King's Theory of Goal Attainment emphasizes the importance of the nurse-patient relationship and the communication and interaction between them to achieve mutually agreed-upon goals. This theory recognizes that both the nurse and the patient have unique perspectives and preferences that should be taken into account when planning and implementing care in the rehabilitation setting. The focus is on the dynamic interpersonal processes that occur during goal setting and attainment, with the aim of promoting optimal health outcomes for the patient. The other options, Rogers' Science of Unitary Human Beings, Neuman's Systems Model, and Orem's Self-Care Deficit Theory, are not specifically focused on the nurse-patient relationship in the same way as King's Theory of Goal Attainment.

Question 46: Correct Answer: B) Providing a quiet and dark sleep environment

Rationale: Providing a quiet and dark sleep environment is essential for promoting sleep in patients. Noise and excessive light can disrupt sleep patterns and hinder restfulness. Sedative medications should be used cautiously in older adults due to their potential adverse effects, such as confusion and falls. Watching television before bedtime can stimulate the brain and make it difficult for the patient to fall asleep. Waking the patient every hour is disruptive and can prevent the patient from getting adequate rest.

Question 47: Correct Answer: A) Providing information on proper bowel and bladder management techniques.

Rationale: When teaching health, wellness, and life skills maintenance to a patient with a spinal cord injury, the CRRN should prioritize providing information on proper bowel and bladder management techniques. This is crucial for maintaining the patient's overall health and preventing complications such as urinary tract infections and constipation. While stress management, mobility improvement, and skin care are also important, addressing bowel and bladder management first ensures the patient's physical well-being and reduces the risk of potential complications.

Question 48: Correct Answer: C) Affordable Care Act (ACA)

Rationale: The Affordable Care Act (ACA) was enacted in 2010 to improve access to healthcare and provide affordable health insurance options for individuals and families. It offers financial assistance programs such as Medicaid expansion and tax credits, especially for individuals with low income and limited resources. The ACA aims to reduce healthcare costs and increase healthcare coverage, making it the appropriate legislation to address the family's concerns about rising medical expenses. The Americans with Disabilities Act (ADA) focuses on prohibiting discrimination based on disability, while the Occupational Safety and Health Act (OSHA) ensures safe and healthy working conditions. The Emergency Medical Treatment and Active Labor Act (EMTALA) mandates that all individuals receive appropriate emergency medical care, regardless of their ability to pay.

Question 49: Correct Answer: D) Flush the tube with water before and after medication administration.

Rationale: When providing nutrition using a nasogastric tube, it is essential to flush the tube with water before and after medication administration. Flushing the tube helps ensure proper medication delivery and prevents clogging. Option A is incorrect as the tube is inserted through the patient's nose, not mouth. Option B is incorrect because listening for air sounds is not the appropriate method to verify tube placement. Option C is incorrect as bolus feeding should not be administered continuously, but rather in intermittent or cyclic feedings as prescribed.

Question 50: Correct Answer: C) Exercise

Rationale: Exercise is a coping strategy that involves engaging in physical activity to manage stress and anxiety. Regular exercise has been shown to have numerous psychological benefits, including the release of endorphins, which help improve mood and reduce stress. Physical activity also promotes relaxation and helps individuals feel more in control of their emotions. While meditation, distraction, and deep breathing are also coping strategies, exercise specifically focuses on the use of physical activity as a tool for stress management and overall well-being.

Question 51: Correct Answer: C) Neurologic assessment

Rationale: As a CRRN, one of the essential skills is the ability to perform a comprehensive neurologic assessment. This includes assessing Mrs. Johnson's level of consciousness, cranial nerve function, motor and sensory function, and coordination. By regularly evaluating her neurologic status, the CRRN can detect any changes or improvements in her condition, which can guide the rehabilitation plan and interventions. Assessing cardiac, wound, and psychosocial aspects are also important, but for optimizing management of a neurological condition, a neurologic assessment takes priority.

Question 52: Correct Answer: D) Maintaining seizure precautions

Rationale: The nurse should prioritize maintaining seizure precautions for Mr. Johnson. Seizure precautions involve providing a safe environment that minimizes the risk of injury during a seizure. This includes padding the side rails of the bed, ensuring the bed is in the lowest position, removing any potential hazards from the patient's environment, and maintaining constant observation. Fall precautions may be necessary for patients at risk of falling due to factors unrelated to seizures. Administering antiepileptic medications is important for seizure control but does not directly address safety concerns. Assessing for impaired judgment is an important aspect of patient care but is not specific to Mr. Johnson's safety in relation to seizures.

Question 53: Correct Answer: A) "The Passy Muir valve will help me speak more clearly."

Rationale: The Passy Muir valve is an adaptive equipment device used for patients with dysphagia. It is not intended to improve balance, memory, or walking ability. Its purpose is to improve speech and communication by allowing air to flow through the vocal cords while blocking the tracheostomy tube. This enables patients to speak more clearly and effectively.

Patients who understand this function of the Passy Muir valve demonstrate a correct understanding of its purpose and potential benefits.

Question 54: Correct Answer: C) Token economy

Rationale: Token economy is a behavioral management technique that involves using tokens or rewards to reinforce positive behaviors. In this technique, individuals are given tokens or points when they exhibit desired behaviors, which can then be exchanged for rewards or privileges. Token economy aims to increase the frequency of positive behaviors by providing immediate reinforcement. This technique is commonly used in rehabilitation settings to promote desirable behaviors and help individuals develop skills to manage their behavior. Other options such as time-out, restraints, and seclusion are not based on positive reinforcement and are usually used as last-resort interventions for managing challenging behaviors.

Question 55: Correct Answer: B) Using non-verbal communication such as gestures and facial expressions.

Rationale: The most effective approach to communication with a patient who has expressive aphasia is to use non-verbal communication techniques such as gestures and facial expressions. This allows the patient to still express their needs and concerns, even if they are unable to speak fluently. Using complex medical terminology may confuse the patient further and hinder effective communication. Ignoring her attempts to communicate can lead to frustration and negatively impact her rehabilitation. Similarly, encouraging her to give up on speaking and relying solely on writing can limit her overall communication abilities. Therefore, option B is the correct answer as it promotes effective communication with Mrs. Taylor.

Question 56: Correct Answer: D) "I frequently isolate myself from family and friends because I don't want them to see me struggling."

Rationale: Isolation and withdrawal from support systems are considered unhealthy coping mechanisms. These behaviors may hinder the patient's ability to effectively manage stress and find emotional support. Options A, B, and C reflect healthy coping strategies such as seeking support from others who have experienced similar situations, engaging in pleasurable activities, and utilizing relaxation techniques to reduce anxiety. It is important for the nurse to identify unhealthy coping mechanisms to provide appropriate interventions and support to promote optimal psychosocial patterns and stress management skills in patients and their caregivers.

Question 57: Correct Answer: B) "You may experience difficulty conceiving, but there are assisted reproductive options available to you if you wish to have children."

Rationale: It is important for the nurse to provide accurate information and reassurance to the patient. Option A is incorrect because while fertility may be affected, it does not guarantee infertility. Option C is incorrect because fertility can be impacted by spinal cord injuries. Option D is incorrect because it may give false hope to the patient. Option B is the most appropriate response as it acknowledges the potential difficulties but offers hope and informs the patient about available assisted reproductive options if she desires to have children in the future.

Question 58: Correct Answer: B) Diagnosis

Rationale: The nursing process consists of five phases: Assessment, Diagnosis, Outcomes Identification, Planning, Implementation, and Evaluation. In the Diagnosis phase, the nurse analyzes the collected data to identify the client's health needs and formulates a nursing diagnosis. This involves identifying actual or potential problems, risks, or strengths based on the assessment data. The nurse uses critical thinking skills and knowledge of nursing models and theories to categorize the client's health problems and develop a nursing care plan. This phase sets the foundation for planning

and implementing appropriate interventions to achieve desired outcomes.

Question 59: Correct Answer: A) Frontal lobe

Rationale: The frontal lobe is responsible for cognitive functions, such as comprehension, problem-solving, decision-making, and communication. Damage to this area can result in difficulties with comprehension and communication, as seen in Mr. Johnson's case. The temporal lobe is primarily involved in auditory processing, the occipital lobe is responsible for visual processing, and the parietal lobe plays a role in integrating sensory information. While these lobes may be affected in certain situations, the symptoms described in the scenario suggest involvement of the frontal lobe.

Question 60: Correct Answer: A) Quad cane

Rationale: A quad cane would be the most appropriate assistive device for Mr. Thompson to improve his balance during walking. Quad canes offer a wider base of support compared to standard canes, providing increased stability and balance. Given the mild left-sided weakness resulting from the stroke, a quad cane would offer the necessary support and prevent falls during ambulation. Wheelchairs, walkers, and crutches are not specifically designed to address balance issues and may not be as effective in Mr. Thompson's case.

Question 61: Correct Answer: A) Consuming caffeine-rich beverages before bedtime.

Rationale: Consuming caffeine-rich beverages, such as coffee or energy drinks, close to bedtime can disrupt sleep as caffeine is a stimulant. It can interfere with falling asleep and staying asleep. Following a consistent sleep routine (option B) and engaging in regular physical exercise (option C) can actually promote better sleep. Having a quiet and dark environment in the bedroom (option D) is also conducive to good sleep hygiene. However, in this scenario, the patient's sleep difficulties may be related to consuming caffeine before bedtime, hence making option A the correct answer.

Question 62: Correct Answer: D) Assessing Mrs. Johnson's ability to perform ADLs.

Rationale: In the assessment phase of the nursing process, the rehabilitation nurse should first assess Mrs. Johnson's ability to perform ADLs. This includes activities such as walking, dressing, and bathing, which are essential for her independence and overall functioning. By assessing her ADL abilities, the nurse can identify her specific needs and determine the appropriate interventions and goals for her rehabilitation plan. Although developing a plan of care is important, it is not the initial step in the assessment phase. Administering medications for pain management and assessing cognitive function are also important aspects of care but may not be the priority in this scenario.

Question 63: Correct Answer: C) Instructing the patient to prioritize tasks and take frequent rest breaks

Rationale: Patients with limited activity tolerance, such as those with chronic fatigue syndrome, require strategies to conserve energy. Prioritizing tasks and taking frequent rest breaks can help prevent excessive fatigue and maintain overall energy levels. Deep breathing exercises may be beneficial for relaxation, but they do not directly address energy conservation. High-intensity aerobic exercises and rigorous physical therapy sessions may exacerbate fatigue and should be avoided in patients with limited activity tolerance. Therefore, option C is the most appropriate intervention to conserve energy for this patient.

Question 64: Correct Answer: A) Encouraging the patient to increase fiber intake and drink plenty of fluids

Rationale: Encouraging the patient to increase fiber intake and drink plenty of fluids promotes regular bowel movements and prevents constipation. Adequate fluid intake helps soften the stool, while fiber adds bulk and promotes peristalsis. Administering a laxative without consulting the healthcare provider is not appropriate as it may have adverse effects or interact with other medications. Limiting fluid intake can lead to dehydration and bladder distention, exacerbating the patient's condition. Prescribing a high-protein diet may be beneficial for muscle strength but does not directly address constipation.

Question 65: Correct Answer: C) Direct the daughter to the facility's medical records department to complete the appropriate paperwork for access.

Rationale: In order to protect patient privacy and ensure compliance with HIPAA regulations, healthcare facilities require individuals to complete the appropriate paperwork to access a patient's medical records. This process helps to verify that the person requesting access has the legal right to do so and protects against unauthorized release of patient information. Providing immediate access or relying solely on verbal permission would violate patient privacy rights and legal obligations. Informing the daughter about the appropriate process for accessing medical records is the correct action to take in this situation.

Question 66: Correct Answer: B) To enhance functional abilities and independence

Rationale: Assistive technology and adaptive equipment play a vital role in rehabilitation nursing by enhancing a patient's functional abilities and promoting independence. These technologies and equipment are designed to assist individuals with disabilities or impairments in performing everyday tasks such as eating, dressing, communication, and mobility. They can include specialized devices like walkers, wheelchairs, communication boards, hearing aids, and computer software. By utilizing these tools, patients can regain or improve their independence, leading to an improved quality of life. While assistive technology may indirectly contribute to improving communication skills, its primary purpose is to enhance independence and functional abilities. Emotional support and medication administration are separate aspects of patient care.

Question 67: Correct Answer: C) Provide education for the patient and family on safety measures, such as installing grab bars in the bathroom.

Rationale: Providing education for the patient and family on safety measures, such as installing grab bars in the bathroom, is a crucial aspect of developing a plan of care for a patient with balance difficulties. This intervention promotes patient-centered care by addressing the patient's specific needs and goals related to safety and independence at home. Encouraging the patient to participate in physical therapy sessions and initiating a home exercise program are important components of the plan, but they do not directly address the patient's safety concerns. Requesting a consultation with a psychologist may be beneficial for addressing emotional well-being, but it is not the most appropriate action to include in the plan of care for this particular scenario.

Question 68: Correct Answer: C) The patient and healthcare provider collaborate in decision-making based on the patient's values and goals.

Rationale: Patient-centered care in rehabilitation nursing emphasizes the partnership between the healthcare provider and the patient. It recognizes the importance of incorporating the patient's preferences, values, and goals into the decision-making process. This approach fosters a collaborative relationship where the patient actively participates in the development of their individualized care plan. By involving the patient in decision-making, healthcare providers can ensure that the care provided aligns with the patient's unique needs and promotes their overall well-being during the rehabilitation process. This patient-centered approach enhances communication, trust, and shared decision-making between the healthcare team and the patient, ultimately leading to improved outcomes and patient satisfaction.

Question 69: Correct Answer: B) Coping theory

Rationale: In this scenario, the nurse is using the coping theory. Coping theory focuses on helping individuals develop effective strategies to manage stressful situations, such as the emotional challenges that can arise after a stroke. By providing emotional support and encouraging expression of feelings and concerns, the nurse is assisting the patient in coping with her current situation. Developmental theory focuses on the stages of human development, stress theory explores the impact of stress on individuals, and self-esteem theory examines individuals' perception of their self-worth, which are not the primary concepts being addressed in this scenario.

Question 70: Correct Answer: A) Adequate fluid intake

Rationale: Adequate fluid intake is a non-pharmacological intervention that can help optimize a patient's elimination patterns. Fluids help in softening the stool and preventing constipation. It is important to encourage patients to drink an adequate amount of fluids, especially water, to promote regular bowel movements and prevent complications related to constipation. Administration of laxatives (Option B) would be a pharmacological intervention, which may be considered when non-pharmacological measures are ineffective. Physical restraints (Option C) and sedative medications (Option D) are not appropriate interventions for optimizing elimination patterns and may actually contribute to the problem.

Question 71: Correct Answer: A) Prospective Payment System (PPS)

Rationale: Medicare uses the Prospective Payment System (PPS) for reimbursement of inpatient rehabilitation facilities (IRFs). Under this system, IRFs are paid based on a predetermined rate that takes into account the patient's diagnosis and characteristics, rather than reimbursing based on the actual costs incurred. The PPS encourages cost-effective care and supports the delivery of patient-centered services by focusing on the patient's needs and functional outcomes. The Fee-for-Service (FFS) system is a traditional payment model that reimburses providers based on the services rendered. The Diagnosis-Related Group (DRG) system is used by Medicare for reimbursement of acute care hospitals. Capitation is a payment model in which providers receive a fixed amount per patient enrolled, regardless of the services provided.

Question 72: Correct Answer: C) Implementing intermittent self-catheterization to ensure complete bladder emptying.

Rationale: For a patient with incomplete bladder emptying due to a neurogenic bladder, intermittent self-catheterization is the most appropriate intervention. This technique allows the patient to manually empty the bladder at regular intervals, ensuring complete emptying and preventing urinary retention. Encouraging the patient to wait for the urge to void may not be effective in cases of neurogenic bladder dysfunction. Anticholinergic medications are commonly used to treat overactive bladder, not incomplete bladder emptying. Timed voiding may be more suitable for patients with bladder control issues related to cognitive impairment or functional limitations.

Question 73: Correct Answer: B) Advocating for patient rights and informed consent

Rationale: A CRRN should have the skill to advocate for patient rights and ensure informed consent is obtained. This skill is crucial in upholding the ethical principles and legal requirements involved in patient care. Advocacy includes protecting patients' rights, promoting autonomous decision-making, and ensuring patients are well-informed about their treatment options. By advocating for patient rights and informed consent, CRRNs contribute to an environment that respects patients' autonomy and fosters a culture of shared decision-making between the healthcare team and patients. This skill is vital in navigating the complex legislative, economic, ethical, and legal issues within rehabilitation nursing practice.

Question 74: Correct Answer: B) Assess the patient's ability to perform activities of daily living (ADLs) independently.

Rationale: Before discharging a patient from rehabilitation, it is crucial to assess their ability to perform ADLs independently. This assessment helps determine if the patient can safely manage their self-care needs at home. By evaluating their ability to perform tasks such as bathing, dressing, and toileting without assistance, the rehabilitation nurse can ensure that the patient will be able to function well after discharge. Providing comprehensive written discharge instructions (option A) is important, but assessing ADL independence takes priority. Consultation with a physical therapist regarding mobility aids (option C) may be necessary, but it is not the immediate step to be taken. While a follow-up appointment with the orthopedic surgeon (option D) is important, it does not directly address the patient's readiness for discharge.

Question 75: Correct Answer: B) Demonstrate techniques for compensatory head movements to improve visual field.

Rationale: Optic neuritis, a common symptom of MS, can lead to visual disturbances and decreased visual field. Teaching Ms. Smith compensatory head movements will allow her to optimize her visual field by using eye movements and head turns. It is a practical and effective strategy to enhance her visual perception and functional abilities. Providing written material on eye examinations, discussing nutrition and hydration, and encouraging support group participation are valuable interventions but focus on different aspects of visual health and MS management.

Question 76: Correct Answer: C) Spiritual practices

Rationale: Spiritual practices, such as healing touch, involve the use of touch to promote relaxation and pain relief in patients. It is a traditional modality that recognizes the connection between the mind, body, and spirit. By incorporating healing touch into care, the nurse can provide a non-pharmacological approach to addressing patients' needs. This modality can help patients reduce stress, enhance their well-being, and improve their overall quality of life. While botanicals, medications, and mindfulness are also important aspects of traditional and alternative modalities, they do not specifically focus on healing touch like spiritual practices do.

Question 77: Correct Answer: A) The combination of antispasmodics and anticholinergics can lead to increased sedation and confusion.

Rationale: Antispasmodic medications work by reducing muscle spasms and promoting muscle relaxation. Anticholinergic medications, on the other hand, block the effects of acetylcholine, a neurotransmitter. When combined, these medications can have an additive effect on the central nervous system, leading to increased sedation and confusion. It is important for the healthcare provider to carefully monitor the patient for potential adverse effects and adjust the medication regimen accordingly. In this case, the combination of antispasmodics and anticholinergics can potentially increase the sedation and confusion experienced by the patient.

Question 78: Correct Answer: A) Understanding the ethical principles and standards that guide nursing practice.

Rationale: A Certified Rehabilitation Registered Nurse (CRRN) must have a profound understanding of the ethical principles and standards that shape nursing practice. This knowledge enables them to provide patient-centered care while respecting autonomy, justice, veracity, and beneficence. Ethical decision-making involving patients, families, and interdisciplinary teams is a crucial responsibility of a CRRN. Although knowledge of economic principles, advocacy, and legal obligations are important for a comprehensive nursing

practice, they are not the primary focus of the 'Skill in:' under the given topic.

Question 79: Correct Answer: D) Offer Katherine small, frequent meals throughout the day

Rationale: Following a spinal cord injury, patients may experience decreased appetite, altered swallowing function, and impaired mobility. Offering Katherine small, frequent meals throughout the day is the most appropriate intervention as it promotes adequate nutrition and minimizes the risk of aspiration. A high-calorie, high-protein diet (Option A) may be necessary for some patients, but it is important to assess Katherine's specific nutritional needs before implementing this intervention. Encouraging Katherine to drink at least 2 liters of water daily (Option B) is essential for hydration, but it does not address her nutritional needs directly. Eating meals while lying in a supine position (Option C) increases the risk of aspiration and should be avoided.

Question 80: Correct Answer: C) "I will handle all the decision-making for my mother to reduce her stress."

Rationale: Teaching self-advocacy skills to patients and caregivers is an essential aspect of rehabilitation nursing. Encouraging patients and their families to actively participate in decision-making, communicate preferences and concerns, ask questions, and express opinions about care promotes a patient-centered approach and empowers patients to become active participants in their own care. However, in this scenario, the daughter's statement suggesting that she will handle all the decision-making for her mother indicates a need for further teaching. It is important to educate the family about the importance of involving the patient in decision-making and promoting independence and autonomy.

Question 81: Correct Answer: D) Standardized assessment tools improve the accuracy and consistency of data collection for effective patient care planning.

Rationale: Standardized assessment tools play a crucial role in rehabilitation nursing practice by enhancing the accuracy and consistency of data collection. These tools provide objective information about the patient's condition, promoting evidence-based decision making and improving patient care planning. By using standardized assessment tools, healthcare professionals can gather reliable data that can be compared over time, across settings, and among different populations. This allows for better evaluation of patient progress and outcomes. Additionally, standardized assessment tools facilitate interprofessional collaboration by providing a common language for communication and documentation among healthcare team members. Therefore, option D is the correct answer.

Question 82: Correct Answer: B) Sarah shares Mr. Roberts' progress and updates with the team during weekly team meetings.

Rationale: Effective collaboration and communication among the interdisciplinary team members are crucial for achieving patient-centered goals. By sharing Mr. Roberts' progress and updates during team meetings, Sarah ensures that all team members are informed and can contribute their expertise to his care. This allows the team to assess the effectiveness of the current plan, make necessary modifications, and set new goals if needed. Collaboration and sharing of information foster a holistic and patient-centered approach to care, ensuring that all team members are working together towards the same objectives.

Question 83: Correct Answer: C) Encouraging the patient to perform regular hand hygiene.

Rationale: Regular hand hygiene is considered one of the most effective infection control practices. It helps to decrease the transmission of microorganisms between the patient, healthcare providers, and the environment. It is important to educate patients, especially those with limited mobility, about the importance of proper hand hygiene techniques and provide them with the necessary supplies. Isolating the patient in a private room may not be warranted unless they have a specific infection that requires isolation precautions. Prophylactic antibiotics should only be used when clinically indicated to prevent infection. Wearing masks and gloves when interacting with the patient is important for healthcare providers but does not directly minimize the risk of infection for the patient.

Question 84: Correct Answer: B) Home healthcare services
Rationale: At this stage, Mrs. Johnson has made substantial progress in her recovery, but still requires some assistance with activities of daily living and ongoing therapy. Home healthcare services would provide her with personalized care in the comfort of her own home, allowing her to continue working towards her rehabilitation goals while receiving assistance with any remaining functional limitations. Assisted living facilities are typically suited for individuals who require minimal assistance, while skilled nursing facilities are more appropriate for patients with complex medical needs. Outpatient rehabilitation may be considered if Mrs. Johnson is able to travel to a facility for therapy sessions but may not provide comprehensive care comparable to home healthcare services.

Question 85: Correct Answer: C) Rehabilitation Acts
Rationale: The Rehabilitation Acts, including the Rehabilitation Act of 1973 and the Americans with Disabilities Act (ADA), ensure equal access to employment opportunities for individuals with disabilities. These acts prohibit discrimination against qualified individuals with disabilities and require employers to provide reasonable accommodations to enable individuals with disabilities to perform their job duties. The Rehabilitation Acts also require federally-funded programs and activities to be accessible to individuals with disabilities. Medicare and Medicaid are health insurance programs providing medical coverage for eligible individuals. HIPAA (Health Insurance Portability and Accountability Act) focuses on safeguarding the privacy and security of individuals' health information. Therefore, the correct answer is C) Rehabilitation Acts.

Question 86: Correct Answer: B) Berg Balance Scale
Rationale: The Berg Balance Scale is a standardized assessment tool used to evaluate a patient's functional mobility and risk of falls. It consists of 14 tasks that assess the patient's ability to maintain balance during various activities. As Mr. Johnson has had a stroke and is likely to have impaired mobility and balance, the Berg Balance Scale would be an appropriate tool to assess his functional abilities. The Mini-Mental State Examination (MMSE) is used to assess cognitive function, the Confusion Assessment Method (CAM) is used to detect delirium in older adults, and the Glasgow Coma Scale (GCS) is used to assess the level of consciousness in patients with acute brain injuries. These tools are not specifically designed to assess mobility and activities of daily living (ADLs).

Question 87: Correct Answer: A) Encouraging Ms. Anderson to set achievable goals for her rehabilitation process.
Rationale: Supporting self-efficacy and self-concept is essential for patients like Ms. Anderson who are struggling with feelings of low self-esteem and dependency. Encouraging her to set achievable goals for her rehabilitation process will enhance her sense of control and competence. By setting small and attainable goals, Ms. Anderson will experience successful outcomes, thereby improving her self-efficacy. This, in turn, will positively influence her self-concept and overall psychological well-being. It is crucial for the nurse to provide emotional support and facilitate empowerment through goal setting to promote self-efficacy and self-concept in patients undergoing rehabilitation.

Question 88: Correct Answer: A) Providing an interpreter to assist in communicating with Sarah.
Rationale: Option A is the correct answer because it demonstrates cultural competence and promotes effective communication. As a CRRN, it is important to recognize and respect cultural diversity, including language barriers. By providing an interpreter, the nurse ensures clear and accurate communication between Sarah and the healthcare team, improving the patient's safety and satisfaction. Relying solely on non-verbal communication (Option B) may lead to misunderstanding or misinterpretation of Sarah's needs. Asking Sarah to bring a family member to translate (Option C) assumes that she has a family member who is available and proficient in both languages, which may not be the case. Assuming Sarah can understand English without any assistance (Option D) disregards her individual needs and inhibits effective communication.

Question 89: Correct Answer: A) A smart home system
Rationale: A smart home system would be the most appropriate device to recommend to Rachel as it can assist her in various daily activities. Smart home systems are integrated networks of devices and appliances that can be controlled remotely, providing convenience and independence for individuals with disabilities. These systems can include voice-activated controls for lighting, heating, and other household tasks, as well as home security features. This technology can greatly enhance Rachel's ability to manage her daily activities and maintain her independence, making it the optimal option for her. Wearable fitness trackers, personal response devices, and telehealth monitoring systems do not directly address Rachel's needs in the same way a smart home system does.

Question 90: Correct Answer: B) "I will make sure to do the exercises at least three times a day."
Rationale: Performing passive range of motion exercises three times a day may increase the risk of fatigue and overexertion, which can lead to further impairments. The recommended frequency for passive range of motion exercises is two to three times a day, with proper rest intervals in between. It is important to educate the patient on the appropriate frequency and limitations to prevent complications and promote optimal recovery.

Question 91: Correct Answer: C) When the patient's psychosocial needs are not being addressed adequately
Rationale: As a CRRN, it is essential to identify and address the psychosocial needs of patients. If the patient's psychosocial needs are not being adequately met, it may be necessary to facilitate a referral to a mental health professional. This referral can help ensure that the patient receives appropriate support and interventions to address any underlying mental health concerns. Options A and B are partial answers because they only address specific signs or symptoms, while option D is more patient-driven and may not capture all instances of referral necessity. Option C, however, encompasses the overall criterion for facilitating a referral when the patient's psychosocial needs are not adequately met.

Question 92: Correct Answer: C) Baclofen
Rationale: Baclofen, a centrally acting skeletal muscle relaxant, is commonly used in the management of muscle spasms associated with MS. It acts by enhancing the inhibitory neurotransmitter gamma-aminobutyric acid (GABA) in the central nervous system, leading to decreased muscle spasticity. Amantadine is primarily used in the management of Parkinson's disease and influenza, while Gabapentin is an antiepileptic drug used for neuropathic pain and seizures. Sertraline is an antidepressant medication used in the treatment of major depressive disorder and anxiety disorders, but it does not have direct antispasmodic effects.

Question 93: Correct Answer: D) Assessing urinary and bowel functions

Rationale: Assessing urinary and bowel functions is a crucial skill for a CRRN in optimizing the patient's elimination patterns. By regularly assessing these functions, the nurse can identify any abnormalities or issues, such as urinary or bowel incontinence, constipation, or urinary retention. Assessments may include observing the patient's voiding and bowel habits, checking for signs of infections or obstructions, and reviewing medication and dietary factors that may affect elimination. These assessments enable the nurse to develop appropriate interventions, such as implementing a bladder or bowel training program, providing medications, or recommending dietary modifications. Overall, assessing urinary and bowel functions plays a vital role in maintaining the patient's optimal elimination patterns and promoting their overall well-being.

Question 94: Correct Answer: B) Teach her relaxation techniques such as deep breathing and guided imagery.

Rationale: Teaching Ms. Anderson relaxation techniques such as deep breathing and guided imagery can help her manage her pain effectively. These techniques promote relaxation and reduce stress, which can help alleviate pain. Encouraging excessive use of painkillers (option A) is not recommended as it may lead to dependence and potential side effects. Advising Ms. Anderson to avoid physical activity (option C) would hinder her recovery and may lead to complications. Engaging in high-intensity exercises (option D) is not appropriate during the rehabilitation phase and may increase the risk of injury. Therefore, teaching relaxation techniques is the most suitable intervention to address Ms. Anderson's concerns.

Question 95: Correct Answer: B) Recognize the severity of the statement and initiate suicide precautions.

Rationale: The statement made by Mr. Anderson expressing feelings of hopelessness and questioning the point of living indicates a potential risk for self-harm. As a nurse, it is essential to take all signs of suicidal ideation seriously. Initiating suicide precautions, such as removing potentially harmful objects from the patient's environment, closely monitoring the patient, and involving the mental health team, is necessary to ensure the safety and well-being of the patient.

Question 96: Correct Answer: A) Prioritizing the patient's autonomy and self-determination.

Rationale: When advocating for a patient, it is crucial for the nurse to prioritize the patient's autonomy and self-determination. This means respecting the patient's right to make decisions about their own healthcare and ensuring that their preferences and concerns are heard and respected. The nurse should not impose their own personal beliefs and values upon the patient. Additionally, they should not blindly follow the recommendations of the healthcare team without considering the patient's individual needs and wishes. Ignoring the patient's concerns and preferences goes against the principles of advocacy and person-centered care. By prioritizing the patient's autonomy and self-determination, the nurse promotes patient-centered care and upholds the patient's rights.

Question 97: Correct Answer: C) Nurse Jane reviews the clinical practice guidelines and adapts them to fit the patient's unique needs.

Rationale: The correct use of clinical practice guidelines involves reviewing and considering the recommendations outlined in the guidelines, but also taking into account the unique needs and preferences of the patient. Adapting the guidelines to fit the individual patient's situation is important for providing patient-centered care. Consulting the patient's family (option A) is important for involving them in the care but does not directly address the use of guidelines. Ignoring the guidelines (option B) ignores evidence-based practice. Strictly

following the guidelines without any adaptation (option D) may not fully address the patient's individual needs. Therefore, option C is the correct answer.

Question 98: Correct Answer: D) Pain

Rationale: Pain is a significant factor that can affect sleep and rest patterns. Mr. Johnson, being a patient with a spinal cord injury, is likely to experience pain, which can interfere with his ability to fall asleep and stay asleep. Pain may also cause frequent awakenings during the night, further disrupting his sleep. It is crucial for the nurse to assess and manage Mr. Johnson's pain effectively to promote restful sleep. While diet, sleep habits, and alcohol can influence sleep, in this scenario, pain is the most relevant factor considering Mr. Johnson's condition.

Question 99: Correct Answer: C) Conduct a family meeting to discuss the goals and expectations of the rehabilitation process.

Rationale: Involving the patient and caregiver in the plan of care is essential for effective rehabilitation. Conducting a family meeting allows for open communication between the healthcare team, patient, and caregiver. This meeting provides an opportunity to discuss the goals, expectations, and preferences of the rehabilitation process, ensuring that the plan of care is patient-centered and addresses the specific needs of Mrs. Thompson. Providing written educational materials (option A) is important but does not actively involve the patient and caregiver in decision-making. Assigning a nursing assistant (option B) may meet physical needs but does not address the need for involvement and collaboration. Restricting visitation hours (option D) may inhibit communication and support from the caregiver, leading to decreased patient and caregiver participation in the plan of care.

Question 100: Correct Answer: A) Utilizing the ethical decision-making framework

Rationale: When faced with an ethical dilemma, the nurse can implement the strategy of utilizing the ethical decision-making framework. This involves collaborating with the interprofessional team and considering their perspectives. By involving the team in the decision-making process, the nurse can gain a diverse range of insights and ensure that all relevant perspectives are taken into account. Seeking guidance from a supervisor or manager (option B) may be helpful, but it does not specifically address collaboration with the interprofessional team. Seeking legal advice (option C) may be necessary in some instances, but it does not focus on interprofessional collaboration. Seeking input from the patient's family (option D) is important, but it does not specifically address collaborating with the interprofessional team. Therefore, the correct option is A.

Question 101: Correct Answer: C) Cognitive theory

Rationale: Cognitive theory, proposed by Jean Piaget, focuses on the understanding and development of an individual's thought processes, including perception, memory, problem-solving, and decision-making. It emphasizes that individuals actively construct knowledge through their experiences and interactions with the environment. This theory highlights the importance of mental processes in understanding human behavior and how individuals acquire and use information. On the other hand, psychosocial theory (A) emphasizes the influence of social interactions on an individual's psychological development, behavioral theory (B) focuses on observable behaviors and the concept of conditioning, and moral theory (D) addresses the development of ethical reasoning and decision-making abilities.

Question 102: Correct Answer: A) Aggressive behavior

Rationale: A safety concern regarding harm to self and others in patients with psychosocial disorders is aggressive behavior. Patients may exhibit physical or verbal aggression towards themselves or others, putting everyone's safety at risk. It is important for rehabilitation nurses to identify triggers and implement appropriate interventions such as de-escalation techniques, therapeutic communication, and environment modifications to ensure the safety of all individuals involved. Aggressive behavior can lead to physical harm, emotional distress, and hinder the patients' overall rehabilitation progress. By addressing and managing aggressive behavior, nurses can create a safe and therapeutic environment for both the patients and the healthcare team.

Question 103: Correct Answer: A) Administering a self-report sleep diary

Rationale: Administering a self-report sleep diary is the most appropriate method to evaluate the effectiveness of sleep and rest interventions for Mrs. Johnson. This method allows the patient to report their sleep patterns, subjective experiences, and any disturbances or improvements in sleep quality accurately. It provides valuable insights into the patient's perspective and enables healthcare professionals to assess changes in sleep patterns over time. Monitoring vital signs during sleep, conducting a subjective interview, or observing sleep behavior through video surveillance may provide supplementary information but cannot capture Mrs. Johnson's personal experiences and perceptions regarding her sleep and rest.

Question 104: Correct Answer: C) Theta waves

Rationale: During NREM (Non-Rapid Eye Movement) sleep, the brain exhibits predominantly Theta waves. These waves are slower in frequency and higher in amplitude compared to the Alpha waves present in wakefulness and relaxation. Beta waves are characteristic of active waking state, while Gamma waves are associated with intense cognitive activity. Theta waves are commonly seen during early stages of sleep and are indicative of the transition from wakefulness to deeper sleep. The knowledge of different brain wave patterns during sleep stages is essential for understanding the physiology of sleep and diagnosing sleep disorders.

Question 105: Correct Answer: A) Ability to navigate and comply with legislative requirements

Rationale: As a Certified Rehabilitation Registered Nurse (CRRN), it is crucial to have the ability to navigate and comply with legislative requirements. This skill ensures that the nurse is knowledgeable about the laws and regulations that govern the healthcare industry and can work within those guidelines to promote a safe environment of care. By understanding and adhering to legislative requirements, CRRNs can not only protect the rights of patients but also minimize risks for both patients and staff. This skill includes staying up to date with changes in legislation, such as patient privacy laws, and implementing proper protocols to comply with them. Overall, this skill is essential in creating a safe and compliant healthcare environment.

Question 106: Correct Answer: A) Gait belt

Rationale: The nurse should prioritize the use of a gait belt when assisting a patient with bed mobility and transferring to a wheelchair. A gait belt is a safety device that is placed around the patient's waist to provide a secure grip and support during these activities. It helps to maintain the patient's safety and reduces the risk of falls or injuries. A transfer board is used for lateral transfers between surfaces, such as from a bed to a wheelchair, but it may not provide sufficient support for a patient with limited mobility. A Hoyer lift is typically used for patients with significant mobility limitations or weight-bearing restrictions. A knee immobilizer is not appropriate for assisting with bed mobility or transfers.

Question 107: Correct Answer: B) The Self-Care Deficit Theory

Rationale: The Self-Care Deficit Theory, developed by Dorothea Orem, is most applicable in Sarah's case. This theory emphasizes the importance of identifying the patient's self-care needs and assisting them in meeting those needs. After a spinal cord injury, individuals often experience limitations in their ability to perform self-care activities. By applying the Self-Care Deficit Theory, the nurse can assess Sarah's self-care abilities and provide interventions to promote independence and enhance her self-care skills. This theory is particularly significant in rehabilitation nursing, as it guides nurses in facilitating the patient's transition from dependent care to self-care.

Question 108: Correct Answer: A) Continuous assessment and evaluation of outcomes

Rationale: Continuous assessment and evaluation of outcomes is an essential component of quality improvement processes in nursing practice. By regularly monitoring and analyzing outcomes, nurses can identify areas for improvement and implement necessary changes to enhance patient care. This process involves the systematic collection of data, the identification of trends or patterns, and the development of strategies to address any identified gaps or concerns. Assigning blame to individuals for errors is counterproductive and does not promote a culture of learning and improvement. Ignoring feedback from patients and colleagues can lead to missed opportunities for enhancing quality of care. Lastly, following outdated evidence-based guidelines may not reflect current best practices, therefore hindering the improvement process.

Question 109: Correct Answer: B) Coping involves using adaptive strategies to effectively deal with stressors.

Rationale: Coping refers to the cognitive and behavioral efforts made to manage the demands of stressors. It is an adaptive process that involves using various strategies to effectively deal with stressful situations. Coping strategies can be problem-focused (e.g., problem-solving, seeking social support) or emotion-focused (e.g., relaxation techniques, positive reframing). Coping is not about completely eliminating stress or avoiding all stressors but rather developing skills to manage stress effectively. Using adaptive strategies helps individuals to maintain psychological well-being and minimize the negative impact of stress on their health.

Question 110: Correct Answer: C) Managing his medication

Rationale: Instrumental activities of daily living (IADL) refer to more complex tasks that are necessary for independent living. These activities include managing finances, shopping, cooking, housekeeping, and managing medication. In this scenario, managing the medication is an IADL because it requires cognitive skills and the ability to follow a medication regimen. Dressing, bathing, and feeding oneself are examples of activities of daily living (ADL), which are basic self-care tasks.

Question 111: Correct Answer: A) The Rancho Los Amigos Scale assesses the patient's level of consciousness and cognitive function.

Rationale: The Rancho Los Amigos Scale is a measurement tool commonly used in rehabilitation settings to assess and document the cognitive functions of patients with acquired brain injuries. It consists of eight levels, ranging from the lowest level of complete unawareness to the highest level of purposeful and appropriate behavior. Each level describes the patient's level of consciousness, cognitive abilities, and behavior patterns. By using this scale, healthcare professionals can monitor the progress and recovery of patients with brain injuries and tailor their treatment plans accordingly. Therefore, option A is the correct answer as it accurately describes the purpose of the Rancho Los Amigos Scale.

Question 112: Correct Answer: B) Rehabilitation emphasizes the achievement of optimal physical functioning.

Rationale: Rehabilitation is a holistic approach that aims to enhance the overall well-being and functional independence of individuals with disabilities or impairments. The primary goal of rehabilitation is to help patients achieve their highest possible level of physical, psychological, and social functioning. While addressing the underlying condition is important, rehabilitation focuses on optimizing physical functionality through a multidisciplinary approach involving therapies, assistive devices, and patient-centered goals. It is not solely focused on curing the medical condition or eliminating pain, although pain management may be a part of the rehabilitation process.

Question 113: Correct Answer: D) The Commission on Accreditation of Rehabilitation Facilities (CARF)

Rationale: The Commission on Accreditation of Rehabilitation Facilities (CARF) is an independent, nonprofit organization that accredits a wide range of rehabilitation facilities. CARF sets standards and evaluates rehabilitation programs and services to ensure they meet or exceed quality benchmarks. This accreditation is important as it demonstrates that a facility has met certain criteria and is committed to providing high-quality care. The other options listed, including the American Nurses Association (ANA), the Centers for Medicare and Medicaid Services (CMS), and the National Council of State Boards of Nursing (NCSBN), are not responsible for accrediting rehabilitation facilities.

Question 114: Correct Answer: B) Decreased energy

Rationale: Substance abuse often leads to decreased energy levels. Individuals who abuse substances may experience fatigue, lack of motivation, and decreased ability to concentrate. This symptom is commonly seen in various substance use disorders, such as alcohol or drug abuse. It is important for rehabilitation nurses to be aware of these symptoms to provide appropriate care and interventions for individuals with substance abuse disorders.

Question 115: Correct Answer: C) Cerebellum

Rationale: The cerebellum is responsible for coordinating voluntary movement, balance, and posture. When this area of the brain is affected, patients often experience difficulties with motor skills and coordination, as seen in this patient. The medulla oblongata controls vital functions like breathing and heart rate, while the pons is involved in relaying information between the cerebrum and cerebellum. The frontal lobe is responsible for cognition, judgment, and decision-making. In this scenario, the intact cognition, judgment, sensation, and perception indicate that the frontal lobe is not affected, pointing towards a cerebellar lesion as the most likely location of the patient's impairment.

Question 116: Correct Answer: D) Patient's physical limitations

Rationale: When assessing safety risks for patients, the certified rehabilitation registered nurse should prioritize the patient's physical limitations. This includes evaluating the patient's mobility, balance, strength, and coordination. By understanding the patient's physical abilities and limitations, the nurse can identify potential hazards or barriers to their safety, such as the need for assistive devices, modifications to the environment, or patient-specific precautions. Assessment of socioeconomic background, religious beliefs, and cultural practices are important but may be secondary considerations unless directly impacting the patient's physical safety. The primary focus is on identifying and addressing the physical risks to promote a safe environment of care.

Question 117: Correct Answer: C) Orem's Self-Care Deficit Theory

Rationale: Orem's Self-Care Deficit Theory focuses on the patient's ability to perform self-care activities and the nurse's role in assisting with this care. In the case of Maria, who has a brain injury, she may have limitations in performing certain self-care activities. Orem's theory can guide the CRRN in assessing Maria's self-care deficits, setting goals, and planning interventions to promote her independence in self-care. Maslow's Hierarchy of Needs is a broader theory that can be applicable in various settings but may not specifically address the self-care deficits of an individual patient. The Health Belief Model and Swanson's Theory of Caring may have some relevance but are not as directly applicable to this scenario as Orem's Self-Care Deficit Theory.

Question 118: Correct Answer: A) A reacher

Rationale: A reacher is an instrumental adaptive equipment that helps individuals with limited upper body mobility to grasp and retrieve objects. It is useful for performing self-care tasks such as picking up items from the floor, reaching for objects on higher shelves, or dressing independently. While a walker, weighted pen, and shower chair may be beneficial in other situations, they are not specifically designed to address limited upper body mobility for self-care tasks. Therefore, option A is the most appropriate choice for this scenario.

Question 119: Correct Answer: D) Pharynx

Rationale: The pharynx is responsible for the propulsion of food into the esophagus during swallowing. It is located behind the nasal cavity, mouth, and larynx. The epiglottis is a flap of cartilage that prevents food from entering the airway by covering the opening of the larynx. The uvula is a small hanging structure at the back of the throat that plays a role in closing off the nasal passage during swallowing. While the esophagus is the tube that carries food from the pharynx to the stomach, it does not actively push the food during swallowing.

Question 120:

Correct Answer: A) Physical stressor

Rationale: Mr. Smith's accident and resulting paralysis has resulted in physical changes and challenges. The loss of mobility and independence can be extremely stressful for individuals and can have a significant impact on their overall well-being. Physical stressors refer to any physical demands or changes that can cause stress on the body. In this case, Mr. Smith's paralysis represents a physical stressor as it affects his physical abilities and requires him to adapt to new physical limitations. While psychological, emotional, and social stressors may also be present, physical stressors are the primary focus in this scenario.

Question 121: Correct Answer: D) Rehabilitation nurse

Rationale: The rehabilitation nurse plays a pivotal role in coordinating the patient's care within the interdisciplinary team. They ensure that all interventions are implemented effectively, promoting patient-centered goals. The rehabilitation nurse collaborates with other team members and closely monitors the patient's progress, adjusting the care plan as needed. This includes coordinating with physical therapists, speech-language pathologists, and occupational therapists to provide comprehensive and coordinated care. With their specialized knowledge and expertise, rehabilitation nurses ensure that all aspects of the patient's rehabilitation are addressed and that the goals of the interdisciplinary team are met.

Question 122: Correct Answer: C) The patient and the interdisciplinary team collaborate to modify the goals based on the patient's progress and preferences.

Rationale: In patient-centered care, the patient's preferences and progress play a significant role in the goal-setting process. The collaboration between the patient and the interdisciplinary team ensures that the goals are realistic, relevant, and tailored to the patient's individual needs. It promotes shared decision-making and empowers the patient in their rehabilitation journey. Options A, B, and D all involve making goal adjustments without the necessary collaboration between the patient and the interdisciplinary team, which contradicts the principles of patient-centered care.

Question 123: Correct Answer: A) To evaluate the quality and appropriateness of patient care

Rationale: Utilization review processes in rehabilitation nursing are designed to assess and monitor the quality and appropriateness of patient care. This involves reviewing the medical necessity of treatments and services, ensuring that they align with established guidelines and standards. The main goal is to optimize patient outcomes and promote cost-effective care delivery. By evaluating and assessing the utilization of resources, healthcare facilities can identify any discrepancies or areas for improvement, ultimately leading to enhanced patient care and better allocation of resources. Utilization review processes are crucial in maintaining high-quality care while balancing the economic considerations of healthcare delivery.

Question 124: Correct Answer: B) Time-limited

Rationale: An effective goal in the rehabilitation setting should be time-limited, meaning it has a specific timeframe for achievement. This helps to create a sense of urgency and motivation for both the patient and the rehabilitation team. A time-limited goal provides a clear target and helps in tracking progress. Goals that are too broad or general may lack specificity, hindering the ability to measure progress. Additionally, vague and immeasurable goals make it challenging to determine whether they have been achieved. While goals may need to be modified over time, a subject to complete change may hinder progress and accountability.

Question 125: Correct Answer: C) Assess and respect the patient's cultural and spiritual beliefs, integrating them into the plan of care.

Rationale: When providing care, it is essential to acknowledge and respect the patient's cultural and spiritual beliefs. This promotes holistic care and enhances patient-centeredness. By assessing the patient's cultural and spiritual background, the nurse can understand their needs, preferences, and values, leading to the development of an individualized plan of care. Integrating the patient's cultural and spiritual beliefs in the plan of care fosters a therapeutic relationship, promotes trust, and increases the likelihood of positive health outcomes. Disregarding or prioritizing the nurse's own beliefs over the patient's could result in culturally insensitive care and hamper the patient's healing process.

Question 126: Correct Answer: B) An ombudsperson acts as a mediator to resolve conflicts between patients and healthcare providers.

Rationale: The role of an ombudsperson in healthcare settings is to act as a neutral mediator in resolving conflicts between patients and healthcare providers. They listen to the concerns of both parties and help facilitate effective communication and resolution of the issues. The ombudsperson does not represent either the patient or the healthcare organization but works towards finding a fair and equitable solution. This role ensures that the ethical principles of patient autonomy, beneficence, and justice are upheld while addressing conflicts and grievances.

Question 127: Correct Answer: A) The nursing process involves assessing the patient's elimination needs, providing appropriate interventions, and evaluating the outcomes.

Rationale: The nursing process is a systematic approach used by registered nurses to provide individualized care. In relation to optimizing a patient's elimination patterns, the nursing process involves assessing the patient's elimination needs, such as frequency, consistency, and any associated symptoms. Based on the assessment, appropriate interventions can be implemented, which may include dietary modifications, medication administration, and toileting schedules. Finally, the outcomes of the interventions are evaluated to determine their effectiveness and make any necessary adjustments to the plan of care. Therefore, option A is the correct answer as it accurately describes the role of the nursing process in optimizing a patient's elimination patterns.

Question 128: Correct Answer: B) Immediately remove the clutter and ensure that the emergency call bell is within reach of the patient.

Rationale: Ensuring a safe environment is crucial in promoting patient and staff well-being. In this scenario, the cluttered pathways and unavailability of the emergency call bell pose potential risks to the patient's safety. The best action to address this concern is to immediately remove the clutter and ensure that the emergency call bell is within the patient's reach. This not only minimizes the risk but also promotes the patient's ability to seek assistance promptly when needed. Informing the patient's family (option A) and documenting the concern (option C) are important actions but should not be the primary response in addressing an immediate safety issue. Ignoring the concern (option D) is not a responsible or ethical response.

Question 129: Correct Answer: D) The nurse asks Mr. Johnson about his social support system and sources of stress.

Rationale: Assessing the functional health patterns involves gathering information about various aspects of a patient's life, including physical, cognitive, emotional, and social domains. In this scenario, the nurse is implementing this knowledge by asking Mr. Johnson about his social support system and sources of stress. This information helps the nurse understand the impact of these factors on Mr. Johnson's rehabilitation process and overall well-being. While options A, B, and C are important assessments, they do not specifically address the knowledge of functional health patterns as described in this scenario.

Question 130: Correct Answer: A) Providing a balanced diet rich in fiber and fluids

Rationale: Providing a balanced diet rich in fiber and fluids is an essential intervention for optimizing bladder and bowel management. Fiber-rich foods promote regular bowel movements, prevent constipation, and maintain bowel health. Adequate fluid intake helps to prevent dehydration and supports overall bowel and bladder function. Administering laxatives on a daily basis (option B) may lead to dependence and should be avoided unless medically necessary. Restricting fluid intake (option C) can contribute to dehydration and can exacerbate bladder and bowel problems. Encouraging the patient to suppress the urge to void or defecate (option D) is not recommended as it can lead to urinary retention and constipation.

Question 131: Correct Answer: A) The NDNQI is a database that collects and analyzes data related to nursing-sensitive quality indicators.

Rationale: The National Database of Nursing Quality Indicators (NDNQI) is a comprehensive nursing quality measurement program. It collects and analyzes data from participating healthcare organizations to identify areas for improvement in nursing-sensitive quality indicators. The NDNQI provides valuable benchmarking data and allows organizations to compare their performance with national norms. It helps healthcare facilities in establishing evidence-based practices and implementing quality improvement initiatives. The database focuses on various aspects of nursing care, such as pressure ulcers, falls, medication errors, patient satisfaction, and nurse staffing levels. Monitoring and analyzing these indicators can lead to enhanced patient outcomes and improved nursing care.

Question 132: D) Providing Mrs. Adams with a bedside commode for easy access.

Correct Answer: B) Encouraging Mrs. Adams to empty her bladder every 4 hours.

Rationale: Encouraging Mrs. Adams to empty her bladder every 4 hours is the most appropriate intervention to promote continence. Regular voiding helps prevent urinary stasis and reduces the risk of urinary tract infections. Limiting fluid intake may lead to dehydration and can have negative effects on overall health. Administering a diuretic may increase urine production but does not address the issue of incontinence. Providing a bedside commode is a good option for patients with limited mobility, but it does not directly address the goal of promoting continence.

Question 133: Correct Answer: B) Assessment
Rationale: The nursing process is a systematic framework used by nurses to provide comprehensive patient care. In the context of promoting optimal psychosocial patterns and coping and stress management skills, the first step in the nursing process is assessment. This involves gathering relevant information about the patient's psychosocial and emotional well-being, coping mechanisms, and stressors. By conducting a thorough assessment, the nurse can identify areas of concern and develop an individualized plan of care. Evaluation comes after the planning and implementation phases to determine the effectiveness of the interventions. Diagnosis and planning follow the assessment phase in the nursing process.

Question 134: Correct Answer: C) Inform the physician and request proper consent from the patient or family members.
Rationale: It is essential for Mrs. Johnson, as a CRRN, to advocate for her patients' rights and ensure the provision of ethical and legal care. The use of physical restraints requires obtaining informed consent from the patient or their family members, as it involves potentially restrictive measures to ensure patient safety. By informing the physician and requesting proper consent, Mrs. Johnson ensures compliance with legal and regulatory requirements, promoting patient autonomy and dignity. It is crucial to involve the patient and their family in decision-making processes to respect their rights and preferences.

Question 135: Correct Answer: C) Bluetooth-enabled devices for monitoring sleep quality
Rationale: Bluetooth-enabled devices, such as sleep trackers or smartwatches, can provide valuable data on sleep quality, duration, and patterns, which can be used to optimize the patient's sleep and rest patterns. These devices can monitor factors like heart rate, movement, and sleep stages, allowing healthcare professionals to identify areas for improvement and tailor interventions accordingly. While virtual reality headsets, robotic assistance devices, and 3D printers have their uses in rehabilitation, they are not specifically designed to optimize sleep and rest patterns.

Question 136: Correct Answer: D) Utilization review involves monitoring the medical necessity and efficiency of healthcare services.
Rationale: Utilization review is a process commonly used in healthcare to monitor the medical necessity and efficiency of healthcare services. It involves reviewing the documentation and appropriateness of a patient's care to ensure that services provided are necessary and delivered in the most efficient manner possible. This helps ensure that resources are used appropriately and cost-effectively, while still meeting the patient's needs. Utilization review plays a crucial role in managing healthcare costs, determining reimbursement, and promoting patient-centered and cost-effective care.

Question 137: Correct Answer: C) Epworth Sleepiness Scale
Rationale: The Epworth Sleepiness Scale is a reliable and validated tool that measures a person's general level of sleepiness. It assesses the effectiveness of sleep and rest interventions by quantifying the individual's likelihood of falling asleep in various situations (e.g., watching TV, reading). The higher the score, the higher the person's daytime sleepiness. This tool helps healthcare professionals evaluate the impact of interventions on improving sleep quality and overall

alertness in patients. While pain assessment, pressure sore risk, and fall risk are important considerations in patient care, they do not directly evaluate the effectiveness of sleep and rest interventions.

Question 138: Correct Answer: A) Explaining the benefits of nonpharmacological pain management techniques
Rationale: For a patient like Mrs. Thompson, who complains of pain in her left arm and shoulder, the nurse should prioritize teaching her about nonpharmacological pain management techniques. These techniques, such as relaxation exercises, heat therapy, and guided imagery, can provide pain relief and minimize the need for opioid pain medication with potential side effects. By educating the patient about these techniques, the nurse empowers her to actively participate in managing her pain and promotes a holistic approach to her care. It is important to prioritize nonpharmacological interventions whenever possible to minimize the risk of drug dependence and adverse effects.

Question 139: Correct Answer: D) Assessment
Rationale: The nursing process consists of five steps: assessment, diagnosis, planning, implementation, and evaluation. In this scenario, assessing Sarah's physical, psychological, and social needs falls under the assessment step. Assessment involves gathering information about the patient's health status to identify actual or potential problems. This step helps the nurse to understand the patient's condition and determine the appropriate care interventions. Once the assessment is complete, the nurse can proceed to the diagnosis step to identify specific problems and plan the care accordingly.

Question 140: Correct Answer: A) Providing Mark with a personal response device
Rationale: Providing Mark with a personal response device would be the most appropriate strategy to prevent falls in this scenario. A personal response device, such as a wearable pendant or wristband, allows Mark to call for help immediately if he experiences a fall or any other emergency. This can help reduce the risk of injury and ensure timely assistance is provided. While alarms, helmets, and padding can also be important safety measures, they may not directly address Mark's risk of falls caused by his right-sided weakness.

Question 141: Correct Answer: A) Roy's Adaptation Model
Rationale: Roy's Adaptation Model is based on the belief that individuals strive to adapt to changes in their internal and external environments to maintain biological, psychological, and social integrity. This model focuses on promoting patient adaptation by assessing and implementing interventions to aid in their ability to adapt and maintain independence in daily activities. In Jennifer's case, the focus on her ability to adapt and regain balance and coordination aligns with the principles of Roy's Adaptation Model. Orem's Self-Care Deficit Model focuses on assisting patients in meeting their self-care needs, Neuman's Systems Model focuses on the prevention and management of stressors, and Leininger's Culture Care Diversity and Universality Theory focuses on providing culturally congruent care.

Question 142: Correct Answer: C) Educating patients and caregivers about coping techniques
Rationale: Educating patients and caregivers about coping techniques is a crucial strategy to promote healthy adaptation to role and relationship changes. This education should include information about the emotional and psychological challenges that may arise, effective communication skills, stress management techniques, and available resources for support. By equipping patients and caregivers with coping strategies, they can develop resilience, enhance their ability to adjust to new roles and responsibilities, and reduce the impact of stressors associated with the changes. Counseling services and peer support groups can also be beneficial, but

they should not be the sole strategy for addressing role and relationship changes.

Question 143: Correct Answer: D) Maslow's Hierarchy of Needs

Rationale: Maslow's Hierarchy of Needs is a nursing model that categorizes human needs into a hierarchical structure. It emphasizes the importance of meeting the patient's basic physiological needs, such as food, water, and shelter, followed by safety needs, love and belonging needs, esteem needs, and finally self-actualization needs. This model recognizes that individuals must have their lower-level needs met before they can strive for higher-level needs. As a rehabilitation registered nurse, understanding Maslow's Hierarchy of Needs enables you to prioritize interventions and provide holistic care that addresses the patient's various levels of needs during the rehabilitation process.

Question 144: Correct Answer: B) To determine the amount of residual urine in the bladder

Rationale: A bladder scan is a non-invasive procedure used to assess the amount of urine left in the bladder after voiding. It is performed by using ultrasound technology to measure the bladder's volume. This information helps healthcare providers determine if there is any residual urine present, which can be indicative of urinary retention. By identifying the amount of residual urine, healthcare providers can make appropriate interventions to prevent complications such as urinary tract infections. The purpose of a bladder scan is not to measure the size and shape of the bladder (Option A), assess the type and severity of urinary incontinence (Option C), or evaluate the effectiveness of bladder training exercises (Option D).

Question 145: Correct Answer: D) "I will provide Mr. Smith with non-slip socks to wear to minimize the risk of falls."

Rationale: Providing non-slip socks to Mr. Smith will help reduce the risk of falls by providing him with better traction while walking. Option A is incorrect because placing a fall risk sign on the door does not directly prevent falls. Option B is incorrect because sleeping with the lights on may disrupt Mr. Smith's sleep and does not specifically address fall prevention. Option C is incorrect because keeping the call bell out of Mr. Smith's reach may lead to delayed assistance and compromise patient safety.

Question 146: Correct Answer: A) Develop an interdisciplinary communication tool to enhance collaboration.

Rationale: Developing an interdisciplinary communication tool to enhance collaboration is the best strategy for the nurse to integrate quality improvement processes into nursing practice. Effective communication and collaboration between team members can significantly reduce errors and improve patient care outcomes. By implementing a structured tool for documentation and communication, all team members will have access to the same information and can effectively coordinate care. This strategy promotes consistency, reduces misunderstandings, and encourages the sharing of critical patient information among healthcare professionals. Implementing standardized protocols for medication administration, increasing the frequency of team meetings, or conducting annual performance evaluations, while important in their own right, may not directly address the issue of inconsistencies in documentation and communication.

Question 147: Correct Answer: B) Skilled nursing facility

Rationale: Given Mr. Smith's current condition, including weakness, balance issues, and coordination difficulties, a skilled nursing facility would be the most suitable setting for his ongoing rehabilitation needs. Skilled nursing facilities offer specialized care and therapy services to individuals who require a higher level of care than can be provided in an assisted living facility or through home health care. These facilities provide 24-hour nursing care, access to physical, occupational, and speech therapy, and can assist with activities of daily living. Adult day care centers do not typically provide the level of rehabilitation services required for Mr. Smith's condition.

Question 148: Correct Answer: A) Centers for Medicare and Medicaid Services (CMS)

Rationale: The Centers for Medicare and Medicaid Services (CMS) is the federal agency responsible for overseeing the quality measurement efforts in healthcare. It plays a crucial role in promoting high-quality care and ensuring patient safety through various initiatives such as the Hospital Quality Reporting Program and the Quality Payment Program. CMS has developed numerous quality measures to assess the performance of healthcare providers, enabling the evaluation and improvement of care delivery. By actively monitoring and enforcing quality standards, CMS aims to enhance the overall quality of care provided to Medicare and Medicaid beneficiaries.

Question 149: Correct Answer: A) Bed alarms

Rationale: Bed alarms are safety devices that alert healthcare providers when a patient attempts to get out of bed independently. They are used as an alternative to physical restraints, promoting patient safety without restricting their movements. Bed alarms help minimize the risk of falls and injuries while allowing the patient some freedom of movement. Side rails, on the other hand, are physical restraints that can limit a patient's mobility and should only be used when necessary. Posey vests and lap belts are also physical restraints that restrict a patient's movement, making them inappropriate alternatives to restraints. It is crucial for CRRNs to be aware of the various safety devices and their appropriate use to promote a safe environment of care for patients and staff.

Question 150: Correct Answer: A) Physical health status

Rationale: In assessing potential for harm to self and others, the priority assessment is to evaluate the physical health status of the individual. This is important because physical health conditions or changes can significantly affect a person's ability to cope with stress and can contribute to increased risk of self-harm or harm to others. By assessing physical health status, the nurse can identify any medical conditions or symptoms that may require immediate intervention or further evaluation. This assessment helps determine the level of medical support needed to address potential risks and develop appropriate interventions.

CRRN Practice Questions (SET 2)

Question 1: When collaborating with private, community, and public resources, which of the following would be the most appropriate action for a Certified Rehabilitation Registered Nurse (CRRN) to take?
A) Work independently without seeking assistance from external resources.
B) Refer the patient to online support groups for additional resources.
C) Collaborate with local rehabilitation facilities to provide comprehensive care.
D) Encourage the patient to rely solely on their healthcare insurance coverage.

Question 2: Which of the following is an essential component of patient-centered care?
A) Providing care based on healthcare provider preferences
B) Focusing only on the physical aspects of care
C) Ignoring patient values and preferences
D) Engaging patients in decision-making and respecting their choices

Question 3: In a rehabilitation facility, the registered nurse is responsible for developing staffing patterns and policies to provide optimal care for patients. Which staffing pattern would best promote cost-effective, patient-centered care?
A) Increasing the number of registered nurses on the unit.
B) Hiring more nursing assistants to provide direct patient care.
C) Assigning a higher nurse-to-patient ratio during high-acuity shifts.
D) Utilizing floating staff from different units to fill staffing gaps.

Question 4: While providing care to a patient in a rehabilitation center, the nurse notices that the patient is withdrawn and avoids eye contact. Which therapeutic communication technique would be most appropriate to use in this situation?
A) Focusing on the patient's physical appearance
B) Offering advice and solutions to the patient's problems
C) Using open-ended questions to encourage the patient to express feelings
D) Avoiding silence and filling the silence with unnecessary conversation

Question 5: Which of the following is an example of an acute illness?
A) Chronic obstructive pulmonary disease (COPD)
B) Hypertension
C) Kidney failure
D) Influenza

Question 6: Mary is a 45-year-old woman who recently had a stroke. She is now undergoing rehabilitation and is experiencing urinary incontinence. The rehabilitation team has recommended implementing interventions for bladder management. As a Certified Rehabilitation Registered Nurse (CRRN), which intervention would be most appropriate for Mary?
A) Restricting fluid intake to reduce urinary frequency and urgency
B) Encouraging Mary to perform Kegel exercises to strengthen pelvic floor muscles
C) Administering pharmacological agents to suppress bladder contractions

D) Providing adaptive equipment such as adult diapers for Mary to manage her incontinence

Question 7: You are a Certified Rehabilitation Registered Nurse (CRRN) working in a rehabilitation facility. A 65-year-old male patient with a history of stroke has been making progress in his rehabilitation program but is experiencing severe difficulty swallowing. The patient's condition has not improved despite interventions such as speech therapy and modified diets. The patient's family is concerned about his worsening condition and requests a referral to a specialist. Which action would be most appropriate at this time?
A) Ignore the family's request for a referral and continue with the current interventions.
B) Discuss the family's concerns with the healthcare team and consider referring the patient to a specialist in dysphagia management.
C) Inform the family that referrals are not necessary in their current situation.
D) Suggest alternative therapies such as acupuncture or herbal remedies to the family.

Question 8: Mr. Johnson is a 45-year-old patient who recently suffered a spinal cord injury resulting in paralysis from the waist down. He will be discharged home soon and will require ongoing care and support. Which community resource would be most appropriate for Mr. Johnson to assist with his rehabilitation and daily living needs?
A) Social Security Administration
B) Department of Parks and Recreation
C) Public Health Department
D) Department of Motor Vehicles

Question 9: A patient with a spinal cord injury is experiencing difficulty in coping with the new changes in their daily life. Which nursing intervention would be most appropriate for addressing the psychosocial needs of the patient?
A) Providing education on adaptive techniques for performing daily activities.
B) Administering medication to alleviate physical discomfort.
C) Encouraging the patient to discuss their fears and concerns with a support group.
D) Assisting the patient with physical therapy exercises to regain mobility.

Question 10: Mr. Johnson, a 48-year-old patient with a spinal cord injury, is being discharged from the rehabilitation unit to his home. As part of his care plan, the nurse is responsible for teaching him about managing his health, wellness, and life skills at home. Which of the following statements by Mr. Johnson indicates a correct understanding of the teaching?
A) "I should avoid physical activities and exercise to prevent further injury."
B) "I will rely on my caregiver to perform all the daily activities for me."
C) "I will follow a balanced diet and maintain a healthy weight to prevent complications."
D) "I don't need to follow any precautions or safety measures at home."

Question 11: A patient with chronic pain secondary to a spinal cord injury is experiencing high levels of

stress. The nurse suggests using biofeedback as a coping mechanism. Which statement made by the patient indicates a correct understanding of biofeedback?
A) "Biofeedback is a technique that involves focusing on pleasant memories to distract from the pain."
B) "Biofeedback uses electronic devices to measure and display physiological functions to improve self-awareness and self-regulation."
C) "Biofeedback involves listening to calming music to promote relaxation and reduce stress levels."
D) "Biofeedback is a form of meditation that involves deep breathing and progressive muscle relaxation."

Question 12:   Ms. Johnson, a 63-year-old female, has recently suffered a stroke and is receiving rehabilitation care at the hospital. The interdisciplinary team is working together to develop a care plan that incorporates relevant research, nursing models, and theories into Ms. Johnson's individualized patient-centered rehabilitation care. Which nursing model would be most appropriate to guide the team in providing holistic and comprehensive care to Ms. Johnson?
A) Maslow's Hierarchy of Needs Model
B) Roy Adaptation Model
C) Orem's Self-Care Deficit Theory
D) Watson's Theory of Human Caring

Question 13:   Ms. Johnson, a Certified Rehabilitation Registered Nurse (CRRN), is working in a rehabilitation facility. She is responsible for managing current and projected resources in a cost-effective manner. She has been asked to implement a new electronic documentation system that will help streamline patient care processes and reduce paper waste. Which of the following is a potential benefit of implementing this system?
A) Increased staff workload and reduced efficiency
B) Increased risk of errors and decreased patient safety
C) Improved accuracy and accessibility of patient information
D) Decreased cost savings and increased resource utilization

Question 14:   Mr. Davis, a 45-year-old patient, has recently been diagnosed with a chronic and debilitating illness. He seems to be in a state of shock, constantly asking, "Why is this happening to me?" Which stage of grief and loss is Mr. Davis most likely experiencing?
A) Acceptance
B) Bargaining
C) Denial
D) Anger

Question 15:   Mrs. Johnson, a 65-year-old patient, is admitted to a rehabilitation facility following a stroke. The healthcare team is assessing her nutritional status and giving recommendations to ensure optimal nutrition and hydration. Which of the following actions by the nurse best promotes Mrs. Johnson's nutritional needs?
A) Encouraging Mrs. Johnson to eat a high-protein diet to promote wound healing.
B) Limiting Mrs. Johnson's fluid intake to prevent urinary incontinence.
C) Providing Mrs. Johnson with whole milk to increase her calorie intake.
D) Assisting Mrs. Johnson to sit in an upright position during meals.

Question 16:   Ms. Johnson, a 43-year-old patient, is admitted to the rehabilitation unit following a stroke. She has weakness on the right side of her body and difficulty swallowing. The nurse is planning to assist Ms. Johnson with her meal. Which of the following adaptive equipment would be most appropriate for Ms. Johnson to facilitate independent feeding?
A) Curved utensils
B) Weighted utensils
C) Nonslip mats
D) Scoop plates

Question 17:   Samantha, a 55-year-old Caucasian woman, has been admitted to the rehabilitation unit after undergoing a below-the-knee amputation due to complications from diabetes. She has been experiencing anxiety and spiritual distress since the surgery. The nurse is preparing to provide holistic care that incorporates cultural awareness and spiritual values. Question: Which action by the nurse demonstrates the incorporation of cultural awareness and spiritual values into Samantha's plan of care?
A) Providing culturally appropriate food options during meals
B) Encouraging Samantha to participate in physical therapy sessions to improve her mobility
C) Assisting Samantha with personal hygiene and dressing changes
D) Exploring Samantha's spiritual beliefs and offering support from a chaplain or spiritual care provider

Question 18:   Sarah, a 45-year-old female, is admitted to the rehabilitation unit following a traumatic brain injury. She is married and has two teenage children. Sarah's husband expresses concerns about the changes he has observed in Sarah since the injury, particularly her emotional lability and forgetfulness. The nurse recognizes the importance of providing education and support not only to Sarah but also to her family. Which nursing intervention is most appropriate in this situation?
A) Provide Sarah's husband with information about community support groups for traumatic brain injury caregivers.
B) Encourage Sarah's husband to take on the role of primary caregiver without seeking outside help.
C) Minimize the involvement of Sarah's children in her rehabilitation process to protect them from emotional distress.
D) Dismiss Sarah's husband's concerns as a normal reaction to the stress of caregiving.

Question 19:   Mr. Smith, a 45-year-old male, is admitted to the rehabilitation unit following a spinal cord injury at level T4. Which of the following statements regarding altered bowel function in patients with a T4 spinal cord injury is correct?
A) The patient will have complete loss of voluntary control over the external anal sphincter.
B) The patient will experience increased sensitivity to gastric distension.
C) The patient may have difficulty initiating bowel movements due to parasympathetic stimulation.
D) The patient will experience frequent involuntary contractions of the rectal muscles.

Question 20:   Mitchell is a 52-year-old patient who has been admitted to the rehabilitation unit following a stroke. The nurse is creating a plan of care to optimize Mitchell's sleep and rest patterns. Which intervention should the nurse prioritize?
A) Administering a sedative medication before bedtime
B) Implementing a routine sleep schedule
C) Encouraging napping throughout the day
D) Limiting fluid intake after dinner

Question 21: Mr. Johnson, a 45-year-old patient with multiple sclerosis, is admitted to the rehabilitation unit. He has been experiencing urinary incontinence and wants to regain control over his bladder function. Which intervention will be most appropriate for Mr. Johnson to improve his bladder control?
A) Encouraging Mr. Johnson to consume caffeinated beverages throughout the day
B) Instructing Mr. Johnson to hold urine for as long as possible before voiding
C) Implementing a scheduled self-catheterization program for Mr. Johnson
D) Advising Mr. Johnson to avoid drinking fluids to reduce urine production

Question 22: Which assessment findings would indicate a need for nursing intervention to optimize a patient's ability to communicate effectively?
A) The patient frequently avoids eye contact.
B) The patient speaks softly and mumbles during conversations.
C) The patient demonstrates difficulty understanding written instructions.
D) The patient frequently interrupts and speaks over others.

Question 23: Mr. Johnson is a 72-year-old male patient admitted to the rehabilitation unit following a stroke. He has right-sided weakness and expressive aphasia. The nurse is implementing safety interventions to prevent falls. Which of the following interventions is most appropriate for this patient?
A) Reorient the patient frequently to enhance spatial awareness.
B) Use non-behavioral restraints to restrict the patient's movement.
C) Assign a sitter to be with the patient at all times.
D) Provide a quiet and dimly lit environment to decrease sensory stimulation.

Question 24: Mrs. Adams, a 70-year-old patient, has been admitted to the rehabilitation unit after undergoing a total hip replacement surgery. She is experiencing pain and has difficulty with mobility. As the nurse responsible for her care, you are implementing the nursing process to provide patient-centered care. During the assessment phase, you gather information about Mrs. Adams' pain level, medication history, and mobility limitations. Which of the following actions best demonstrates the use of the nursing process to deliver cost-effective patient-centered care for Mrs. Adams?
A) Requesting a complete blood count (CB
C) to assess for infection.
B) Initiating physical therapy sessions twice a day to improve mobility.
C) Administering pain medication as ordered to manage Mrs. Adams' pain.
D) Collaborating with the healthcare team to develop an individualized care plan.

Question 25: What religious practice involves abstaining from food and drink from sunrise to sunset during the holy month of Ramadan?
A) Hinduism
B) Buddhism
C) Islam
D) Sikhism

Question 26: Which clinical sign is commonly associated with sensorimotor deficits in patients?
A) Hyperreflexia
B) Hypoactive bowel sounds
C) Increased coordination
D) Normal muscle tone

Question 27: Mrs. Thompson, a 74-year-old patient, was admitted to a rehabilitation facility following a hip replacement surgery. She has Medicare insurance and is concerned about her coverage for rehab services. As a Certified Rehabilitation Registered Nurse (CRRN), you explain to her about the Prospective Payment System (PPS) for Medicare beneficiaries. Question: Which of the following statements about the Prospective Payment System (PPS) for Medicare beneficiaries is correct?
A) PPS reimburses healthcare providers based on the actual costs incurred for delivering care.
B) PPS uses a fee-for-service model, where providers receive reimbursement for each individual service.
C) PPS determines reimbursement rates based on the patient's length of stay and specific diagnosis-related groups (DRGs).
D) PPS applies only to inpatient hospital stays and does not cover post-acute care services.

Question 28: Sarah, a 35-year-old patient, has recently been admitted to a rehabilitation center for spinal cord injury. She is keen on exploring alternative modalities to assist in her recovery process. As her nurse, you are discussing different options with her. Which alternative modality is based on the concept of using therapeutic touch to promote healing and relaxation?
A) Acupuncture
B) Meditation
C) Aromatherapy
D) Healing touch

Question 29: Sarah, a 60-year-old patient with end-stage renal disease, is admitted to the rehabilitation unit after a recent kidney transplant. She has a triple lumen catheter in place for hemodialysis access. The nurse notices that the catheter dressing is loose and soiled with blood. Which action should the nurse prioritize in managing Sarah's triple lumen catheter dressing?
A) Clean the dressing with sterile saline and replace it with a sterile dressing.
B) Remove the dressing and inspect the catheter insertion site for signs of infection.
C) Notify the healthcare provider and request an order to resecure the catheter dressing.
D) Reinforce the dressing with additional tape to prevent further displacement.

Question 30: Mrs. Johnson, a 65-year-old patient with a history of heart failure, is admitted with exacerbation of dyspnea and fatigue. Her vital signs show tachypnea and decreased oxygen saturation. The healthcare provider suspects acute respiratory distress syndrome (ARDS) and orders initiation of assisted ventilation. Which of the following statements accurately describes the goals of assisted ventilation in patients with ARDS?
A) To maintain normal oxygen saturation levels and prevent further lung damage
B) To decrease the workload of the heart and increase cardiac output
C) To improve lung compliance and decrease airway resistance
D) To provide long-term ventilatory support to eliminate the need for spontaneous breathing

Question 31: What is the primary purpose of using personal response devices in a rehabilitation setting?
A) To monitor vital signs
B) To enhance communication between patients and healthcare providers
C) To administer medications
D) To prevent falls

Question 32: A 55-year-old patient, Mr. Jensen, is admitted to the rehabilitation unit after a stroke. He has left-sided weakness and difficulty with mobility. The physical therapist recommends passive range of motion (ROM) exercises for his affected limbs. As the nurse, which of the following goals related to ROM exercises is the most appropriate for Mr. Jensen?
A) Increase muscle strength
B) Improve joint flexibility
C) Enhance cardiovascular endurance
D) Enhance coordination and balance

Question 33: Mrs. Anderson, a 68-year-old patient, recently suffered a stroke and is currently undergoing rehabilitation therapy. The nursing staff is implementing the Self-care Deficit Nursing Theory (SCDNT) to guide her care. According to this theory, which of the following actions should the nurse prioritize to assist Mrs. Anderson in meeting her self-care needs?
A) Assessing Mrs. Anderson's mobility and balance.
B) Administering pain medication as needed.
C) Providing emotional support and encouragement.
D) Assisting with activities of daily living (ADLs).

Question 34: Damage to which brain structure is most commonly associated with deficits in cognition and judgment?
A) Hippocampus
B) Cerebellum
C) Prefrontal cortex
D) Amygdala

Question 35: Ms. Anderson, a 72-year-old female patient, has been admitted to the rehabilitation unit following a stroke. As a Certified Rehabilitation Registered Nurse (CRRN), you are responsible for providing appropriate care and adhering to rehabilitation standards and the scope of practice. While reviewing the patient's plan of care, you notice that the patient has been prescribed a medication that is not commonly used in stroke rehabilitation. What should you do in this situation?
A) Administer the medication as prescribed without question.
B) Discuss the medication prescription with the prescriber to ensure its appropriateness.
C) Consult with the interdisciplinary team before administering the medication.
D) Discontinue the medication without informing anyone.

Question 36: You are a Certified Rehabilitation Registered Nurse (CRRN) working in a rehabilitation facility. You have been assigned to care for a patient, Mr. Smith, who sustained a severe traumatic brain injury in a car accident. Mr. Smith is non-verbal and requires total assistance with his personal care. His family is actively involved in his care and expresses concerns about his nutrition. They want to ensure that he receives the appropriate nutrition and hydration to aid in his recovery. However, Mr. Smith does not have a designated healthcare proxy or advance directives in place. What is the most appropriate action for the nurse to take in this situation?

A) Respect the family's wishes and provide Mr. Smith with supplemental nutrition and hydration.
B) Contact the healthcare facility's ethics committee for guidance.
C) Consult with the facility's legal department to understand the legal implications.
D) Advocate for Mr. Smith's right to make decisions about his own care.

Question 37: Ms. Johnson, a 55-year-old patient, is admitted to a rehabilitation center after suffering a stroke. As a rehabilitation nurse, you are aware of the importance of using nursing models and theories as a framework for your practice. Which nursing model or theory would be most suitable for guiding your care of Ms. Johnson?
A) Maslow's Hierarchy of Needs
B) Orem's Self-Care Deficit Theory
C) Watson's Theory of Human Caring
D) Roy's Adaptation Model

Question 38: Which of the following is a safety risk factor that should be minimized in a rehabilitation setting?
A) Poorly maintained equipment
B) Adequate staffing levels
C) Regular safety training for staff
D) Encouraging patient independence

Question 39: Which skill is essential for a Certified Rehabilitation Registered Nurse (CRRN) when addressing legislative, economic, ethical, and legal issues in patient care?
A) Critical thinking and problem-solving
B) Patient assessment and care planning
C) Effective communication and collaboration
D) Evidence-based practice and research utilization

Question 40: Which of the following factors should a Rehabilitation Registered Nurse consider when assessing a patient's sleep and rest patterns?
A) Age and gender of the patient
B) Social and environmental factors
C) Medications the patient is taking
D) Education level of the patient

Question 41: A 45-year-old male patient recently suffered a traumatic brain injury and is undergoing rehabilitation. The patient has been making progress in his therapy sessions, but has been experiencing emotional challenges such as anxiety and depression. The rehabilitation nurse determines that it would be beneficial for the patient to receive additional support from a mental health professional. Which professional resource should the nurse recommend for this patient?
A) Neurologist
B) Teacher
C) Case manager
D) Psychologist

Question 42: Which of the following assistive devices is commonly used by individuals with weakened lower extremities to assist with walking and maintain balance?
A) Crutches
B) Hearing aids
C) Wheelchair
D) Prosthetic limb

Question 43: Elizabeth, a 52-year-old woman, sustained a spinal cord injury resulting in paraplegia. She has completed her inpatient rehabilitation program

successfully and is ready for discharge. As a Certified Rehabilitation Registered Nurse (CRRN), you are responsible for assessing barriers to Elizabeth's community reintegration. Which of the following is an example of a social barrier to community reintegration?
A) Inaccessible public transportation options
B) Lack of caregiver support at home
C) Difficulty using assistive devices
D) Cognitive impairments

Question 44: A rehabilitation unit is implementing a quality improvement process to reduce patient falls. The team has identified a need for a structured approach to guide their efforts and has decided to utilize the Plan, Do, Check, Act (PDCA) model. The team is currently in the planning phase, gathering data and information to identify potential causes of falls. As a Certified Rehabilitation Registered Nurse (CRRN), you are asked to explain the PDCA model to the team. Question: Which of the following statements best describes the Plan, Do, Check, Act (PDC
A) model?
A) The PDCA model is a continuous improvement framework that involves four stages: planning, doing, checking, and acting.
B) The PDCA model is a problem-solving approach that uses statistical analysis to identify causes and solutions.
C) The PDCA model is a lean approach that focuses on eliminating waste and increasing efficiency in processes.
D) The PDCA model is a Six Sigma methodology that uses data-driven decision-making for process improvement.

Question 45: When utilizing the nursing process to deliver cost-effective patient-centered care, the nurse should always consider:
A) Legislative standards and guidelines
B) Economic concerns and financial resources
C) Ethical principles and moral obligations
D) Legal issues and liability concerns

Question 46: Which factors should the rehabilitation registered nurse consider when optimizing the patient's sleep and rest patterns?
A) Pain level, anxiety, and medication side effects
B) Social support, cultural beliefs, and nutritional status
C) Physical activity, spiritual practices, and social interactions
D) Cardiac status, respiratory rate, and bowel elimination

Question 47: Which of the following is a barrier to community reintegration for individuals with disabilities?
A) Financial constraints
B) Adequate transportation
C) Supportive social network
D) Accessible recreational facilities

Question 48: You are a Certified Rehabilitation Registered Nurse (CRRN) working with an interdisciplinary team to provide patient-centered care. During a team meeting, a physical therapist suggests a new treatment approach for a patient with a spinal cord injury. As the CRRN, how should you respond to the physical therapist's suggestion?
A) Accept the suggestion without question, as the physical therapist is the expert in this area.
B) Reject the suggestion immediately, as it goes against your own expertise and experience.
C) Listen to the suggestion and ask for more information before making a decision.
D) Disregard the suggestion, as it is not within the scope of practice for a physical therapist.

Question 49: Which intervention should a Certified Rehabilitation Registered Nurse (CRRN) prioritize to address the safety concern of dysphagia in a patient?
A) Encouraging the patient to eat rapidly to avoid choking
B) Providing small, frequent meals throughout the day
C) Allowing the patient to eat in a reclined position
D) Offering foods with mixed textures in the same meal

Question 50: When documenting services provided as a Certified Rehabilitation Registered Nurse (CRRN), which of the following is NOT an important consideration?
A) Accuracy and completeness
B) Timeliness
C) Inclusion of personal opinions
D) Using approved medical abbreviations

Question 51: Which step of the nursing process involves the identification and documentation of actual or potential problems?
A) Assessment
B) Diagnosis
C) Planning
D) Implementation

Question 52: Which of the following strategies would be most effective in teaching self-advocacy skills to patients and caregivers?
A) Providing pamphlets and educational materials on self-advocacy
B) Conducting role-playing scenarios to practice assertiveness skills
C) Assigning a knowledgeable nurse to advocate on behalf of the patient
D) Encouraging passive communication to avoid confrontation

Question 53: What is the recommended teaching intervention to prevent constipation in individuals with a spinal cord injury?
A) Encouraging a diet high in fiber and fluids
B) Limiting fluid intake to prevent bowel overstimulation
C) Encouraging a sedentary lifestyle to minimize bowel movement
D) Recommending the use of laxatives regularly

Question 54: Mr. Johnson is a 72-year-old patient who was recently admitted to the rehabilitation unit after suffering a stroke. As part of his rehabilitation, the nurse is implementing interventions to promote optimal nutrition. Which intervention would be most appropriate for Mr. Johnson?
A) Encouraging Mr. Johnson to eat large meals three times a day to meet his nutritional needs.
B) Administering total parenteral nutrition (TPN) to provide all of Mr. Johnson's nutritional needs.
C) Consult a speech therapist to assess Mr. Johnson's swallowing ability and recommend modifications to his diet as needed.
D) Providing Mr. Johnson with a high-fat, low-fiber diet to maintain his energy levels.

Question 55: Ms. Adams, a 60-year-old patient, is admitted to the rehabilitation unit following a stroke. As a rehabilitation nurse, which skill is most important for you to demonstrate when collaborating with the interdisciplinary team to achieve patient-centered goals?
A) Documentation skills

B) Medication administration skills
C) Communication and teamwork skills
D) Technical nursing skills

Question 56: Sarah is a CRRN working in a rehabilitation facility. She is knowledgeable about the legislative, economic, ethical, and legal issues related to promoting a safe environment of care for patients and staff. While ensuring the safety of patients and staff, Sarah understands that it is essential to comply with legal regulations and ethical standards. Which of the following best describes an example of an ethical issue that Sarah might encounter in her practice?
A) Ensuring the facility follows fire safety regulations
B) Reporting suspected abuse to the appropriate authorities
C) Maintaining patient confidentiality and privacy
D) Adhering to infection control and prevention measures

Question 57: Which of the following is NOT a goal of involving and educating support systems in rehabilitation nursing?
A) Enhancing the patient's psychological and emotional well-being
B) Improving the patient's functional abilities
C) Promoting independence and self-care skills
D) Minimizing the involvement of family members in the rehabilitation process

Question 58: Which of the following is an example of a community resource that can support patients with physical disabilities?
A) Public transportation services
B) Grocery store coupons
C) Personal care products
D) Online support groups

Question 59: Which device is used to deliver pain relief through electrical stimulation to the affected area?
A) TENS unit
B) Baclofen pump
C) LVAD
D) Intrathecal drug delivery system

Question 60: Mr. Adams, a 55-year-old male, has recently suffered a stroke and is undergoing rehabilitation in a skilled nursing facility. The interdisciplinary team is evaluating his progress and adjusting his goals accordingly. The team finds that Mr. Adams is experiencing difficulty with feeding himself independently due to weakness in his upper extremities. Which of the following should be the primary goal adjustment for Mr. Adams at this stage?
A) Increase the number of therapy sessions per week.
B) Modify the nutritional plan to include pureed or soft foods.
C) Provide adaptive equipment to assist with self-feeding.
D) Refer Mr. Adams to a speech-language pathologist for swallowing evaluation.

Question 61: Ms. Rodriguez, a Hispanic patient, has been admitted to the rehabilitation unit following a stroke. As a Certified Rehabilitation Registered Nurse (CRRN), you understand the importance of considering cultural and religious practices related to dietary habits. Which statement is most accurate regarding Ms. Rodriguez's cultural dietary preferences?
A) Ms. Rodriguez would prefer a high-fat, low-fiber diet.
B) Ms. Rodriguez would prefer a vegetarian diet due to her cultural practices.
C) Ms. Rodriguez would prefer a diet rich in spicy foods.
D) Ms. Rodriguez would prefer a diet similar to the standard American diet.

Question 62: Which of the following statements about bladder retraining is correct?
A) Bladder retraining is a technique used to increase the frequency of urination.
B) Bladder retraining is recommended for patients with urinary incontinence.
C) Bladder retraining involves delaying urination whenever the urge arises.
D) Bladder retraining is contraindicated in patients with bladder overactivity.

Question 63: Carol, a 45-year-old patient, was admitted to the rehabilitation unit following a traumatic brain injury. As the nurse, you are responsible for optimizing Carol's care and management of her neurological condition. During your assessment, you notice that Carol has difficulty speaking and understanding spoken language. She also exhibits right-sided weakness and has difficulty performing self-care activities independently. Which nursing diagnosis would be most appropriate for Carol?
A) Impaired physical mobility
B) Impaired verbal communication
C) Impaired social interaction
D) Impaired memory

Question 64: Amy, a Certified Rehabilitation Registered Nurse (CRRN), is caring for a patient in a rehabilitation center. The patient, Mr. Johnson, has recently suffered a severe stroke and is unable to communicate effectively. While reviewing Mr. Johnson's medical records, Amy comes across a note from another nurse stating that Mr. Johnson's family members have requested that he not be informed about his prognosis, as they believe it may worsen his mental state. Which of the following actions should Amy take in this situation?
A) Respect the family's wishes and refrain from disclosing prognosis information to Mr. Johnson.
B) Disregard the family's wishes and inform Mr. Johnson about his prognosis.
C) Discuss the situation with the healthcare team and seek their guidance.
D) Suggest involving an ethics committee to make a decision about disclosing the prognosis.

Question 65: Which agency is responsible for accrediting rehabilitation facilities and programs in the United States?
A) CARF
B) APS
C) SSA
D) OSHA

Question 66: Skill in the Certified Rehabilitation Registered Nurse (CRRN) exam primarily focuses on:
A) Interpretation of economic policies
B) Enforcing ethical principles
C) Understanding legal regulations
D) Analyzing legislative procedures

Question 67: Which factor plays a significant role in determining an individual's cultural beliefs, values, and behaviors?
A) Environmental factors
B) Societal factors
C) Familial factors
D) Gender factors

Question 68: Which class of medications is commonly used to manage spasticity in patients with neurological disorders?
A) Antihistamines
B) NSAIDs
C) Opioids
D) Antispasmodics

Question 69: Mr. Johnson, a 55-year-old patient, has recently been admitted to the rehabilitation unit after a traffic accident resulting in a lower limb injury. He has been experiencing difficulty sleeping and complains of feeling restless and fatigued during the day. The nurse recognizes the importance of promoting sleep and rest for Mr. Johnson's recovery. Which teaching intervention would be most appropriate to help improve Mr. Johnson's sleep and rest patterns?
A) Encouraging consumption of caffeinated beverages in the evening
B) Promoting daytime napping for longer durations
C) Implementing a regular bedtime routine
D) Encouraging engaging in stimulating activities close to bedtime

Question 70: Mrs. Johnson, a 65-year-old patient with chronic low back pain, has been referred to the rehabilitation unit. As her nurse, you are conducting an initial assessment. Which of the following statements accurately describes chronic pain?
A) Chronic pain is localized, lasts for a short duration, and is usually caused by tissue injury.
B) Chronic pain subsides on its own without any intervention or treatment.
C) Chronic pain persists for more than three months and may not have an identifiable cause.
D) Chronic pain is usually sharp and well-defined in nature.

Question 71: Jane, a 45-year-old patient, is admitted to the rehabilitation unit following a spinal cord injury. She reports having difficulty with bowel movements since the injury. As the rehabilitation nurse, which intervention should you prioritize to optimize Jane's elimination patterns?
A) Encourage Jane to increase her fluid intake.
B) Implement a regular toileting schedule for Jane.
C) Administer a laxative to facilitate bowel movements.
D) Instruct Jane to increase her fiber intake.

Question 72: Which of the following is an example of a physiological stressor?
A) A difficult exam
B) A car accident
C) A breakup in a relationship
D) A severe illness

Question 73: When collaborating with the interdisciplinary team, which action by the Certified Rehabilitation Registered Nurse (CRRN) is most effective in promoting effective communication?
A) Providing written instructions to team members
B) Using medical jargon to ensure accuracy and precision
C) Assuming the role of the team leader in all situations
D) Actively listening to team members' input and perspectives

Question 74: When providing care for a culturally diverse population, the nurse should prioritize:
A) Implementing evidence-based interventions
B) Using the same approach for all patients
C) Minimizing the use of interpreters
D) Avoiding cultural assessments

Question 75: Which statement accurately describes enteral nutrition?
A) The administration of nutrition directly into the gastrointestinal tract.
B) The administration of nutrition through a central venous catheter.
C) The administration of nutrition through a peripheral intravenous line.
D) The administration of nutrition through inhalation.

Question 76: A 55-year-old patient, Mr. Smith, is admitted with a diagnosis of a stroke affecting the right side of his brain. The nurse is performing a neurological assessment to evaluate the patient's sensorimotor deficits. Which of the following clinical signs would the nurse expect to find in the patient?
A) Weakness on the left side of the body
B) Difficulty with balance and coordination
C) Decreased sensation on the right side of the body
D) Impaired fine motor skills on the right hand

Question 77: Which nursing model or theory focuses on the belief that personal experiences, beliefs, and culture influence a person's health and wellness?
A) Orem's Self-Care Model
B) Roy's Adaptation Model
C) Peplau's Interpersonal Theory
D) Leininger's Transcultural Nursing Model

Question 78: Ms. Johnson, a 55-year-old patient, has recently been admitted to the rehabilitation unit following a spinal cord injury. The patient is experiencing urinary retention and has been using an indwelling catheter for the past week. The nurse is providing education to the patient and her caregiver about bladder management. Which statement made by the caregiver indicates a correct understanding of bladder management education?
A) "We will need to perform intermittent catheterization every 4 hours to prevent urinary tract infections."
B) "The indwelling catheter should not be changed regularly, as it may cause more harm."
C) "It is best to restrict fluid intake to minimal amounts to reduce the frequency of catheterization."
D) "We should avoid emptying the urinary drainage bag regularly to prevent accidental dislodgement of the catheter."

Question 79: Which theory focuses on the development of an individual's self-concept and self-esteem?
A) Developmental theory
B) Coping theory
C) Stress theory
D) Grief and loss theory

Question 80: When applying the nursing process to provide individualized patient-centered rehabilitation care, which step involves analyzing the data collected and identifying the client's actual or potential problems?
A) Assessment
B) Diagnosis
C) Planning
D) Evaluation

Question 81: Which of the following is a key step in analyzing quality and utilization data?
A) Collecting data from various sources
B) Ignoring outliers in the data

C) Relying solely on subjective opinions
D) Using only qualitative data

Question 82: What teaching strategy would be most appropriate when working with a patient who has neurological deficits related to memory impairment?
A) Visual aids and cues
B) Verbal explanations and demonstrations
C) Written instructions and handouts
D) Group discussion and brainstorming sessions

Question 83: Mrs. Johnson, a 48-year-old female, has recently been admitted to the rehabilitation unit after a spinal cord injury. The healthcare team is implementing the rehabilitation nursing practice model for her care. As a rehabilitation registered nurse, which of the following skills falls under the category of "Skill in:" communication?
A) Assessment and Documentation
B) Advocacy and Collaboration
C) Education and Training
D) Therapeutic Communication and Counseling

Question 84: Mrs. Smith, a 45-year-old patient with a spinal cord injury, is struggling with role and relationship changes after her injury. As a Certified Rehabilitation Registered Nurse (CRRN), what strategy would you recommend to promote her adjustment and coping?
A) Encourage her to isolate herself from friends and family to focus on self-care.
B) Provide education and resources on support groups for individuals with spinal cord injuries.
C) Discourage Mrs. Smith from expressing her emotional concerns.
D) Avoid discussing the changes in roles and relationships to prevent further distress.

Question 85: Mr. Thompson, a 45-year-old male, has been admitted to the rehabilitation unit following a motor vehicle accident resulting in severe physical injuries. He has a history of substance abuse and has been diagnosed with depression. During the initial assessment, the nurse observes that Mr. Thompson appears sad and withdrawn. He expresses feelings of guilt and worthlessness, stating that his accident was punishment for his past mistakes. Which nursing intervention would be most appropriate for Mr. Thompson?
A) Encouraging reliance on pain medication to alleviate emotional distress
B) Providing opportunities for therapeutic communication and active listening
C) Setting strict limitations on visitors to prevent potential stressors
D) Suggesting holistic therapies such as acupuncture to treat depression effectively

Question 86: Which model is used in process improvement to guide the continuous improvement of systems and processes?
A) Plan, Do, Check, Act (PDCA)
B) Six Sigma Approach
C) Lean Approach
D) None of the above

Question 87: Which ethical principle emphasizes the importance of being truthful and honest with patients?
A) Autonomy
B) Beneficence

C) Nonmaleficence
D) Veracity

Question 88: Tracy, a Certified Rehabilitation Registered Nurse (CRRN), is responsible for analyzing quality and utilization data in a rehabilitation facility. She notices that the average length of stay (LOS) for patients with spinal cord injuries has increased significantly over the past month. What should Tracy do in this situation?
A) Ignore the increase in LOS as it could be due to random variation.
B) Discuss the situation with the healthcare team and develop a plan to address the increase in LOS.
C) Inform the administration about the increase in LOS without investigating further.
D) Discharge the current spinal cord injury patients earlier to reduce the LOS.

Question 89: When providing care to a patient at the rehabilitation facility, the nurse should consider which community resource that helps facilitate the patient's transition to the next level of care?
A) Vocational rehabilitation programs
B) Annual physical examinations
C) Home exercise equipment
D) Financial planning services

Question 90: Which entity enforces legislation and regulations related to healthcare practices in the United States?
A) The American Nurses Association (ANA)
B) The State Health Department
C) The Centers for Medicare and Medicaid Services (CMS)
D) The National Institute of Health (NIH)

Question 91: You are a Certified Rehabilitation Registered Nurse (CRRN) working in a rehabilitation unit, and you have been assigned to care for Mr. Smith, a patient with traumatic brain injury. Mr. Smith has been demonstrating aggressive behaviors towards staff and other patients, which is impacting the overall safety of the unit. As part of your role in promoting a safe environment, you decide to implement behavior management techniques to de-escalate Mr. Smith's aggression. What is one important approach you should use when applying behavior management techniques to de-escalate Mr. Smith's aggression?
A) Isolate Mr. Smith in a locked room for a specific duration.
B) Physically restrain Mr. Smith until he calms down.
C) Engage in active listening and calmly communicate with Mr. Smith.
D) Administer a sedative medication to Mr. Smith.

Question 92: Which of the following is an essential component of safe patient handling practices?
A) Using manual lifting techniques
B) Utilizing mechanical lifting equipment
C) Assigning patient handling tasks to untrained staff
D) Encouraging patient self-mobilization

Question 93: Which statement demonstrates the use of therapeutic communication?
A) "You should be happy that you survived the accident."
B) "Tell me more about how you're feeling."
C) "Stop crying, it's not that bad."
D) "I know exactly how you feel."

Question 94: Which intervention involves the use of a mind-body technique that allows individuals to gain control over their physiological responses to stressors?

A) Biofeedback
B) Cognitive behavioral therapy
C) Complementary alternative medicine
D) Pharmacology

Question 95: Which model of healthcare team emphasizes collaboration, communication, and shared decision-making among team members?
A) Interdisciplinary team
B) Multidisciplinary team
C) Transdisciplinary team
D) Unidisciplinary team

Question 96: John, a 40-year-old patient with a spinal cord injury, is receiving rehabilitation services in a residential facility. The nurse observes that he frequently experiences autonomic dysreflexia, characterized by sudden onset of severe hypertension, bradycardia, and throbbing headache. Which intervention would be appropriate to manage autonomic dysreflexia in John?
A) Administer a beta-blocker medication to lower blood pressure
B) Place John in a supine position with legs elevated
C) Loosen tight clothing and check for any restrictive devices
D) Administer a vasodilator medication to lower blood pressure

Question 97: When assisting a client in using adaptive equipment for eating, which action should the nurse prioritize?
A) Ensuring the equipment is clean and sanitized properly
B) Assessing the client's ability to self-feed
C) Demonstrating the correct use of the adaptive equipment
D) Providing emotional support and encouragement

Question 98: An 80-year-old patient, Mr. Johnson, has recently suffered a stroke and is experiencing difficulties with his speech. The patient's family has expressed concerns about his limited ability to communicate effectively. As the Certified Rehabilitation Registered Nurse (CRRN), what is your primary goal in implementing communication interventions for Mr. Johnson?
A) Minimizing the use of nonverbal communication techniques.
B) Facilitating independence in expressing basic needs.
C) Eliminating all forms of written communication.
D) Focusing solely on augmentative and alternative communication methods.

Question 99: The rehabilitation unit you work in is preparing for an upcoming audit conducted by a regulatory agency. As a certified rehabilitation registered nurse (CRRN), you need to ensure that the unit complies with all the necessary regulations. Which of the following is an important step to prepare for a regulatory agency audit?
A) Providing specialized training to the nursing staff only
B) Limiting the audit preparation to management personnel
C) Ensuring that documentation is complete, accurate, and up-to-date
D) Restricting patient access during the audit process

Question 100: A patient with chronic pain reports difficulty sleeping at night. Which nursing intervention would be most appropriate to optimize the patient's sleep and rest patterns?
A) Administer a sedative medication at bedtime
B) Encourage the patient to limit daytime napping

C) Provide a relaxing environment by dimming lights and reducing noise
D) Encourage the patient to engage in vigorous physical exercise before bedtime

Question 101: As a Certified Rehabilitation Registered Nurse (CRRN), you must possess the skill to incorporate ethical considerations and legal obligations that affect nursing practice. While providing care to patients, you encounter a scenario where a patient diagnosed with a severe brain injury is deemed incapable of making decisions. The patient's family members are divided on the decision to withdraw life-sustaining treatment. As the CRRN, what should be your immediate action?
A) Make the decision to withdraw life-sustaining treatment based on the family's majority vote.
B) Seek guidance from the healthcare facility's ethics committee to determine the best course of action.
C) Appoint yourself as the decision-maker due to your expertise as a CRRN.
D) Respect the autonomy of the patient's family and continue providing all necessary life-sustaining treatment.

Question 102: When applying the nursing process to optimize a patient's functional ability, which step should the nurse prioritize?
A) Assessment
B) Diagnosis
C) Planning
D) Evaluation

Question 103: Mrs. Smith is a 68-year-old patient who sustained a spinal cord injury resulting in paraplegia. She has been receiving rehabilitation therapy in an inpatient rehabilitation facility for the past 6 weeks. During a team meeting, Mrs. Smith expresses her concern about transitioning back home and resuming her daily activities. As the Certified Rehabilitation Registered Nurse (CRRN), what is your role in promoting Mrs. Smith's community reintegration and transition to the next level of care?
A) Collaborating with the physical therapist to develop a home exercise program for Mrs. Smith
B) Assisting Mrs. Smith in identifying community resources for individuals with disabilities
C) Educating Mrs. Smith and her family about adaptive equipment and assistive devices
D) Coordinating with the social worker to arrange transportation services for Mrs. Smith

Question 104: Which of the following is an essential component of rehabilitation standards and scope of practice for Certified Rehabilitation Registered Nurses (CRRN)?
A) Administering medications and performing invasive procedures
B) Conducting psychotherapy sessions for patients with mental health disorders
C) Collaborating with interdisciplinary teams for holistic patient care
D) Prescribing physical exercises and therapy modalities

Question 105: When assessing a patient's readiness for discharge, which of the following factors should the nurse consider?
A) Patient's insurance coverage
B) Patient's rehabilitation goals
C) Availability of family and caregiver support
D) Hospital's bed availability

Question 106: Which of the following is an example of an adaptive equipment used for rehabilitation purposes?
A) Smartwatch
B) Virtual reality headset
C) Smartphone
D) Cane

Question 107: Which nursing intervention is an example of an energy conservation strategy to promote sleep and rest in a rehabilitation setting?
A) Encourage the patient to ambulate independently in the room.
B) Assist the patient with dressing and grooming activities.
C) Allow the patient to rest in a well-lit room during the day.
D) Modify the patient's schedule to incorporate multiple therapy sessions.

Question 108: Mr. Johnson, a 45-year-old patient, has been admitted to the rehabilitation unit following a severe traumatic brain injury. The rehabilitation team is discussing the scope of practice for a Certified Rehabilitation Registered Nurse (CRRN). Which of the following tasks is within the scope of practice for a CRRN?
A) Prescribing medications for pain management
B) Administering physical therapy sessions
C) Developing individualized treatment plans
D) Performing surgical procedures on patients

Question 109: When participating in team and patient caregiver conferences, the role of the Certified Rehabilitation Registered Nurse (CRRN) is to:
A) Provide the medical history of the patient
B) Evaluate the patient's progress in therapy sessions
C) Advocate for the patient's preferences and goals
D) Suggest the need for additional diagnostic tests

Question 110: Which measurement tool is commonly used to assess the level of consciousness and cognitive function in patients with brain injuries?
A) Rancho Los Amigos Scale
B) Glasgow Coma Scale
C) Mini Mental State Examination
D) ASIA Scale

Question 111: When dealing with ethical dilemmas in nursing practice, which ethical theory places emphasis on the duty to adhere to moral rules and principles, regardless of the outcome?
A) Utilitarianism
B) Virtue ethics
C) Deontology
D) Ethical relativism

Question 112: Sarah is a 60-year-old patient with diabetes who has been recently admitted to a rehabilitation facility following a lower limb amputation. She has been placed on a modified diet to manage her blood glucose levels. As a CRRN, which of the following diet types should you implement for Sarah?
A) High protein diet
B) Low sodium diet
C) Renal diet
D) Diabetic diet

Question 113: Which of the following interventions is most important to implement for a patient with impaired judgment?

A) Providing handrails in all areas of the patient's living environment.
B) Educating the patient about the importance of safety precautions.
C) Assigning a nursing staff member to provide constant supervision.
D) Encouraging the patient to use assistive devices for mobility.

Question 114: Which of the following interventions promotes the respiratory function of a patient with a musculoskeletal impairment?
A) Encouraging the use of an incentive spirometer
B) Administering sedatives to promote relaxation
C) Restricting fluid intake to minimize coughing
D) Applying cold packs to the chest area

Question 115: Which of the following should be included in documentation to support regulatory requirements?
A) Patient's social security number
B) Nursing interventions provided
C) Personal opinions about the patient
D) Non-relevant medical information

Question 116: Which level of care focuses on providing comprehensive, intensive, interdisciplinary rehabilitation services to individuals with disabling conditions?
A) Assisted living
B) Hospice care
C) Acute rehab
D) Home care

Question 117: Ms. Thompson, a Certified Rehabilitation Registered Nurse (CRRN), is working in a rehabilitation facility. She is reviewing the scope of practice for rehabilitation nursing. Which of the following best describes the scope of practice for a CRRN?
A) Administering medications and performing advanced procedures
B) Creating rehabilitation plans and overseeing multidisciplinary care teams
C) Conducting research studies and analyzing data
D) Providing triage in emergency departments and managing critical care patients

Question 118: Which organization is responsible for the creation and maintenance of the National Database of Nursing Quality Indicators?
A) World Health Organization (WHO)
B) Centers for Disease Control and Prevention (CDC)
C) Agency for Healthcare Research and Quality (AHRQ)
D) Institute of Medicine (IOM)

Question 119: You are a Certified Rehabilitation Registered Nurse (CRRN) working with a patient named John, who recently sustained a spinal cord injury and is transitioning from an acute care hospital to a rehabilitation center. During your assessment, John expresses concern about his housing situation when he is discharged from the rehabilitation center. He mentions that he currently lives in a two-story house and wonders if there are any community resources available to help with housing modifications or finding accessible housing. What would be your best response to address John's concern?
A) "I'm sorry, but there are no community resources available for housing modifications or finding accessible housing."

B) "Let me contact our social worker who can provide you with information about community resources that can assist with housing modifications or finding accessible housing."
C) "You will need to start looking for a new place to live right away since the rehabilitation center doesn't provide any support with housing modifications or finding accessible housing."
D) "Housing modifications and accessible housing are not important for your recovery. You should focus on your rehabilitation exercises instead."

Question 120: Which federal legislation protects the rights of individuals with disabilities, including those receiving rehabilitation services?
A) Americans with Disabilities Act (ADA)
B) Occupational Safety and Health Act (OSHA)
C) Health Insurance Portability and Accountability Act (HIPAA)
D) Emergency Medical Treatment and Labor Act (EMTALA)

Question 121: Charles is a 45-year-old patient who recently suffered a severe traumatic brain injury (TBI) in a motor vehicle accident. Upon assessment and observation, the certified rehabilitation registered nurse (CRRN) identified impaired physical mobility related to TBI as a nursing diagnosis for Charles. Which of the following interventions is most appropriate for addressing impaired physical mobility in Charles?
A) Encouraging Charles to ambulate independently as soon as possible to regain strength and coordination.
B) Implementing a range of motion exercises to maintain joint flexibility and prevent contractures.
C) Providing frequent repositioning and turning every 2 hours to prevent pressure ulcers.
D) Administering medications to control pain and inflammation associated with the TBI.

Question 122: Mrs. Johnson, an elderly patient, has been admitted to the rehabilitation unit following a hip replacement surgery. The nurse is assessing her for potential safety concerns. Which of the following measures should the nurse prioritize to prevent falls in Mrs. Johnson?
A) Placing a restraint device on Mrs. Johnson's bed.
B) Keeping the bedrails raised at all times.
C) Providing a bedside commode for Mrs. Johnson.
D) Encouraging Mrs. Johnson to stay in bed as much as possible.

Question 123: Jane, a 45-year-old patient, has been diagnosed with a spinal cord injury and is undergoing rehabilitation. Her husband, Michael, has been actively involved in her care and attends all therapy sessions. During a family meeting, the nurse explains the importance of involving and educating support systems during the rehabilitation process. The nurse emphasizes that involving support systems can enhance the patient's progress and overall well-being. In this context, what is the primary goal of involving and educating support systems for a patient like Jane?
A) To decrease the burden on healthcare professionals
B) To improve the patient's adherence to treatment plans
C) To minimize the need for allied health professionals
D) To maintain the privacy and independence of the patient

Question 124: Samantha is a 55-year-old patient who recently underwent a stroke and is receiving rehabilitation therapy. During the assessment, the nurse observes that Samantha smokes cigarettes regularly. What action should the nurse take?

A) Advise Samantha to quit smoking immediately
B) Ignore Samantha's smoking habit as it does not affect her current health status
C) Encourage Samantha to smoke fewer cigarettes per day
D) Educate Samantha about the dangers of smoking, but respect her decision to continue

Question 125: When discussing the legal implications of healthcare-related policies and documents, the Health Insurance Portability and Accountability Act (HIPA
A) ensures which of the following?
A) The right to refuse medical treatment
B) The protection of patients' medical information
C) The provision of insurance coverage for all individuals
D) The establishment of advance directives

Question 126: During a rehabilitation session, a patient with a below-knee amputation expresses frustration with using a conventional prosthetic limb. The patient mentions difficulty in performing daily activities and desires to explore technological options. As the Certified Rehabilitation Registered Nurse (CRRN), you suggest exploring the use of computer-supported prosthetics to assist the patient. Which of the following is a benefit of using computer-supported prosthetics for individuals with lower limb amputations?
A) Increased risk of falls and injuries
B) Limited ability to customize and adjust the prosthetic
C) Improved balance and stability during walking
D) Inability to use the prosthetic in different environments

Question 127: A patient is admitted to the rehabilitation unit with a diagnosis of spinal cord injury at level C6. The nurse is responsible for ensuring that the patient's care respects the legislative, economic, ethical, and legal issues surrounding the provision of care. Which action demonstrates the nurse's skill in legislative and regulatory management of care?
A) Educating the patient about the potential complications of a spinal cord injury.
B) Collaborating with the interdisciplinary team to develop an individualized care plan.
C) Ensuring that the patient's privacy is maintained by closing curtains during personal care.
D) Adhering to infection control practices when inserting a urinary catheter.

Question 128: Which of the following is NOT a risk factor for patient falls in a rehabilitation setting?
A) Advanced age
B) Impaired gait
C) Use of assistive devices
D) Adequate lighting

Question 129: A patient is admitted to the rehabilitation unit following a stroke. The nurse is assessing the patient's functional health patterns. Which of the following areas should the nurse specifically assess to evaluate the patient's ability to perform activities of daily living (ADLs)?
A) Nutritional-Metabolic pattern.
B) Sleep-Rest pattern.
C) Self-Perception-Self-Concept pattern.
D) Activity-Exercise pattern.

Question 130: Which diet is recommended for individuals with renal impairment?
A) Cardiac diet
B) Diabetic diet
C) Renal diet

D) Dysphagia diet

Question 131: John, a 60-year-old male, has recently been discharged from a rehabilitation facility following a stroke. He is currently living alone and is financially struggling as he was the sole breadwinner for his family. His daughter, who lives in another city, wants to provide financial assistance to him. What resources can the nurse suggest to John that may help him with his financial situation?
A) Applying for government assistance programs
B) Finding a part-time job to supplement his income
C) Seeking financial advice from a professional
D) Borrowing money from friends and family

Question 132: Which team member is responsible for coordinating the transition of care for a patient in rehabilitation?
A) Physical therapist
B) Social worker
C) Registered nurse
D) Occupational therapist

Question 133: Which of the following conditions is characterized by excessive fluid retention?
A) Dehydration
B) Hypovolemia
C) Hypertonicity
D) Edema

Question 134: A patient with a diagnosis of multiple sclerosis (MS) is experiencing fatigue and decreased activity tolerance. The patient is scheduled to attend physical therapy sessions twice a week. During the physical therapy session, the nurse would incorporate which of the following strategies to promote activity tolerance and conserve the patient's energy?
A) Encourage the patient to engage in high-intensity exercises to build endurance.
B) Instruct the patient to continuously exercise without taking rest breaks.
C) Teach the patient deep breathing and relaxation techniques before and after exercise.
D) Discourage the use of assistive devices to challenge the patient's abilities.

Question 135: Mr. Johnson, a 45-year-old patient with Parkinson's disease, has been experiencing difficulty in writing legibly. The nurse recommends the use of assistive technology to improve his writing ability. Which assistive technology or adaptive equipment would be most suitable for Mr. Johnson?
A) Hearing aid
B) Reading glasses
C) Writing guide
D) Bedside commode

Question 136: When implementing interventions for skin integrity, which factor should the Certified Rehabilitation Registered Nurse (CRRN) prioritize?
A) Moisture reduction
B) Nutrition and hydration
C) Skin assessment
D) Pressure relief

Question 137: Which organ releases insulin to regulate blood sugar levels in the body?
A) Liver
B) Pancreas
C) Stomach

D) Kidneys

Question 138: Ms. Johnson, a 60-year-old patient with a history of a stroke, has been admitted to a rehabilitation facility. As a Certified Rehabilitation Registered Nurse (CRRN), you are actively involved in collaborating with the interdisciplinary team to achieve patient-centered goals. Which of the following is NOT a role of the rehabilitation nurse in this team?
A) Assessing the patient's rehabilitation needs and developing an individualized care plan.
B) Coordinating and providing direct care to the patient, including physical therapy and medication administration.
C) Communicating and collaborating with the patient's family and caregivers to ensure continuity of care.
D) Conducting research and contributing to evidence-based practice for improved patient outcomes.

Question 139: Which of the following is a key characteristic of evidence-based research?
A) It is based on opinions and personal experiences.
B) It focuses on maintaining traditional practices.
C) It relies on anecdotal evidence.
D) It incorporates scientific evidence and clinical expertise.

Question 140: Which assessment method can the nurse utilize to evaluate a patient's ability for effective communication?
A) Observing non-verbal cues
B) Conducting a physical examination
C) Reviewing laboratory test results
D) Collecting a patient's medical history

Question 141: Ms. Johnson, a 45-year-old female patient, has been admitted to the rehabilitation unit following a spinal cord injury. The nurse is assessing her elimination patterns. Which of the following findings would require immediate intervention?
A) The patient reports difficulty initiating urination and incomplete bladder emptying.
B) The patient reports occasional constipation and tends to strain during bowel movements.
C) The patient reports having a regular bowel movement pattern of once every two to three days.
D) The patient reports experiencing occasional episodes of urinary incontinence during coughing or sneezing.

Question 142: Mrs. Johnson, a 45-year-old patient with a spinal cord injury, is at risk for developing autonomic dysreflexia. The nurse is providing education to Mrs. Johnson and her family about preventing this complication. Which teaching intervention should the nurse prioritize?
A) Encouraging adequate fluid intake
B) Promoting regular bowel movements
C) Emphasizing the importance of proper bladder management
D) Instructing the patient to have regular skin checks

Question 143: Emma is a rehabilitation nurse who wants to apply quality measurement tools in her practice. She is responsible for collecting data on patient outcomes to assess the effectiveness of the rehabilitation interventions. Which of the following quality measurement tools should Emma use?
A) SWOT analysis
B) Root cause analysis
C) Nursing-sensitive indicators
D) Failure mode and effects analysis

Question 144: During a team conference, the rehabilitation team is discussing the discharge planning for Ms. Johnson, a 65-year-old patient who suffered a stroke and has left-sided weakness. The patient and her daughter, who is her primary caregiver, are present in the conference. The team agrees that Ms. Johnson requires further therapy and assistance with daily living activities at a skilled nursing facility before she can safely return home. The nurse's role in this conference is to:

A) Offer a dissenting opinion and suggest that Ms. Johnson should be discharged directly home with home health services.

B) Keep silent and observe the discussion without actively engaging or providing input.

C) Advocate for Ms. Johnson's preferences and actively participate in the discussion.

D) Disregard the patient and caregiver's input, as they may be unfamiliar with the options available.

Question 145: Which of the following best describes the scope of practice for a Certified Rehabilitation Registered Nurse (CRRN)?

A) Providing direct patient care during the acute phase of illness or injury.

B) Administering medications and performing advanced procedures independently.

C) Collaborating with interdisciplinary teams to develop and implement individualized care plans.

D) Conducting research studies and publishing findings in scholarly journals.

Question 146: Which of the following medications should be closely monitored for potential adverse effects on patient safety?

A) Anticoagulants
B) Acetaminophen
C) Antihistamines
D) Antibiotics

Question 147: Which tool is commonly used to assess an individual's risk for developing pressure ulcers?

A) FLACC scale
B) Braden scale
C) Wong-Baker FACES scale
D) CAGE questionnaire

Question 148: Mary, a 45-year-old patient, has been admitted to a rehabilitation facility following a stroke. As a Certified Rehabilitation Registered Nurse (CRRN), you are responsible for promoting a safe environment of care for patients and staff. Which of the following actions will help minimize safety risk factors for Mary?

A) Conducting regular safety inspections of the patient's room.

B) Providing Mary with assistive devices such as handrails and non-slip mats.

C) Ensuring that Mary's medications are within reach on her bedside table.

D) Ignoring potential hazards if they don't appear to be immediate threats.

Question 149: Ms. Johnson, a Certified Rehabilitation Registered Nurse (CRRN), is working in a rehabilitation center. She notices that there have been several incidents of medication errors in the facility. She decides to implement a quality improvement process to address this issue. Which of the following steps should Ms. Johnson take as part of the quality improvement process?

A) Assess the current medication administration policies and protocols in the facility

B) Ignore the incidents as they may be isolated cases

C) Delegate the task of addressing the issue to a nursing assistant

D) Implement disciplinary action against the staff involved in the incidents

Question 150: Which step of the nursing process involves gathering information about the patient's present health condition and past medical history?

A) Assessment
B) Diagnosis
C) Planning
D) Evaluation

ANSWERS WITH DETAILED EXPLANATION (SET 2)

Question 1: Correct Answer: C) Collaborate with local rehabilitation facilities to provide comprehensive care.
Rationale: Collaborating with local rehabilitation facilities is an essential action for a CRRN when working with private, community, and public resources. By collaborating with these facilities, the nurse can ensure that the patient receives comprehensive care that addresses their rehabilitation needs. This collaboration allows for the sharing of expertise, resources, and support systems that can enhance the patient's overall well-being and recovery. Working independently without seeking assistance from external resources (Option A) is not an appropriate approach as it may limit the quality and effectiveness of care. Referring the patient to online support groups (Option B) is valuable, but it may not provide the comprehensive care needed. Encouraging the patient to rely solely on healthcare insurance coverage (Option D) neglects the importance of collaborating with diverse resources to meet the patient's needs.

Question 2: Correct Answer: D) Engaging patients in decision-making and respecting their choices
Rationale: Patient-centered care involves actively involving patients in their healthcare decisions and respecting their choices. It emphasizes tailoring care to meet the unique needs, values, and preferences of individual patients. Providing care based solely on healthcare provider preferences, focusing only on physical aspects, or disregarding patient values and preferences goes against the principles of patient-centered care. By engaging patients in decision-making and respecting their choices, healthcare providers can ensure that care is aligned with patients' goals, values, and preferences, leading to improved patient satisfaction, compliance, and outcomes.

Question 3: Correct Answer: C) Assigning a higher nurse-to-patient ratio during high-acuity shifts.
Rationale: By assigning a higher nurse-to-patient ratio during high-acuity shifts, the registered nurse ensures that patients receive appropriate care without compromising their safety. During periods of increased acuity, patients may require closer monitoring and more complex interventions. By assigning more nurses to manage these patients, the nurse can provide timely interventions and prevent adverse events. This staffing pattern promotes cost-effective, patient-centered care by maximizing resources while ensuring patient safety and quality outcomes. Increasing the number of registered nurses on the unit or hiring more nursing assistants may improve staffing levels but may not address the acuity of patients. Utilizing floating staff from different units may not have the required expertise to manage high-acuity patients.

Question 4: Correct Answer: C) Using open-ended questions to encourage the patient to express feelings
Rationale: The patient's withdrawn behavior and avoidance of eye contact might indicate feelings of anxiety, fear, or discomfort. By using open-ended questions, the nurse can encourage the patient to express their feelings, thoughts, and concerns without imposing any judgments or restrictions. This technique allows the patient to share their experiences at their own pace and promotes a therapeutic environment that fosters trust and open communication. Focusing on the patient's physical appearance may not address the underlying emotional issues. Offering advice and solutions may diminish the patient's autonomy and hinder their ability to express themselves. Avoiding silence and filling it with unnecessary conversation may be overwhelming for the patient and prevent them from sharing their thoughts and feelings.

Question 5: Correct Answer: D) Influenza
Rationale: An acute illness refers to a condition that develops suddenly and lasts for a short period. Influenza, commonly known as the flu, is an example of an acute illness. It is characterized by a sudden onset of symptoms such as fever, body aches, cough, sore throat, and fatigue. In contrast, chronic illnesses like COPD, hypertension, and kidney failure are long-term conditions that require ongoing management and may have a gradual onset. It is important for rehabilitation nurses to differentiate between acute and chronic illnesses to provide appropriate care and intervention strategies for patients.

Question 6: Correct Answer: B) Encouraging Mary to perform Kegel exercises to strengthen pelvic floor muscles
Rationale: In the given scenario, Mary is experiencing urinary incontinence following a stroke. The most appropriate intervention for bladder management in this case would be to encourage Mary to perform Kegel exercises. Kegel exercises help strengthen the pelvic floor muscles, which can improve urinary control. Restricting fluid intake may lead to dehydration and is not a suitable long-term solution. Pharmacological agents should be used cautiously and only if non-invasive interventions are ineffective. Providing adaptive equipment such as adult diapers should be considered when other interventions fail to improve urinary control.

Question 7: Correct Answer: B) Discuss the family's concerns with the healthcare team and consider referring the patient to a specialist in dysphagia management.
Rationale: Given the patient's worsening condition and the lack of improvement with current interventions, it is essential to address the family's concerns and explore additional avenues for the patient's care. By discussing the concerns with the healthcare team and considering a referral to a specialist in dysphagia management, the appropriate course of action can be identified. This demonstrates the nurse's commitment to facilitating appropriate referrals and ensures that the patient receives the specialized care required to improve his swallowing difficulties. Ignoring the family's request (Option A) or suggesting alternative therapies (Option D) may not address the patient's needs effectively, while informing the family that referrals are not necessary (Option C) disregards their valid concerns and may inhibit the patient's progress in rehabilitation.

Question 8: Correct Answer: A) Social Security Administration
Rationale: The Social Security Administration can provide financial assistance and benefits for individuals with disabilities, such as Mr. Johnson. They can help him access resources such as disability benefits, Medicaid, and vocational rehabilitation services. This will support him in his rehabilitation journey and help with his daily living needs. The Department of Parks and Recreation, Public Health Department, and Department of Motor Vehicles do not offer services specific to Mr. Johnson's situation and needs.

Question 9: Correct Answer: C) Encouraging the patient to discuss their fears and concerns with a support group.
Rationale: Encouraging the patient to discuss their fears and concerns with a support group can help promote optimal psychosocial patterns and coping skills. Support groups provide a safe space for individuals with similar experiences to share their feelings, learn from others, and receive emotional support. This intervention addresses the patient's psychosocial needs by offering them an outlet to express their emotions and cope with the changes in their life. Providing education on adaptive techniques (option A) and engaging in physical therapy exercises (option D) are essential interventions for addressing functional needs but may not specifically target the patient's psychosocial well-being. Administering medication (option B) may help manage

physical discomfort but does not directly address the psychosocial aspects of coping and stress management.

Question 10: Correct Answer: C) "I will follow a balanced diet and maintain a healthy weight to prevent complications."

Rationale: It is important for patients with spinal cord injuries to maintain a healthy lifestyle to prevent complications. Following a balanced diet and maintaining a healthy weight can help reduce the risk of pressure ulcers, improve bowel and bladder function, and promote overall well-being. Physical activities and exercises are also essential for maintaining strength and independence. Relying solely on a caregiver for daily activities may hinder the patient's ability to regain independence. Additionally, following safety measures and precautions at home is crucial to prevent accidents and promote a safe environment.

Question 11: Correct Answer: B) "Biofeedback uses electronic devices to measure and display physiological functions to improve self-awareness and self-regulation."

Rationale: Biofeedback is a technique that uses electronic devices to measure and display physiological functions such as heart rate, blood pressure, and muscle tension. By providing real-time feedback, it helps individuals become aware of their body's responses and learn to self-regulate. This can be useful for managing stress, pain, and other psychophysiological conditions. Option A is incorrect as it describes distraction rather than biofeedback. Option C is incorrect as it describes relaxation techniques rather than biofeedback. Option D is incorrect as it describes meditation techniques rather than biofeedback.

Question 12: Correct Answer: B) Roy Adaptation Model

Rationale: The Roy Adaptation Model focuses on the patient's ability to adapt to their environment and promote health and well-being through four adaptive modes: physiological, self-concept, role function, and interdependence. This model emphasizes the nurse's role in assessing the patient's adaptive responses and intervening to promote adaptation. As Ms. Johnson is in need of rehabilitation care following a stroke, the Roy Adaptation Model would be most appropriate to guide the team in providing comprehensive care that addresses her physiological, psychological, and social needs during the recovery process.

Question 13: Correct Answer: C) Improved accuracy and accessibility of patient information

Rationale: By implementing an electronic documentation system, Ms. Johnson can ensure improved accuracy and accessibility of patient information. Electronic systems allow for more efficient tracking and storage of patient data, reducing the risk of errors and improving overall patient safety. This system also enables better communication and coordination among healthcare providers, leading to increased efficiency and ultimately saving costs. By digitizing patient records, the facility can reduce the reliance on paper, contributing to reduced waste and environmental impact. Therefore, implementing this system is a cost-effective approach that benefits both patients and the facility.

Question 14: Correct Answer: C) Denial

Rationale: Mr. Davis's constant questioning and disbelief about his diagnosis indicate that he is in the denial stage of grief and loss. During this stage, individuals may experience shock, numbness, and denial as they struggle to accept the reality of their situation. They may refuse to acknowledge their illness or delay seeking appropriate care. It is important for the rehabilitation nurse to provide support, educate the patient about their condition, and help them gradually move towards acceptance and adaptive coping strategies.

Question 15: Correct Answer: D) Assisting Mrs. Johnson to sit in an upright position during meals.

Rationale: Assisting Mrs. Johnson to sit in an upright position during meals promotes optimal digestion and prevents aspiration. This position facilitates swallowing, reduces the risk of choking, and enhances the absorption of nutrients. Encouraging her to eat a high-protein diet is important for wound healing but does not specifically address optimal nutrition and hydration. Limiting fluid intake can lead to dehydration, while providing whole milk may be contraindicated due to Mrs. Johnson's health condition. Therefore, the correct action is to assist Mrs. Johnson in maintaining an upright position during meals to promote optimal nutrition and hydration.

Question 16: Correct Answer: B) Weighted utensils

Rationale: Weighted utensils would be most appropriate for Ms. Johnson to facilitate independent feeding. The weight in the utensils provides additional stability, making it easier for the patient to control and manipulate the utensils despite her weakness and coordination difficulties. Curved utensils are typically used for individuals with limited hand mobility or arthritis. Nonslip mats are used to prevent plates and bowls from sliding during mealtime, but they do not directly address Ms. Johnson's swallowing difficulties. Scoop plates are designed for patients with limited coordination or the use of only one hand, which is not the case for Ms. Johnson. Weighted utensils would best support her feeding independence while accommodating her current physical limitations.

Question 17: Correct Answer: D) Exploring Samantha's spiritual beliefs and offering support from a chaplain or spiritual care provider

Rationale: In order to incorporate cultural awareness and spiritual values in the plan of care, the nurse should explore Samantha's spiritual beliefs and offer support from a chaplain or spiritual care provider. This demonstrates a holistic approach to care that acknowledges and respects Samantha's spiritual needs. Providing culturally appropriate food options (option A) may be important, but it does not directly address her spiritual distress. Encouraging participation in physical therapy (option B) and assisting with personal hygiene and dressing changes (option C) are important aspects of care, but they do not specifically address her spiritual distress. Therefore, option D is the correct answer.

Question 18: Correct Answer: A) Provide Sarah's husband with information about community support groups for traumatic brain injury caregivers.

Rationale: Providing education and support to the family is crucial in addressing the psychosocial needs of both the patient and the caregivers. In this scenario, Sarah's husband expresses concerns about the changes he has observed in Sarah since the injury. By providing information about community support groups for traumatic brain injury caregivers, the nurse acknowledges the husband's concerns and offers him an opportunity to connect with others who are facing similar challenges. This support network can provide emotional support, coping strategies, and valuable resources to navigate the caregiving process. It is important to empower the husband with information that can facilitate his role as a caregiver and enhance the overall well-being of both Sarah and her family.

Question 19: Correct Answer: A) The patient will have complete loss of voluntary control over the external anal sphincter.

Rationale: A spinal cord injury at level T4 results in paraplegia, affecting the lower extremities and the trunk below the level of injury. This level of injury also causes a complete loss of voluntary control over the external anal sphincter, leading to neurogenic bowel dysfunction. The patient will require programs consisting of scheduled bowel evacuation, digital stimulation, suppositories, and/or enemas to achieve regular bowel movements. Options B, C, and D are incorrect statements as they do not correlate with the altered bowel function associated with a T4 spinal cord injury.

Question 20: Correct Answer: B) Implementing a routine sleep schedule

Rationale: Implementing a routine sleep schedule is the priority intervention to optimize Mitchell's sleep and rest patterns. Establishing a consistent bedtime routine helps regulate the sleep-wake cycle and promotes better sleep quality. Administering a sedative medication may lead to dependency and should be used cautiously. Encouraging napping throughout the day can disrupt nighttime sleep, and limiting fluid intake after dinner alone may not address the complex factors influencing sleep patterns after a stroke. Therefore, prioritizing a routine sleep schedule is the most appropriate intervention in this scenario.

Question 21: Correct Answer: C) Implementing a scheduled self-catheterization program for Mr. Johnson

Rationale: Implementing a scheduled self-catheterization program will assist Mr. Johnson in regaining control over his bladder function. This intervention involves teaching him how to insert a urinary catheter at specific intervals to empty the bladder completely, reducing the instances of incontinence. It is a safe and effective technique commonly used for patients with neurological conditions, such as multiple sclerosis, who have difficulty controlling their urination. It allows for the management of urine retention, regular emptying of the bladder, and restoration of bladder control. Encouraging him to consume caffeinated beverages, holding urine for extended periods, or reducing fluid intake are not appropriate interventions for improving bladder control.

Question 22: Correct Answer: C) The patient demonstrates difficulty understanding written instructions.

Rationale: Difficulty understanding written instructions can indicate a deficit in the patient's ability to comprehend and process information, which can hinder effective communication. Nursing intervention may involve providing alternative forms of communication, such as visual aids or verbal instructions, to enhance understanding. Options A, B, and D may also indicate communication challenges, but they do not directly address the optimization of the patient's ability to understand written instructions. Therefore, option C is the correct answer.

Question 23: Correct Answer: C) Assign a sitter to be with the patient at all times.

Rationale: Assigning a sitter to be with the patient at all times is the most appropriate safety intervention for a patient with right-sided weakness and expressive aphasia. This intervention ensures constant supervision and assistance, reducing the risk of falls and providing immediate help in case of any emergency or need. The other options may not be as effective or appropriate for this patient. Reorienting the patient frequently may not address the underlying weakness and communication difficulties. Non-behavioral restraints should be avoided unless absolutely necessary due to the associated risks. Providing a quiet and dimly lit environment may not directly address the safety concern of falls.

Question 24: Correct Answer: D) Collaborating with the healthcare team to develop an individualized care plan.

Rationale: Collaborating with the healthcare team to develop an individualized care plan is the best action that demonstrates the use of the nursing process to deliver cost-effective patient-centered care for Mrs. Adams. By involving the healthcare team, including physical therapists and pain management specialists, the nurse ensures that all aspects of Mrs. Adams' care are addressed and coordinated efficiently. This collaborative approach minimizes redundancy, reduces costs, and focuses on meeting Mrs. Adams' specific needs, making it the most patient-centered and cost-effective option. Requesting a CBC may be necessary in certain situations but is not directly related to Mrs. Adams' pain and mobility.

Initiating physical therapy sessions and administering pain medication are important interventions but do not encompass the comprehensive approach of the nursing process.

Question 25: Correct Answer: C) Islam

Rationale: Ramadan is a religious practice observed by Muslims worldwide. During this month, individuals fast from sunrise to sunset, abstaining from food and drink. This practice is meant to promote self-discipline, empathy for those less fortunate, and spiritual reflection. It is important for rehabilitation registered nurses to be aware of this cultural and religious practice, as it may impact a patient's dietary habits and medication administration during the fasting hours. By understanding and respecting the religious beliefs and practices of patients, nurses can provide culturally sensitive care and support their nutritional needs accordingly.

Question 26: Correct Answer: A) Hyperreflexia

Rationale: Sensorimotor deficits often result in an abnormal response in reflexes. Hyperreflexia, which is an exaggerated reflex response, is a common clinical sign of sensorimotor deficits. It is characterized by an overactive response in reflexes such as deep tendon reflexes, which may result in exaggerated movements or jerking of muscles. This is due to damage or dysfunction in the sensory or motor pathways of the nervous system. Hypoactive bowel sounds (option B) may be present in other conditions but are not directly associated with sensorimotor deficits. Increased coordination (option C) is unlikely in the presence of sensorimotor deficits. Normal muscle tone (option D) may also be present in sensorimotor deficits, but it is not a specific clinical sign.

Question 27: Correct Answer: C) PPS determines reimbursement rates based on the patient's length of stay and specific diagnosis-related groups (DRGs).

Rationale: Option C is the correct answer because under the Prospective Payment System (PPS), reimbursement rates for Medicare beneficiaries are determined based on the patient's length of stay and specific diagnosis-related groups (DRGs). This system helps control costs by assigning a fixed payment amount for each DRG, irrespective of the actual costs incurred by the healthcare provider. This approach promotes cost-effectiveness and standardized care delivery. Options A, B, and D are incorrect because PPS does not reimburse based on actual costs, does not use a fee-for-service model, and applies to both inpatient hospital stays and post-acute care services.

Question 28: Correct Answer: D) Healing touch

Rationale: Healing touch is an alternative modality that involves using gentle touch on or near the body to promote healing and relaxation. It is based on the concept that energy flows through the body and can be manipulated to enhance the body's ability to heal itself. Healing touch can be beneficial for patients with spinal cord injuries as it may help reduce pain, improve sleep, and enhance overall well-being. Acupuncture focuses on the insertion of thin needles into specific points of the body, meditation involves deep relaxation and focus of the mind, and aromatherapy uses essential oils for therapeutic purposes. While these modalities may have their benefits, they are not specifically based on therapeutic touch like healing touch is.

Question 29: Correct Answer: A) Clean the dressing with sterile saline and replace it with a sterile dressing.

Rationale: In this scenario, the nurse should prioritize cleaning the dressing with sterile saline and replacing it with a sterile dressing to maintain catheter site hygiene and prevent infection. A soiled dressing increases the risk of infection and can lead to complications such as catheter-related bloodstream infections. Removing the dressing without proper precautions or resecuring the dressing with additional tape may cause further complications or compromise catheter site integrity. Therefore, option A is the correct answer based on the principles of maintaining catheter care and preventing infection.

Question 30: Correct Answer: A) To maintain normal oxygen saturation levels and prevent further lung damage

Rationale: Assisted ventilation in patients with ARDS aims to maintain normal oxygen saturation levels and prevent further lung damage. ARDS is characterized by severe hypoxemia and increased work of breathing. By providing ventilatory support, assisted ventilation helps deliver adequate oxygen to the tissues and reduces the strain on the patient's respiratory muscles. The primary goal is to ensure adequate oxygenation and prevent complications associated with hypoxemia, such as organ dysfunction. Assisted ventilation is typically initiated in the acute setting and not intended for long-term use. Therefore, option D is incorrect. Additionally, ventilatory support does not directly improve lung compliance or decrease airway resistance (option C). While assisted ventilation may indirectly reduce the workload of the heart, its primary purpose is to address oxygenation and lung function in ARDS (option B is incorrect).

Question 31: Correct Answer: B) To enhance communication between patients and healthcare providers

Rationale: Personal response devices, such as call buttons or nurse call systems, are used in rehabilitation settings to enhance communication between patients and healthcare providers. These devices enable patients to call for assistance when they require help with activities of daily living, are in pain, or have any other immediate needs. By having access to these devices, patients can feel more secure and have quicker access to healthcare providers when necessary. Monitoring vital signs, administering medications, and fall prevention are important aspects of patient care but not the primary purpose of personal response devices in a rehabilitation setting.

Question 32: Correct Answer: B) Improve joint flexibility

Rationale: The goal of passive ROM exercises is to improve joint flexibility. These exercises are performed by the therapist or nurse passively moving the patient's limbs through a full range of motion to prevent contractures and maintain joint mobility. Passive ROM exercises do not focus on increasing muscle strength, enhancing cardiovascular endurance, or improving coordination and balance. These goals may be addressed through other interventions such as active ROM exercises, strength training, aerobic conditioning, and balance training, respectively.

Question 33: Correct Answer: D) Assisting with activities of daily living (ADLs).

Rationale: The Self-care Deficit Nursing Theory (SCDNT) emphasizes assisting individuals in meeting their self-care needs. Assisting with activities of daily living (ADLs) is a fundamental part of self-care. Providing physical assistance and encouraging independence in performing ADLs can enhance Mrs. Anderson's rehabilitation progress and overall well-being. While assessing mobility, administering pain medication, and providing emotional support are important aspects of care, they are not the primary focus according to the SCDNT. The theory prioritizes assisting individuals in performing self-care activities to the extent possible to promote optimal functioning and independence.

Question 34: Correct Answer: C) Prefrontal cortex

Rationale: The prefrontal cortex is primarily responsible for executive functions, such as cognition, judgment, decision-making, and impulse control. Damage to this area, whether due to trauma, stroke, or neurodegenerative diseases, can result in deficits in these cognitive processes. The hippocampus is more involved in memory formation and retrieval, while the cerebellum primarily controls motor coordination. The amygdala is responsible for emotional processing. Therefore, the prefrontal cortex is the most likely

brain structure associated with deficits in cognition and judgment.

Question 35: Correct Answer: B) Discuss the medication prescription with the prescriber to ensure its appropriateness.

Rationale: As a CRRN, it is essential to practice within the scope of rehabilitation nursing and adhere to rehabilitation standards. In this situation, it is crucial to question a medication prescription that deviates from the usual stroke rehabilitation protocols. By discussing the medication prescription with the prescriber, the nurse ensures patient safety and promotes evidence-based practice in rehabilitation. This step allows for a collaborative approach to healthcare, involving the interdisciplinary team's expertise and avoiding potential adverse effects or contraindications specific to the patient's condition.

Question 36: Correct Answer: B) Contact the healthcare facility's ethics committee for guidance.

Rationale: In this situation, the nurse should contact the healthcare facility's ethics committee for guidance. Without a designated healthcare proxy or advance directives, Mr. Smith's autonomy and ability to make decisions about his own care are compromised. The ethics committee can provide guidance on the ethical considerations and legal obligations involved in providing nutrition and hydration for non-verbal patients without clear directives. It is important to involve the ethics committee to ensure that the best interest of the patient is upheld and that the nursing practice aligns with ethical and legal principles. Respecting the family's wishes without proper guidance may not fully address the ethical and legal implications involved in this complex situation.

Question 37: Correct Answer: C) Watson's Theory of Human Caring

Rationale: Watson's Theory of Human Caring emphasizes the importance of building a caring relationship between the nurse and the patient. In the case of Ms. Johnson, who is going through a challenging phase after a stroke, this theory would guide the nurse in providing holistic and compassionate care, fostering a healing environment, and enhancing her overall well-being. The theory aligns with the principles of patient-centered care and emphasizes the nurse's role in promoting healing and restoring the patient's sense of wholeness. This approach can facilitate Ms. Johnson's physical and emotional recovery, allowing her to regain independence and improve her quality of life during rehabilitation.

Question 38: Correct Answer: A) Poorly maintained equipment

Rationale: In a rehabilitation setting, it is crucial to minimize safety risk factors to provide a safe environment for patients and staff. One of these risk factors is poorly maintained equipment. Equipment that is not properly maintained can malfunction or pose a threat to patient safety. Regular maintenance checks and repairs should be carried out to ensure that all equipment is in good working condition. Adequate staffing levels (option B) and regular safety training for staff (option C) are also important measures to promote a safe environment. While encouraging patient independence (option D) is a goal in rehabilitation, it is not directly related to minimizing safety risk factors.

Question 39: Correct Answer: A) Critical thinking and problem-solving

Rationale: When addressing legislative, economic, ethical, and legal issues in patient care, critical thinking and problem-solving skills are essential for a CRRN. These skills enable the nurse to analyze complex situations, gather relevant information, and make informed decisions that comply with legal and ethical standards. By using critical thinking, a CRRN can effectively navigate through legislative and economic factors, considering the impact on patient care. By employing problem-solving skills, they can resolve ethical dilemmas and make decisions that support optimal patient outcomes while adhering to legal guidelines. The ability to think critically and solve problems is vital for a CRRN to provide patient-centered care within the context of legislative, economic, ethical, and legal considerations.

Question 40: Correct Answer: B) Social and environmental factors

Rationale: Assessing a patient's sleep and rest patterns requires consideration of various factors. Among these factors, social and environmental aspects are crucial. These factors may include the patient's living situation, noise levels, the presence of distractions or interruptions, and the availability of a comfortable sleeping environment. By evaluating social and environmental factors, a Rehabilitation Registered Nurse can identify potential barriers to optimal sleep and rest patterns that may hinder the patient's recovery and well-being. Therefore, it is essential for nurses to assess and address these factors in order to optimize the patient's sleep and rest patterns.

Question 41: Correct Answer: D) Psychologist

Rationale: A psychologist specializes in mental health and can provide appropriate support and counseling for the patient's emotional challenges such as anxiety and depression. While a neurologist focuses on the diagnosis and treatment of neurological disorders, a teacher is not qualified to provide mental health support, and a case manager primarily coordinates the patient's care and resources. Therefore, the most appropriate professional resource for this patient is a psychologist, who can address his emotional needs during rehabilitation.

Question 42: Correct Answer: A) Crutches

Rationale: Crutches are commonly used assistive devices for individuals with weakened lower extremities. They provide support and stability during walking, allowing individuals to maintain balance and reduce stress on the lower limbs. Crutches are particularly helpful for individuals with temporary or short-term mobility issues, such as those recovering from lower extremity injuries or surgeries. Hearing aids (option B) are used for hearing impairment, wheelchair (option C) is used for individuals with significant mobility limitations, and a prosthetic limb (option D) is used for individuals with limb amputations. While all these devices are important, crutches specifically address the needs of individuals with weakened lower extremities.

Question 43: Correct Answer: B) Lack of caregiver support at home

Rationale: A social barrier refers to challenges arising from the social environment that impede an individual's reintegration into the community. In this scenario, having a lack of caregiver support at home can significantly hinder Elizabeth's ability to reintegrate into the community. Having a caregiver to assist with daily activities, provide emotional support, and ensure her safety and well-being is essential for Elizabeth's successful community reintegration. Inaccessible public transportation options (choice A) would be considered an environmental barrier. Difficulty using assistive devices (choice C) is a personal barrier. Cognitive impairments (choice D) fall under the category of health-related barriers. However, in this scenario, the lack of caregiver support is the primary social barrier affecting Elizabeth's community reintegration.

Question 44: Correct Answer: A) The PDCA model is a continuous improvement framework that involves four stages: planning, doing, checking, and acting.

Rationale: The PDCA (Plan, Do, Check, Act) model is a widely used continuous improvement framework. It involves four stages: planning, doing, checking, and acting. In the planning phase, data and information are gathered, potential causes are identified, and a plan is developed. In the doing phase, the plan is implemented on a small scale to test its

effectiveness. In the checking phase, data is collected and analyzed to evaluate the outcomes and determine if any adjustments are needed. In the acting phase, changes are made based on the results of the previous stages to improve the process further. The PDCA model provides a structured approach to process improvement and fosters a culture of continuous learning and improvement.

Question 45: Correct Answer: B) Economic concerns and financial resources

Rationale: When utilizing the nursing process, the nurse must take economic concerns and financial resources into account to deliver cost-effective patient-centered care. This includes considering the patient's ability to afford healthcare services, availability of insurance coverage, and the cost-effectiveness of treatment options. By considering economic factors, the nurse can ensure that the care provided is both appropriate and affordable for the patient. Legislative standards and guidelines (Option A) are important to ensure healthcare practices are in line with legal requirements, but they may not directly impact cost-effectiveness. Ethical principles and moral obligations (Option C) guide nursing practice but do not specifically address cost-effectiveness. Legal issues and liability concerns (Option D) pertain to the legal aspects of nursing care, but may not directly influence cost-effectiveness.

Question 46: Correct Answer: A) Pain level, anxiety, and medication side effects

Rationale: To optimize the patient's sleep and rest patterns, the rehabilitation registered nurse should consider factors such as pain level, anxiety, and medication side effects. Pain can significantly disrupt sleep and rest, so appropriate pain management interventions should be implemented. Anxiety can also contribute to sleep disturbances, and addressing anxiety through relaxation techniques or medications can promote better sleep. Medication side effects, such as insomnia or sedation, should be identified and managed accordingly. Considering these factors can help the nurse develop a comprehensive plan to improve the patient's sleep and rest patterns during rehabilitation.

Question 47: Correct Answer: A) Financial constraints

Rationale: Financial constraints can pose a significant barrier to community reintegration for individuals with disabilities. The cost of adaptive equipment, assistive devices, and necessary modifications to their living environment can be substantial. These financial burdens may prevent individuals from accessing the resources and support needed to participate fully in community activities and engage in meaningful occupations. Adequate transportation, a supportive social network, and accessible recreational facilities are important factors that facilitate community reintegration, rather than barriers. However, financial constraints can hinder individuals' ability to access these resources and participate in community life.

Question 48: Correct Answer: C) Listen to the suggestion and ask for more information before making a decision.

Rationale: As a CRRN working with an interdisciplinary team, it is important to value the input and expertise of all team members. In this scenario, the appropriate response is to actively listen to the physical therapist's suggestion and ask for more information. This allows for collaboration and a better understanding of the proposed treatment approach. As the CRRN, you can then make an informed decision based on the patient's specific needs, goals, and the input from the entire team. Effective communication and collaboration are essential for achieving patient-centered goals in rehabilitation care.

Question 49: Correct Answer: B) Providing small, frequent meals throughout the day

Rationale: When addressing the safety concern of dysphagia, it is important for the CRRN to prioritize interventions that promote optimal nutrition and hydration. Providing small, frequent meals throughout the day allows for better control of the swallowing process and minimizes the risk of aspiration. This approach also helps to prevent fatigue during meals. Encouraging the patient to eat rapidly can increase the risk of choking, while allowing the patient to eat in a reclined position may lead to aspiration. Offering foods with mixed textures in the same meal can be challenging for individuals with dysphagia and may increase the risk of choking or aspiration. Therefore, option B is the correct intervention to prioritize in this scenario.

Question 50: Correct Answer: C) Inclusion of personal opinions

Rationale: When documenting services provided, it is crucial to maintain accuracy and completeness to ensure effective communication among healthcare professionals. Timeliness is also important to ensure that the information is recorded in a timely manner. However, it is not appropriate to include personal opinions in documentation as it can introduce bias and subjective information, which may affect the overall quality and credibility of the documentation. It is essential to focus on objective and factual information in order to maintain professionalism and ensure the integrity of the patient's medical record.

Question 51: Correct Answer: B) Diagnosis

Rationale: The nursing process consists of five steps: assessment, diagnosis, planning, implementation, and evaluation. The diagnosis step involves the identification and documentation of actual or potential problems based on the assessment data. It is during this phase that nurses analyze and interpret the data collected to identify the client's healthcare needs. This helps in formulating client-centered goals and developing individualized care plans. Therefore, option B is the correct answer as it represents the step of the nursing process that involves problem identification and documentation.

Question 52: Correct Answer: B) Conducting role-playing scenarios to practice assertiveness skills

Rationale: In order to effectively teach self-advocacy skills to patients and caregivers, conducting role-playing scenarios to practice assertiveness skills is the most impactful approach. This hands-on approach allows individuals to actively engage in simulated situations, enabling them to practice and develop effective communication techniques. By experiencing different scenarios, patients and caregivers can gain confidence in expressing their needs and rights, negotiate effectively, and overcome potential barriers to effective communication. Providing pamphlets and educational materials alone may not facilitate practical application, while assigning a nurse to advocate for the patient can hinder the development of independent self-advocacy skills. Encouraging passive communication may perpetuate ineffective communication patterns and hinder the empowerment of patients and caregivers.

Question 53: Correct Answer: A) Encouraging a diet high in fiber and fluids

Rationale: Individuals with a spinal cord injury are at a higher risk of developing constipation due to decreased bowel motility. Encouraging a diet high in fiber and fluids is an effective teaching intervention to prevent constipation. Fiber helps add bulk to the stool, promoting bowel movements, while an adequate intake of fluids helps maintain hydration and soften the stool. Limiting fluid intake or leading a sedentary lifestyle can aggravate constipation. The regular use of laxatives should be avoided as it can lead to dependency and may disrupt normal bowel function. Therefore, option A is the correct answer in promoting optimal bowel function and preventing constipation in individuals with a spinal cord injury.

Question 54: Correct Answer: C) Consult a speech therapist to assess Mr. Johnson's swallowing ability and recommend modifications to his diet as needed.

Rationale: After experiencing a stroke, Mr. Johnson may have difficulty swallowing, a condition known as dysphagia. It is crucial to consult a speech therapist to assess his swallowing ability and recommend appropriate modifications to his diet if necessary. By doing so, the nurse can ensure that Mr. Johnson receives optimal nutrition without compromising his safety or risking aspiration. Encouraging large meals three times a day (option A) may put Mr. Johnson at risk of choking, while administering TPN (option B) may not be necessary if he is able to take in oral nutrition safely. Providing a high-fat, low-fiber diet (option D) may not be the best option without a comprehensive assessment of his specific nutritional needs.

Question 55: Correct Answer: C) Communication and teamwork skills

Rationale: Communication and teamwork skills are crucial for a rehabilitation nurse when collaborating with the interdisciplinary team to achieve patient-centered goals. Through effective communication, the nurse can ensure the exchange of pertinent information, provide updates on the patient's progress, and address any concerns or ideas. Effective teamwork promotes better coordination and synergy among healthcare professionals, leading to improved patient outcomes and satisfaction. Although documentation, medication administration, and technical nursing skills are important, they alone cannot guarantee the successful collaboration required in a rehabilitation setting.

Question 56: Correct Answer: C) Maintaining patient confidentiality and privacy

Rationale: Maintaining patient confidentiality and privacy is an ethical issue that rehabilitation nurses often encounter in their practice. Rehabilitative care requires trust and respect for patient autonomy, and protecting patient confidentiality is an essential aspect of ethical healthcare practice. By safeguarding patient information and respecting their privacy, healthcare professionals can promote a safe environment that fosters trust and patient-centered care. Adhering to fire safety regulations, reporting suspected abuse, and following infection control measures are important, but they primarily fall within the domain of legislative and legal obligations rather than ethical issues.

Question 57: Correct Answer: D) Minimizing the involvement of family members in the rehabilitation process

Rationale: Involving and educating support systems is an essential aspect of rehabilitation nursing. It aims to enhance the patient's psychological and emotional well-being, improve functional abilities, and promote independence and self-care skills. Family members play a vital role in the rehabilitation process, providing support and assistance to the patient. Thus, minimizing their involvement would be counterproductive to achieving the goals of rehabilitation.

Question 58: Correct Answer: A) Public transportation services

Rationale: Public transportation services are an example of a community resource that can support patients with physical disabilities. Access to reliable and accessible transportation can enable individuals to attend medical appointments, therapy sessions, and engage in community activities. It enhances their independence and promotes their active participation in society. Grocery store coupons, personal care products, and online support groups are not specifically community resources targeted at supporting patients with physical disabilities.

Question 59: Correct Answer: A) TENS unit

Rationale: A TENS unit, or transcutaneous electrical nerve stimulation, is a portable, battery-operated device that is used to deliver pain relief through electrical stimulation to the affected area. It is commonly used for conditions such as back pain, arthritis, and nerve-related pain. The device works by sending small electrical pulses through the skin, which helps to block pain signals and increase endorphin production. Baclofen pump is used to deliver medication directly to the spinal cord for the treatment of spasticity. An LVAD (left ventricular assist device) is used to help the heart pump blood in patients with severe heart failure. An intrathecal drug delivery system is used to deliver medications directly into the spinal fluid.

Question 60: Correct Answer: C) Provide adaptive equipment to assist with self-feeding.

Rationale: The primary goal adjustment for Mr. Adams should be providing adaptive equipment to assist with self-feeding. This will help him regain independence in feeding himself despite the weakness in his upper extremities. Increasing the number of therapy sessions may not directly address the specific issue of self-feeding. Modifying the nutritional plan may be necessary based on the swallowing evaluation by a speech-language pathologist, but it is not the primary goal adjustment at this stage. Referring Mr. Adams to a speech-language pathologist would be appropriate if there are concerns about his swallowing function, but it is not the primary goal adjustment for his self-feeding difficulties.

Question 61: Correct Answer: B) Ms. Rodriguez would prefer a vegetarian diet due to her cultural practices.

Rationale: Dietary preferences can vary across different cultures and religions. In Hispanic culture, vegetarianism is commonly practiced due to cultural preferences and religious influences (e.g., Catholicism, Seventh-day Adventists). By understanding this cultural preference, the Certified Rehabilitation Registered Nurse (CRRN) can collaborate with the healthcare team to provide appropriate dietary options that align with Ms. Rodriguez's cultural and religious beliefs, promoting optimal nutrition and hydration during her rehabilitation journey.

Question 62: Correct Answer: C) Bladder retraining involves delaying urination whenever the urge arises.

Rationale: Bladder retraining is a technique used to help patients regain control over their bladder function. It involves delaying urination whenever the urge arises, gradually increasing the time between voiding episodes. This technique helps to increase the capacity of the bladder and reduce the frequency of urination. Bladder retraining is recommended for patients with symptoms of urinary urgency, frequency, and urge incontinence. It is not contraindicated in patients with bladder overactivity, but it may not be as effective in these cases. Patients should be educated about proper bladder retraining techniques and the importance of adhering to the recommended schedule to achieve optimal results.

Question 63: Correct Answer: B) Impaired verbal communication

Rationale: The patient's difficulty speaking and understanding spoken language, along with right-sided weakness, indicates a neurological deficit affecting communication. This can be attributed to the traumatic brain injury. Impaired verbal communication is the most appropriate nursing diagnosis for Carol in this scenario. The other options, while relevant to rehabilitation nursing, do not directly address the communication issues observed in the patient.

Question 64: Correct Answer: C) Discuss the situation with the healthcare team and seek their guidance.

Rationale: In this scenario, it is crucial for Amy to engage in ethical decision-making. While respecting patient autonomy is important, it is equally important to take into consideration the patient's right to be informed about their medical condition. By discussing the situation with the healthcare team and seeking their guidance, Amy can ensure that the decision made considers both the family's wishes and the patient's right to information. The healthcare team, which may include physicians, psychologists, and social workers, can provide valuable insights and help to resolve any conflicts that arise in regard to disclosing prognosis information to Mr. Johnson. Ultimately, the decision should be made in the best interest of the patient and their overall well-being.

Question 65: Correct Answer: A) CARF

Rationale: CARF (Commission on Accreditation of Rehabilitation Facilities) is an independent, nonprofit organization that accredits rehabilitation facilities and programs in the United States. CARF sets standards for quality and safety, and facilities must meet these standards to earn accreditation. CARF accreditation indicates that a rehabilitation facility or program meets or exceeds established criteria for patient care, safety, and outcomes. APS (Adult Protective Services) is a government agency that investigates abuse, neglect, and exploitation of vulnerable adults. SSA (Social Security Administration) is responsible for administering social security programs, while OSHA (Occupational Safety and Health Administration) ensures safe and healthy working conditions.

Question 66: Correct Answer: C) Understanding legal regulations

Rationale: Skill in understanding legal regulations is crucial for a Certified Rehabilitation Registered Nurse (CRRN). This skill enables the nurse to adhere to the law while managing patient care effectively. Legal regulations may include laws related to privacy, consent, documentation, negligence, malpractice, and more. Rehabilitation nurses must possess a comprehensive understanding of these regulations to ensure the provision of quality care while maintaining legal compliance. While economic policies and legislative procedures may have some relevance, they are not the primary focus in this context. Enforcing ethical principles is important, but legal regulations hold a greater significance in terms of managing care within the boundaries of the law.

Question 67: Correct Answer: C) Familial factors

Rationale: Familial factors, such as upbringing, socialization, and family traditions, heavily influence an individual's cultural beliefs, values, and behaviors. The family unit is responsible for transmitting cultural practices and shaping an individual's worldview from an early age. Cultural beliefs, values, and behaviors are often learned through observation, imitation, and active participation in familial activities and rituals. While environmental, societal, and gender factors may also have an impact, the familial context holds particular significance in shaping an individual's cultural identity. Rehabilitation nurses must be aware of the influence of familial factors to provide culturally sensitive and appropriate care to patients and their families.

Question 68: Correct Answer: D) Antispasmodics

Rationale: Antispasmodics are medications commonly used to manage spasticity in patients with neurological disorders. These medications work by inhibiting the activity of certain neurotransmitters in the central nervous system, thereby reducing abnormal muscle contractions and improving muscle tone. Antihistamines (Option A) are not effective in managing spasticity and are primarily used for allergy relief. NSAIDs (Option B) are non-steroidal anti-inflammatory drugs that mainly provide pain relief but do not directly target spasticity. Opioids (Option C) are potent pain medications and are not typically used to manage spasticity.

Question 69: Correct Answer: C) Implementing a regular bedtime routine

Rationale: Implementing a regular bedtime routine can help establish a consistent sleep schedule and improve sleep quality. It involves encouraging Mr. Johnson to engage in relaxing activities before bed, such as reading a book or listening to calming music, and avoiding stimulating activities, caffeine, and excessive napping close to bedtime. This routine will signal to his body that it is time to prepare for sleep, helping him fall asleep faster and improving his overall rest patterns.

Question 70: Correct Answer: C) Chronic pain persists for more than three months and may not have an identifiable cause.

Rationale: Chronic pain is defined as pain that continues for an extended period, typically lasting for more than three months. It may not have an identifiable cause and can affect various body systems. Unlike acute pain, chronic pain is not an adaptive response to injury and may require multidisciplinary management. It can have a considerable impact on a patient's quality of life and requires comprehensive assessment and intervention strategies. Understanding the nature and characteristics of chronic pain is crucial for rehabilitation nurses in developing appropriate care plans and optimizing pain management for patients like Mrs. Johnson.

Question 71: Correct Answer: B) Implement a regular toileting schedule for Jane.

Rationale: Following a spinal cord injury, neurogenic bowel dysfunction is common, leading to difficulty with bowel movements. Implementing a regular toileting schedule helps stimulate normal bowel function and promote bowel regularity. This intervention involves establishing a routine time for bowel movements, maintaining consistency in toileting techniques, and providing privacy and assistance as needed. Encouraging fluid intake, administering laxatives, and increasing fiber intake may be appropriate interventions for other patients with bowel issues, but in this scenario, prioritizing a regular toileting schedule is essential for optimizing Jane's elimination patterns.

Question 72: Correct Answer: D) A severe illness

Rationale: Physiological stressors are those that affect the physical well-being of an individual. Examples of physiological stressors include severe illness, injury, surgery, or physical pain. These stressors can have a direct impact on the body's physiological functions, leading to increased heart rate, blood pressure, and hormonal changes. In contrast, options A, B, and C are examples of psychological or emotional stressors, which primarily affect an individual's mental state and emotions.

Question 73: Correct Answer: D) Actively listening to team members' input and perspectives

Rationale: Actively listening to team members' input and perspectives is the most effective action by the CRRN in promoting effective communication. It demonstrates respect for others' opinions, encourages open dialogue, and fosters a collaborative and patient-centered approach to care. Providing written instructions may be helpful, but it does not facilitate real-time interaction and may limit opportunities for clarification or discussion. Using medical jargon can alienate team members who may not be familiar with such terminology and hinder effective communication. Assuming the role of the team leader in all situations may undermine the expertise and contributions of other team members, leading to poor collaboration and communication. Therefore, active listening is the key to effective communication and collaboration within the interdisciplinary team.

Question 74: Correct Answer: A) Implementing evidence-based interventions

Rationale: When providing care for a culturally diverse population, it is essential for the nurse to implement evidence-based interventions. This approach ensures that care is based on proven practices that have been shown to be effective across various cultural backgrounds. Using the same approach for all patients (option B) is not recommended as cultural diversity requires an individualized approach to care. Additionally, the use of interpreters (option C) should be encouraged to facilitate effective communication between the nurse and the patient. Lastly, cultural assessments (option D) play a crucial role in gaining an understanding of the patient's cultural beliefs, practices, and preferences, allowing for culturally sensitive care.

Question 75: Correct Answer: A) The administration of nutrition directly into the gastrointestinal tract.

Rationale: Enteral nutrition refers to the delivery of nutrition directly into the gastrointestinal tract. This is typically achieved through the use of a feeding tube. Enteral nutrition is the preferred method when the patient's gastrointestinal tract is functioning and can adequately absorb nutrients. It helps maintain the integrity of the gut mucosa, supports normal immune function, and can be easily adjusted based on the patient's nutritional requirements. Other options such as parenteral nutrition involve bypassing the gastrointestinal tract and delivering nutrition directly into the bloodstream, which is reserved for patients who cannot tolerate enteral nutrition or have non-functioning gastrointestinal tracts. The correct option A accurately describes enteral nutrition and its administration method.

Question 76: Correct Answer: A) Weakness on the left side of the body

Rationale: In a stroke affecting the right side of the brain, the patient is likely to experience sensorimotor deficits on the left side of the body. This is because each side of the brain controls movement and sensation for the opposite side of the body. Therefore, weakness on the left side of the body would be a clinical sign of sensorimotor deficits in this patient. Difficulty with balance and coordination (option B) may also occur due to the involvement of the right side of the brain. Decreased sensation on the right side of the body (option C) is not expected as the stroke is on the right side. Impaired fine motor skills on the right hand (option D) would not be a direct clinical sign in this scenario.

Question 77: Correct Answer: D) Leininger's Transcultural Nursing Model

Rationale: Leininger's Transcultural Nursing Model emphasizes the importance of cultural competence in providing holistic and patient-centered care. This model recognizes that personal experiences, beliefs, and culture significantly impact an individual's health and wellness. By understanding and respecting cultural differences, rehabilitation nurses can develop individualized care plans that meet the unique needs of each patient. This approach promotes effective communication, builds trust, and enhances patient outcomes in the rehabilitation setting.

Question 78: Correct Answer: A) "We will need to perform intermittent catheterization every 4 hours to prevent urinary tract infections."

Rationale: Intermittent catheterization is a recommended technique for bladder management to prevent urinary tract infections in patients with urinary retention. This process involves emptying the bladder regularly using a catheter to avoid the accumulation of urine and reduce the risk of infection. The caregiver's understanding demonstrates the correct knowledge regarding the need for regular catheterization to maintain proper bladder function and prevent complications. Option B is incorrect as an indwelling catheter should be changed regularly to prevent infections. Option C is incorrect as restricting fluid intake may lead to dehydration and other complications. Option D is incorrect as regular emptying of the drainage bag is necessary to prevent excessive stretching and dislodgement of the catheter.

Question 79: Correct Answer: A) Developmental theory

Rationale: Developmental theory, also known as psychosocial theory, focuses on the development of an individual's self-concept and self-esteem throughout different stages of life. This theory, proposed by Erik Erikson, suggests that individuals go through a series of psychosocial stages, and successful resolution of each stage contributes to a healthy self-concept and self-esteem. Coping theory and stress theory, on the other hand, focus more on how individuals adapt and respond to stressors. Grief and loss theory deals specifically with the emotional processes related to dealing with loss. Therefore, the correct answer is A) Developmental theory.

Question 80: Correct Answer: B) Diagnosis

Rationale: The nursing process consists of five steps: Assessment, Diagnosis, Planning, Implementation, and Evaluation. During the diagnosis step, the nurse analyzes the data collected during the assessment phase and identifies the client's actual or potential problems. This analysis helps to determine the client's needs and prioritize the nursing interventions. By accurately diagnosing the client's problems, the nurse can develop an appropriate plan of care and implement interventions effectively. Therefore, option B is the correct answer as it represents the step of analyzing data and identifying problems in the nursing process.

Question 81: Correct Answer: A) Collecting data from various sources

Rationale: Analyzing quality and utilization data requires collecting data from various sources to ensure comprehensive and accurate information. This includes gathering data from electronic health records, patient surveys, healthcare professionals, and administrative databases. By collecting data from multiple sources, healthcare providers can obtain a holistic view of the patient's experience and identify potential areas for improvement. Ignoring outliers in the data (option B) can lead to the omission of important information, while relying solely on subjective opinions (option C) may introduce bias. Similarly, using only qualitative data (option D) may overlook quantitative factors that are crucial for a thorough analysis of quality and utilization.

Question 82: Correct Answer: A) Visual aids and cues

Rationale: When working with patients who have memory impairment, visual aids and cues are the most effective teaching strategy. These individuals may struggle with verbal information processing, making it difficult for them to retain and recall information. Visual aids can help them better understand and remember instructions or concepts. By utilizing visual aids such as diagrams, pictures, charts, and models, patients with memory impairment can rely on visual cues to enhance their comprehension and retention of information. This strategy allows for the integration of visual memory, compensating for deficits in auditory or verbal memory pathways. Overall, visual aids and cues are valuable tools in facilitating learning for patients with neurological deficits related to memory impairment.

Question 83: Correct Answer: D) Therapeutic Communication and Counseling

Rationale: The rehabilitation registered nurse should possess the skill in therapeutic communication and counseling. This involves the ability to effectively communicate and build rapport with patients with complex conditions such as spinal cord injuries. It includes active listening, empathetic responding, and counseling techniques to support patients emotionally and help them develop coping mechanisms. This skill is essential in facilitating the patient's engagement in the rehabilitation process and promoting emotional well-being. Options A, B, and C are also important skills for rehabilitation nurses, but they are not specifically related to communication.

Question 84: Correct Answer: B) Provide education and resources on support groups for individuals with spinal cord injuries.

Rationale: Connecting Mrs. Smith with support groups for individuals with spinal cord injuries can be a beneficial strategy to promote her adjustment and coping. Support groups offer opportunities for individuals to share experiences, gain emotional support, and access resources. It provides a platform for Mrs. Smith to connect with others who can relate to her situation, share coping strategies, and learn from their experiences. By participating in a support group, Mrs. Smith can develop a sense of belonging, reduce isolation, and gain insight into managing role and relationship changes.

Question 85: Correct Answer: B) Providing opportunities for therapeutic communication and active listening

Rationale: Mr. Thompson's symptoms of sadness, guilt, and worthlessness indicate worsening depression. Providing opportunities for therapeutic communication and active listening is essential in assessing his emotional state, identifying potential triggers, and developing an appropriate care plan. It allows the nurse to establish a trusting relationship, validate his feelings, and encourage him to express his emotions. This intervention promotes optimal psychosocial patterns and coping skills, fostering a therapeutic environment for Mr. Thompson's recovery. Option A is incorrect as relying solely on pain medication would not address his underlying emotional distress. Option C is incorrect as social support is crucial for patients with depression, and limiting visitors may exacerbate feelings of isolation. Option D is incorrect as suggesting holistic therapies should be based on individual preferences and evidence-based practice, not blanket recommendations.

Question 86: Correct Answer: A) Plan, Do, Check, Act (PDCA)

Rationale: The Plan, Do, Check, Act (PDCA) is a model used in process improvement to guide the continuous improvement of systems and processes. It involves four stages: planning, where objectives and processes are defined; doing, where the plan is implemented and executed; checking, where performance is monitored and data is collected; and acting, where necessary adjustments and improvements are made based on the data and results obtained. PDCA is a systematic and iterative approach that promotes quality improvement by identifying and eliminating problems and maximizing efficiency. It is widely used in industries and healthcare settings to enhance performance and achieve better outcomes.

Question 87: Correct Answer: D) Veracity

Rationale: Veracity is the ethical principle that encompasses being truthful and honest with patients. It involves providing accurate and complete information to patients, enabling them to make informed decisions about their care. Veracity is essential for establishing trust between healthcare professionals and patients and upholding the principle of autonomy, which empowers patients to have control over their healthcare decisions. By practicing veracity, healthcare professionals demonstrate respect for patients' autonomy and promote open communication and honesty in the delivery of care.

Question 88: Correct Answer: B) Discuss the situation with the healthcare team and develop a plan to address the increase in LOS.

Rationale: Analyzing quality and utilization data is an important responsibility of a CRRN. When Tracy notices a significant increase in the average length of stay (LOS) for patients with spinal cord injuries, it is essential for her to discuss the situation with the healthcare team. By involving the team in the analysis, they can identify potential causes and develop a plan to address the increase in LOS. Ignoring the increase in LOS or simply informing the administration without investigating further would not be proactive approaches. Discharging patients earlier solely to reduce LOS could compromise patient care and outcomes. Therefore, the best course of action is to collaborate with the healthcare team to address the issue.

Question 89: Correct Answer: A) Vocational rehabilitation programs

Rationale: Vocational rehabilitation programs are an essential community resource that can assist patients in their transition to the next level of care. These programs aim to help individuals with disabilities or health conditions acquire or maintain employment and achieve independence in the community. By providing job training, career counseling, and support services, vocational rehabilitation programs play a vital role in reintegrating patients into society. Annual physical examinations, home exercise equipment, and financial planning services are not specifically targeted towards facilitating community reintegration or transition to the next level of care.

Question 90: Correct Answer: C) The Centers for Medicare and Medicaid Services (CMS)
Rationale: The Centers for Medicare and Medicaid Services (CMS) is the entity responsible for administering and enforcing legislation and regulations related to healthcare practices in the United States. CMS oversees the Medicare and Medicaid programs, sets standards for healthcare providers, and ensures compliance with regulations. The American Nurses Association (ANA) is a professional nursing organization that focuses on advocacy and supporting nurses' interests. The State Health Departments play a role in public health initiatives and may implement state-specific regulations. The National Institute of Health (NIH) is a biomedical research agency and does not enforce healthcare regulations.

Question 91: Correct Answer: C) Engage in active listening and calmly communicate with Mr. Smith.
Rationale: Engaging in active listening and calmly communicating with Mr. Smith is an important approach to de-escalate his aggression. By actively listening to his concerns and calmly communicating with him, you can help to diffuse the situation and address any underlying issues or triggers that may be contributing to his aggression. This approach promotes a therapeutic and supportive environment, rather than resorting to isolating or restraining the patient, which can further escalate the situation and potentially compromise his safety. Administering a sedative medication should only be considered as a last resort and under the guidance of a healthcare provider.

Question 92: Correct Answer: B) Utilizing mechanical lifting equipment
Rationale: Safe patient handling practices aim to minimize the risk of injury to both patients and healthcare staff during patient transfers and movements. One essential component is the use of mechanical lifting equipment, such as hoists and transfer aids, which reduce the physical strain on healthcare providers and decrease the likelihood of accidents or patient falls. Using manual lifting techniques (option A) can put the staff at risk of musculoskeletal injuries. Assigning patient handling tasks to untrained staff (option C) can be hazardous and increase the likelihood of errors. While patient self-mobilization (option D) is encouraged when possible, mechanical lifting equipment is still necessary for patients who are unable to mobilize independently.

Question 93: Correct Answer: B) "Tell me more about how you're feeling."
Rationale: Therapeutic communication involves active listening, empathy, and open-ended questions to facilitate patient expression and promote a trusting relationship. Option B demonstrates the use of therapeutic communication by encouraging the patient to share their thoughts and feelings in a non-judgmental and supportive manner. Options A, C, and D lack the essential elements of therapeutic communication as they are dismissive, judgmental, and assume the nurse's understanding of the patient's emotions. It is important for the nurse to create a safe and empathetic environment for effective communication and understanding of the patient's psychosocial needs.

Question 94: Correct Answer: A) Biofeedback
Rationale: Biofeedback is a technique that enables individuals to gain control over their physiological responses by providing real-time feedback on these responses. It helps individuals become more aware of their physical and psychological responses to stress and teaches them techniques to control these responses. By monitoring various body functions such as heart rate, blood pressure, and muscle tension, individuals can learn to recognize and regulate their stress responses. Cognitive behavioral therapy focuses on changing unhealthy thoughts and behaviors, complementary alternative medicine encompasses a range of therapies, and pharmacology involves the use of medications. While these interventions may also be useful in stress management, they are not specifically related to gaining control over physiological responses like biofeedback.

Question 95: Correct Answer: A) Interdisciplinary team
Rationale: An interdisciplinary team is a model of healthcare team that emphasizes collaboration, communication, and shared decision-making among team members. In this model, professionals from different disciplines work together to provide comprehensive and coordinated care to patients. They share their expertise, knowledge, and skills to develop and implement a holistic plan of care. The interdisciplinary team promotes a patient-centered approach, where all team members actively participate in discussions, contribute to treatment planning, and work towards achieving patient-centered goals. This approach ensures that the patient receives the best possible care, as each team member brings their unique perspective and specialized knowledge to the table.

Question 96: Correct Answer: C) Loosen tight clothing and check for any restrictive devices
Rationale: Autonomic dysreflexia is a potentially life-threatening condition that can occur in individuals with spinal cord injuries. It is characterized by a sudden onset of severe hypertension, bradycardia, and throbbing headache. The first step in managing autonomic dysreflexia is to identify and remove the triggering stimulus. In this scenario, loosening tight clothing and checking for any restrictive devices can help alleviate the symptoms. Administering medications such as beta-blockers or vasodilators should only be done after removing the triggering stimulus and under the guidance of a healthcare provider. Placing the patient in a supine position with legs elevated may worsen autonomic dysreflexia as it can increase blood pressure.

Question 97: Correct Answer: C) Demonstrating the correct use of the adaptive equipment
Rationale: When assisting a client in using adaptive equipment for eating, it is essential for the nurse to demonstrate the correct use of the equipment. By doing so, the nurse ensures that the client understands how to effectively and safely utilize the adaptive equipment for a successful eating experience. While ensuring the cleanliness of the equipment is important, demonstrating the correct use takes priority to promote the client's independence and functional ability. Assessing the client's ability to self-feed and providing emotional support are also crucial aspects of care, but they are not the priority when it comes to assisting with adaptive equipment usage for eating.

Question 98: Correct Answer: B) Facilitating independence in expressing basic needs.
Rationale: The primary goal in implementing communication interventions for Mr. Johnson should be to facilitate independence in expressing basic needs. As a CRRN, the nurse aims to optimize the patient's ability to communicate effectively. By focusing on facilitating independence, the nurse helps Mr. Johnson regain the confidence and capability to express his basic needs, enhancing his overall quality of life. Minimizing the use of nonverbal communication

techniques, eliminating all forms of written communication, or solely focusing on augmentative and alternative communication methods may limit Mr. Johnson's ability to express himself and impede his rehabilitation process.

Question 99: Correct Answer: C) Ensuring that documentation is complete, accurate, and up-to-date

Rationale: In preparation for a regulatory agency audit, it is essential to ensure that documentation is complete, accurate, and up-to-date. This includes medical records, nursing assessments, care plans, treatment documentation, and any other relevant documentation. The regulatory agency will thoroughly review the documentation to assess compliance with standards and regulations. By ensuring proper documentation, the rehabilitation unit demonstrates its commitment to providing high-quality care and adherence to regulatory requirements. Providing specialized training to the nursing staff, limiting the audit preparation to management personnel, or restricting patient access during the audit process may not directly address the importance of documentation and may not fully prepare the unit for a successful audit.

Question 100: Correct Answer: C) Provide a relaxing environment by dimming lights and reducing noise

Rationale: Providing a relaxing environment by dimming lights and reducing noise can contribute to a more restful sleep for the patient. It helps create a calm and peaceful atmosphere that promotes relaxation and sleep. Administering sedative medication at bedtime may be necessary in some cases, but it should not be the first line of intervention. Encouraging the patient to limit daytime napping may help regulate their sleep-wake cycle, but it may not directly address the difficulty in sleeping at night. Engaging in vigorous physical exercise before bedtime can have a stimulating effect on the body and may interfere with sleep.

Question 101: Correct Answer: B) Seek guidance from the healthcare facility's ethics committee to determine the best course of action.

Rationale: In situations where patients are incapable of making decisions and conflicts arise within the family regarding treatment plans, it is essential to seek guidance from an ethics committee. Ethical issues and legal obligations may arise when dealing with end-of-life decisions, and it is crucial to involve a multidisciplinary team to evaluate the situation and establish the most appropriate course of action. The ethics committee consists of professionals well-versed in ethical considerations and legal obligations, ensuring that decisions are made in the best interest of the patient and within the legal framework. It is vital for CRRNs to work collaboratively with the ethics committee to promote ethical practice in rehabilitation nursing.

Question 102: Correct Answer: C) Planning

Rationale: Planning is a crucial step in optimizing a patient's functional ability. After performing a comprehensive assessment and making an accurate diagnosis, the nurse develops a plan of care that addresses the patient's specific needs and goals. This involves identifying appropriate interventions, setting realistic targets, and coordinating resources. By prioritizing the planning step, the nurse ensures a systematic approach to address functional limitations and promote the patient's independence and quality of life. Evaluation, the final step of the nursing process, assesses the effectiveness of the interventions implemented during the planning phase. However, without thorough planning, the interventions may not effectively address the patient's functional ability.

Question 103: Correct Answer: B) Assisting Mrs. Smith in identifying community resources for individuals with disabilities

Rationale: As a CRRN, one of your roles in promoting community reintegration and transition to the next level of care is to assist the patient in identifying community resources. This includes providing information about support groups, vocational rehabilitation services, and other agencies that specialize in assisting individuals with disabilities. Collaborating with the physical therapist to develop a home exercise program, educating the patient and family about adaptive equipment, and arranging transportation services are important aspects of rehabilitation, but they do not directly address Mrs. Smith's concern about transitioning back home and resuming her daily activities in the community.

Question 104: Correct Answer: C) Collaborating with interdisciplinary teams for holistic patient care

Rationale: Collaboration with interdisciplinary teams is a crucial aspect of rehabilitation standards and scope of practice for CRRNs. Rehabilitation requires a comprehensive approach involving various healthcare professionals, including physical therapists, occupational therapists, speech therapists, psychologists, social workers, and physicians. CRRNs work collaboratively with these professionals to develop individualized care plans, ensure holistic patient care, and optimize the restoration and preservation of the patient's health and well-being. While CRRNs may administer medications in some cases, it is not the primary focus of their scope of practice. Conducting psychotherapy and prescribing physical exercises and therapy modalities fall under the responsibilities of other healthcare professionals specializing in those areas.

Question 105: Correct Answer: B) Patient's rehabilitation goals

Rationale: When assessing a patient's readiness for discharge, the nurse should consider various factors. One of the most important factors is the patient's rehabilitation goals. The nurse should evaluate if the goals have been achieved or if progress has been made towards those goals. This is crucial in determining if the patient is ready to be discharged and continue their rehabilitation outside the hospital. The other options, such as insurance coverage, availability of family and caregiver support, and hospital's bed availability, are also important factors but do not directly indicate the patient's readiness for discharge. It is essential to prioritize the patient's rehabilitation goals to ensure a successful transition to the next level of care or community reintegration.

Question 106: Correct Answer: D) Cane

Rationale: Adaptive equipment refers to devices specifically designed to assist individuals with disabilities in performing daily activities and improving their functional independence. A cane is a common adaptive equipment used to support balance and help with mobility for individuals with decreased lower extremity strength or stability. Smartwatches, virtual reality headsets, and smartphones are modern technology devices that can have various health-related applications, but they do not specifically fall under the category of adaptive equipment for rehabilitation purposes.

Question 107: Correct Answer: A) Encourage the patient to ambulate independently in the room.

Rationale: Energy conservation strategies aim to minimize energy expenditure and promote adequate rest and sleep. Encouraging the patient to ambulate independently in the room is an example of such a strategy as it promotes engagement in light physical activity, conserving energy for rest and sleep. Assisting the patient with dressing and grooming activities may be helpful but does not directly address energy conservation. Allowing the patient to rest in a well-lit room during the day contradicts the need for a conducive sleep environment. Modifying the patient's schedule to incorporate multiple therapy sessions may lead to increased energy expenditure, hindering rest and sleep.

Question 108: Correct Answer: C) Developing individualized treatment plans

Rationale: As a Certified Rehabilitation Registered Nurse (CRRN), developing individualized treatment plans falls within their scope of practice. CRRNs work closely with the interdisciplinary team to assess the patient's needs, set goals, and create a rehabilitation plan. This plan may include interventions from various disciplines, such as physical therapy, occupational therapy, and speech therapy. Prescribing medications, administering therapy sessions, and performing surgical procedures are not within the scope of practice for a CRRN.

Question 109: Correct Answer: C) Advocate for the patient's preferences and goals

Rationale: The role of the CRRN in team and patient caregiver conferences is to advocate for the patient's preferences and goals. As a rehabilitation nurse, the CRRN ensures that the patient's voice is heard and their individualized needs are addressed in the treatment plan. The CRRN collaborates with the interdisciplinary team to promote patient-centered care and fosters open communication among team members, patients, and caregivers. While providing the medical history and evaluating progress may be part of the nurse's responsibilities, advocating for the patient's preferences and goals is crucial in promoting patient-centered care and optimizing outcomes. Suggesting the need for additional diagnostic tests is typically done by the medical doctor or physician.

Question 110: Correct Answer: B) Glasgow Coma Scale

Rationale: The Glasgow Coma Scale (GCS) is a widely recognized and commonly used measurement tool to assess the level of consciousness and cognitive function in patients with brain injuries. It evaluates eye opening, verbal response, and motor response, assigning scores that indicate the severity of impairment. The Rancho Los Amigos Scale is a measurement tool used to assess the cognitive and behavioral levels of individuals with brain injuries in the rehabilitation phase. The Mini Mental State Examination is a screening tool used to assess cognitive impairment in the elderly. The ASIA Scale is used to assess the extent and severity of neurological impairment in patients with spinal cord injuries.

Question 111: Correct Answer: C) Deontology

Rationale: Deontology is an ethical theory that focuses on the duty to follow moral rules and principles. It emphasizes the importance of acting ethically based on a set of rules or duties, rather than considering the consequences of the action. Nurses who adhere to deontological principles prioritize their moral obligations and responsibilities, even if the outcome may not be favorable. This theory ensures that actions are guided by moral rules and principles, providing a framework for ethical decision-making in nursing practice.

Question 112: Correct Answer: D) Diabetic diet

Rationale: For a patient with diabetes, a diabetic diet is implemented to regulate blood glucose levels. This diet emphasizes portion control, carbohydrate counting, and including a balance of carbohydrates, protein, and fats in the diet. It restricts simple sugars and high glycemic index foods to prevent blood sugar spikes. Considering Sarah's diagnosis of diabetes, a diabetic diet is the most appropriate choice for managing her blood glucose levels while promoting optimal nutrition during her rehabilitation journey.

Question 113: Correct Answer: C) Assigning a nursing staff member to provide constant supervision.

Rationale: The most important intervention for a patient with impaired judgment is assigning a nursing staff member to provide constant supervision. Impaired judgment can put the patient at risk for engaging in unsafe behaviors or making poor decisions regarding their safety. By having a nurse constantly monitor the patient, potential hazards can be identified and prevented. Providing handrails and educating the patient about safety precautions are also important interventions, but they may not be sufficient to ensure the patient's safety given their impaired judgment. Encouraging the use of assistive devices is relevant for mobility but does not directly address the issue of impaired judgment.

Question 114: Correct Answer: A) Encouraging the use of an incentive spirometer

Rationale: Encouraging the use of an incentive spirometer is an appropriate intervention to promote respiratory function in a patient with a musculoskeletal impairment. An incentive spirometer helps the patient to expand their lung capacity, prevent atelectasis, and improve overall respiratory function. Administering sedatives may depress the respiratory system, therefore, it is contraindicated. Restricting fluid intake can lead to dehydration and thickened secretions, impairing respiratory function. Applying cold packs to the chest area may cause vasoconstriction and reduce the effectiveness of coughing and deep breathing, hindering respiratory function. Thus, option A is the correct answer.

Question 115: Correct Answer: B) Nursing interventions provided

Rationale: Documentation to support regulatory requirements must be accurate, objective, and relevant. It should include information such as nursing interventions provided, patient observations, medications administered, and any changes in the patient's condition. Including the patient's social security number would violate patient privacy regulations. Personal opinions about the patient are subjective and not appropriate for documentation. Non-relevant medical information should not be included as it may lead to confusion and clutter the patient's record. Therefore, option B is the correct answer as it aligns with the requirements for documentation supporting regulatory standards.

Question 116: Correct Answer: C) Acute rehab

Rationale: Acute rehab refers to a level of care that provides intensive rehabilitation services for individuals with disabling conditions. This setting is typically located within a hospital and involves a multidisciplinary team approach. Patients in acute rehab receive a high level of medical supervision, therapy, and nursing care to optimize their functional abilities and promote their transition to the next level of care, which may include home care or assisted living. Assisted living, hospice care, and home care do not typically provide the same level of intensive rehabilitation services as acute rehab. Therefore, the correct answer is option C) Acute rehab.

Question 117: Correct Answer: B) Creating rehabilitation plans and overseeing multidisciplinary care teams

Rationale: The scope of practice for a Certified Rehabilitation Registered Nurse (CRRN) includes creating rehabilitation plans and overseeing multidisciplinary care teams. CRRNs are responsible for coordinating and implementing comprehensive care plans for patients with disabilities, chronic illnesses, and injuries. This involves assessing patient needs, collaborating with other healthcare professionals, and developing individualized treatment plans. CRRNs are also involved in educating patients and their families, providing support, and advocating for the needs of individuals with disabilities. While medication administration and advanced procedures may be part of the CRRN's role, it is not the primary focus or the scope of practice. Conducting research studies and managing critical care patients are also outside the scope of practice for a CRRN.

Question 118: Correct Answer: C) Agency for Healthcare Research and Quality (AHRQ)

Rationale: The National Database of Nursing Quality Indicators (NDNQI) is a comprehensive database that collects and analyzes nursing-sensitive quality indicators to help healthcare organizations improve patient care outcomes. The database is created and maintained by the Agency for Healthcare Research and Quality (AHRQ), an agency within the U.S. Department of Health and Human Services. AHRQ's mission is to produce evidence to make healthcare safer, higher quality, more accessible, equitable, and affordable. It is responsible for promoting research and implementing quality improvement processes in healthcare settings. The other options, WHO, CDC, and IOM, are important healthcare organizations but are not directly involved in the creation and maintenance of the NDNQI.

Question 119: Correct Answer: B) "Let me contact our social worker who can provide you with information about community resources that can assist with housing modifications or finding accessible housing."

Rationale: As a CRRN, it is essential to recognize the importance of addressing patients' concerns regarding housing during their transition to the community. By contacting the social worker, who is trained in connecting patients with community resources, the patient can receive information about housing modifications and accessible housing options. Accessible housing is crucial for patients with spinal cord injuries to ensure their safety and independence. By providing this resource, it supports the patient's community reintegration and promotes their successful transition to the next level of care.

Question 120: Correct Answer: A) Americans with Disabilities Act (ADA)

Rationale: The Americans with Disabilities Act (ADA) is a federal legislation that prohibits discrimination against individuals with disabilities in areas of employment, public accommodations, transportation, and telecommunications. It ensures equal rights and opportunities for individuals with disabilities, including those receiving rehabilitation services. The Occupational Safety and Health Act (OSHA) focuses on ensuring safe and healthy working conditions. The Health Insurance Portability and Accountability Act (HIPAA) protects the privacy and security of patient health information. The Emergency Medical Treatment and Labor Act (EMTALA) guarantees that individuals have access to emergency medical services regardless of their ability to pay. However, only the ADA specifically addresses the rights of individuals with disabilities.

Question 121: Correct Answer: B) Implementing a range of motion exercises to maintain joint flexibility and prevent contractures.

Rationale: The most appropriate intervention for addressing impaired physical mobility in a patient with traumatic brain injury (TBI) is to implement a range of motion exercises. These exercises help maintain joint flexibility, prevent contractures, and improve overall physical function. Encouraging independent ambulation may not be suitable immediately after a severe TBI, as the patient may have reduced strength and coordination. Repositioning and turning are important interventions to prevent pressure ulcers but may not directly address impaired physical mobility. Administering pain and anti-inflammatory medications is essential for managing TBI-related symptoms but does not directly address impaired physical mobility. Thus, option B is the correct answer.

Question 122: Correct Answer: C) Providing a bedside commode for Mrs. Johnson.

Rationale: Providing a bedside commode for Mrs. Johnson is the most appropriate measure to prevent falls. It ensures that she can safely use the bathroom without the need to walk alone or use a bedpan. Restraint devices are discouraged due to the associated risks, including pressure injuries and impaired mobility. Keeping the bedrails raised at all times may increase the risk of injury in case of a fall or restrict Mrs. Johnson's mobility. Encouraging Mrs. Johnson to stay in bed as much as possible can lead to complications such as deconditioning and muscle weakness. Therefore, providing a

bedside commode promotes safety and independence while minimizing fall risk.

Question 123: Correct Answer: B) To improve the patient's adherence to treatment plans

Rationale: Involving and educating support systems in the rehabilitation process plays a crucial role in improving the patient's adherence to treatment plans. Support systems, such as the patient's family members, can provide motivation, encouragement, and practical assistance that promotes the patient's active involvement in their rehabilitation. Educating the support systems about the treatment plans, goals, and expected outcomes enhances their understanding and ability to provide appropriate support. This involvement and education help in fostering a collaborative approach and increases the likelihood of the patient following through with the prescribed therapies, leading to better outcomes and progress in rehabilitation.

Question 124: Correct Answer: A) Advise Samantha to quit smoking immediately

Rationale: Smoking has several negative effects on a person's health, and it is especially dangerous for individuals who have had a stroke. Smoking increases the risk of blood clots, reduces the effectiveness of rehabilitation therapies, and can lead to further complications. As a Certified Rehabilitation Registered Nurse, it is crucial to promote the overall well-being and health of the patient. Therefore, advising Samantha to quit smoking is the most appropriate action to take in this situation. By quitting smoking, Samantha can improve her chances of successful rehabilitation and reduce the risk of further health issues.

Question 125: Correct Answer: B) The protection of patients' medical information

Rationale: The Health Insurance Portability and Accountability Act (HIPAA) was enacted to safeguard patients' medical information and ensure their privacy. It establishes guidelines for healthcare providers and organizations to protect and secure patients' health records and other identifiable information. HIPAA regulations also provide patients with control over their medical information, allowing them to grant or deny access to their records. This legislation plays a crucial role in maintaining patient confidentiality and preventing unauthorized release of sensitive medical data, thus ensuring the protection and privacy of patients' medical information.

Question 126: Correct Answer: C) Improved balance and stability during walking

Rationale: Computer-supported prosthetics offer individuals with lower limb amputations improved balance and stability during walking. These technologically advanced prosthetics are designed to mimic natural movements and provide better control while walking. Increased balance and stability can enhance the patient's ability to perform daily activities and improve overall mobility. Options A, B, and D are incorrect as they do not accurately represent the benefits of computer-supported prosthetics and may hinder the patient's rehabilitation process.

Question 127: Correct Answer: B) Collaborating with the interdisciplinary team to develop an individualized care plan.

Rationale: Collaborating with the interdisciplinary team to develop an individualized care plan demonstrates the nurse's skill in legislative and regulatory management of care. This action ensures that the patient's care is in compliance with relevant legislation and regulations by incorporating input from various healthcare professionals and addressing the specific needs and goals of the patient. This collaboration is essential in providing safe, effective, and patient-centered care while adhering to legal and ethical requirements. Educating the patient about potential complications, maintaining privacy, and adhering to infection control practices are important aspects of nursing care, but they do not specifically demonstrate skill in legislative and regulatory management of care.

Question 128: Correct Answer: D) Adequate lighting

Rationale: Adequate lighting is not a risk factor for patient falls in a rehabilitation setting; in fact, it is an important mitigation strategy. Advanced age, impaired gait, and use of assistive devices are all risk factors for falls as they can affect a patient's balance and stability. Poor lighting, on the other hand, can contribute to falls by making it difficult for patients to see obstacles or uneven surfaces. Therefore, ensuring adequate lighting is crucial in creating a safe environment and minimizing the risk of falls.

Question 129: Correct Answer: D) Activity-Exercise pattern.

Rationale: Assessing the patient's ability to perform activities of daily living (ADLs) falls under the Activity-Exercise pattern. This pattern focuses on the patient's physical abilities, mobility, coordination, and ability to participate in activities. After a stroke, patients often experience deficits in their functional abilities, which can impact their independence and overall quality of life. Therefore, it is essential for the nurse to assess the patient's ability to perform ADLs to determine their level of functional impairment and plan appropriate interventions for rehabilitation. By assessing the patient's Activity-Exercise pattern, the nurse can gather information about the patient's current capabilities and set realistic goals for the rehabilitation process.

Question 130: Correct Answer: C) Renal diet

Rationale: A renal diet, also known as a kidney diet, is specifically designed for individuals with renal impairment. This type of diet aims to reduce the workload on the kidneys by restricting foods that are high in sodium, potassium, and phosphorus. It also focuses on consuming adequate amounts of high-quality protein and maintaining a balanced fluid intake. By following a renal diet, individuals with renal impairment can help slow the progression of kidney disease and manage their symptoms effectively. Therefore, option C is the correct answer as it aligns with the dietary needs of individuals with renal impairment.

Question 131: Correct Answer: A) Applying for government assistance programs

Rationale: Given John's financial struggles and being the sole breadwinner for his family, applying for government assistance programs would be a suitable option. These programs can provide financial support to individuals in need, helping John cover his expenses. Additionally, seeking financial advice from a professional may also be beneficial, but it may require additional costs. Finding a part-time job at John's age and health status might not be feasible, and borrowing money from friends and family should be considered as a last resort after exploring other options.

Question 132: Correct Answer: B) Social worker

Rationale: The social worker is responsible for coordinating the transition of care for a patient in rehabilitation. They collaborate with the interdisciplinary team to ensure a smooth transition from the rehabilitation facility to the patient's home or another healthcare setting. The social worker assesses the patient's social and emotional needs, connects them with community resources, and helps develop a discharge plan that meets the patient's goals. They play a vital role in addressing any psychosocial issues and coordinating necessary services, such as home health care or outpatient therapy, to facilitate a successful transition.

Question 133: Correct Answer: D) Edema

Rationale: Edema is the abnormal accumulation of fluid in interstitial spaces, leading to swelling of the affected area. It is characterized by excessive fluid retention and can be caused by various factors such as heart failure, liver disease, kidney disease, or venous insufficiency. Dehydration refers to a deficit of body water, hypovolemia refers to a decreased blood volume, and hypertonicity refers to an increased concentration of solutes in the blood. These conditions are not synonymous with excessive fluid retention seen in edema.

Question 134: Correct Answer: C) Teach the patient deep breathing and relaxation techniques before and after exercise.

Rationale: In patients with MS experiencing fatigue and decreased activity tolerance, incorporating deep breathing and relaxation techniques before and after exercise can help conserve their energy. These techniques promote relaxation and reduce muscle tension, thereby reducing fatigue. Engaging in high-intensity exercises may further contribute to fatigue and worsen the patient's condition. It is important for the patient to take rest breaks during exercise to prevent overexertion. Additionally, the use of assistive devices may be necessary to support the patient's abilities and prevent excessive fatigue during physical therapy sessions.

Question 135: Correct Answer: C) Writing guide

Rationale: A writing guide is an assistive technology that can help individuals with fine motor skill difficulties, such as those caused by Parkinson's disease, to write more legibly. It provides a stable platform and guides the hand, reducing tremors and enabling smoother and clearer writing. For Mr. Johnson, who has difficulty writing legibly due to Parkinson's disease, a writing guide would provide the necessary support and assistance in improving his writing ability. A hearing aid, reading glasses, and a bedside commode are not directly related to addressing difficulties in writing legibly.

Question 136: Correct Answer: D) Pressure relief

Rationale: When implementing interventions for skin integrity, the CRRN should prioritize pressure relief. Pressure ulcers are a common complication that can occur in patients with limited mobility. Pressure relief techniques such as repositioning and using pressure-relieving devices help to reduce the risk of developing pressure ulcers. While other factors like moisture reduction, nutrition, and hydration are important for maintaining skin integrity, they may not be the primary focus when it comes to prevention and management of pressure ulcers. Proper skin assessment is also crucial, but in this case, pressure relief takes precedence in order to prevent the formation of pressure ulcers.

Question 137: Correct Answer: B) Pancreas

Rationale: The pancreas is responsible for releasing insulin, a hormone that helps regulate blood sugar levels in the body. Insulin enables cells to absorb glucose from the bloodstream, allowing it to be used as an energy source. Without insulin, blood sugar levels can become unbalanced, leading to conditions such as diabetes. The liver plays a role in glucose regulation by storing and releasing glucose as needed, but it does not release insulin. The stomach and kidneys are not involved in the production or regulation of insulin.

Question 138: Correct Answer: B) Coordinating and providing direct care to the patient, including physical therapy and medication administration.

Rationale: Providing direct care to the patient, including physical therapy and medication administration, is not primarily the role of the rehabilitation nurse. The rehabilitation nurse is responsible for assessing the patient's rehabilitation needs, developing an individualized care plan, and coordinating the multidisciplinary team's efforts to achieve patient-centered goals. The nurse collaborates with the patient's family and caregivers to ensure continuity of care and may conduct research and contribute to evidence-based practice to improve patient outcomes. However, direct care provision, such as physical therapy and medication administration, is typically undertaken by other members of the interdisciplinary team, such as physical therapists and pharmacists.

Question 139: Correct Answer: D) It incorporates scientific evidence and clinical expertise.

Rationale: Evidence-based research is an approach that combines scientific evidence with clinical expertise and patient values to make informed decisions about patient care. It is not based solely on opinions or personal experiences, but on rigorous scientific research. Rather than relying on maintaining traditional practices, evidence-based research seeks to incorporate the most current and effective interventions. It does not rely on anecdotal evidence, which can be subjective and unreliable. Instead, evidence-based research emphasizes the use of scientifically validated data to guide clinical decision-making, resulting in improved patient outcomes and enhanced quality of care.

Question 140: Correct Answer: A) Observing non-verbal cues

Rationale: Observing non-verbal cues is an essential assessment method that can help the nurse evaluate a patient's ability for effective communication. Non-verbal cues, such as facial expressions, body language, and gestures, provide valuable information about a patient's emotions, needs, and understanding. This assessment method helps the nurse gauge the patient's ability to express themselves and comprehend verbal communication effectively. Conducting a physical examination (Option B) and reviewing laboratory test results (Option C) are important assessments but are not specific to evaluating effective communication. Collecting a patient's medical history (Option D) provides valuable information about the patient's health but does not directly assess their communication abilities.

Question 141: Correct Answer: A) The patient reports difficulty initiating urination and incomplete bladder emptying.

Rationale: Difficulty initiating urination and incomplete bladder emptying suggest urinary retention, which can be a medical emergency and require immediate intervention to prevent bladder distension and potential urinary tract infections. Options B, C, and D may require interventions such as stool softeners for constipation, education on bowel movement regularity, and pelvic floor exercises for urinary incontinence, but they do not indicate immediate risk to the patient's health and safety.

Question 142: Correct Answer: C) Emphasizing the importance of proper bladder management

Rationale: Autonomic dysreflexia is a potentially life-threatening condition that can occur in patients with spinal cord injuries above the T6 level. It is often triggered by bladder distention or urinary tract infections. Therefore, the nurse should prioritize teaching interventions related to proper bladder management. This includes regular catheterization or intermittent self-catheterization to ensure bladder emptying, avoiding bladder overdistention, and promptly treating urinary tract infections. While promoting adequate fluid intake, regular bowel movements, and performing regular skin checks are important interventions, they are not specific to preventing autonomic dysreflexia in this scenario.

Question 143: Correct Answer: C) Nursing-sensitive indicators

Rationale: Nursing-sensitive indicators are quality measurement tools specifically designed to evaluate the impact of nursing care on patient outcomes. These indicators help nurses assess the effectiveness of their interventions and identify areas for improvement. SWOT analysis is a strategic planning tool, while root cause analysis and failure mode and effects analysis are methods used to investigate errors or adverse events. However, these tools do not specifically focus on measuring the quality of nursing care and patient outcomes. Therefore, the most suitable option for Emma in this scenario is nursing-sensitive indicators.

Question 144: Correct Answer: C) Advocate for Ms. Johnson's preferences and actively participate in the discussion.

Rationale: The nurse's role in a team conference is to actively participate and advocate for the patient's preferences and needs. In this scenario, Ms. Johnson and her daughter are

present, indicating their involvement in decision-making. The nurse should facilitate open communication, ensure that the patient's voice is heard, and advocate for their preferences whenever possible. By actively participating in the discussion, the nurse fosters a collaborative approach and helps ensure that the care plan aligns with the patient's goals and needs.

Question 145: Correct Answer: C) Collaborating with interdisciplinary teams to develop and implement individualized care plans.

Rationale: As a Certified Rehabilitation Registered Nurse (CRRN), the scope of practice includes working as part of an interdisciplinary team to provide holistic care to patients with disabilities or chronic conditions. This involves collaborating with professionals from various specialties to develop and implement individualized care plans that address the physical, psychological, and social needs of the patients. The CRRN does not typically provide direct care during the acute phase of illness or injury, administer medications independently, or conduct research studies. Instead, the focus is on optimizing the restoration and preservation of the patient's health and well-being across the lifespan, in line with rehabilitation standards.

Question 146: Correct Answer: A) Anticoagulants

Rationale: Anticoagulants are medications that are used to prevent the formation of blood clots. While they are effective in preventing clotting, they also carry a risk of bleeding, which can be life-threatening. Therefore, it is crucial for rehabilitation registered nurses (RRNs) to closely monitor patients on anticoagulants for any signs or symptoms of bleeding, such as bruising, nosebleeds, or blood in the urine or stool. By closely monitoring patients on anticoagulants, RRNs can intervene early to prevent complications and ensure patient safety. Acetaminophen, antihistamines, and antibiotics, although important medications, do not carry the same level of risk as anticoagulants when it comes to patient safety.

Question 147: Correct Answer: B) Braden scale

Rationale: The Braden scale is a commonly used tool to assess an individual's risk for developing pressure ulcers. It evaluates sensory perception, moisture, activity, mobility, nutrition, and friction/shear. Each category is assigned a score, and the lower the total score, the higher the risk for developing pressure ulcers. The FLACC scale is used to assess pain in nonverbal patients, Wong-Baker FACES scale is used to assess pain intensity in children, and the CAGE questionnaire is used to assess alcoholism. Therefore, option B is the correct answer as it is specifically designed to assess pressure ulcer risk.

Question 148: Correct Answer: B) Providing Mary with assistive devices such as handrails and non-slip mats.

Rationale: Providing Mary with assistive devices such as handrails and non-slip mats will help minimize safety risk factors. These devices can assist Mary in maintaining balance, preventing falls, and promoting independent mobility. Conducting regular safety inspections of the patient's room (option A) is important, but providing assistive devices directly addresses Mary's specific needs. Ensuring that Mary's medications are within reach on her bedside table (option C) may pose a safety risk if she accidentally takes the wrong medication or overdoses. Ignoring potential hazards (option D) goes against the CRRN's role in promoting a safe environment and should never be done.

Question 149: Correct Answer: A) Assess the current medication administration policies and protocols in the facility

Rationale: As a CRRN, Ms. Johnson is responsible for integrating quality improvement processes into nursing practice. Assessing the current medication administration policies and protocols in the facility is an essential step in identifying areas where improvements can be made to prevent medication errors. Ignoring the incidents or delegating the task to a nursing assistant would not address the root cause of the problem. Implementing disciplinary action without investigating the policies and protocols first would not be an appropriate approach. Assessing the current practices will help Ms. Johnson identify areas that need improvement and develop strategies to enhance the quality of care provided in the facility.

Question 150: Correct Answer: A) Assessment

Rationale: The assessment is the first step of the nursing process. It involves gathering data about the patient's current health status, including physical, psychological, social, and environmental factors. This step includes the collection of subjective and objective data through interviews, physical examinations, and reviewing medical records. By obtaining a thorough assessment, the nurse can identify the patient's strengths, limitations, and healthcare needs, which then contribute to the development of an individualized care plan. The assessment process is essential in delivering cost-effective, patient-centered care as it forms the foundation for clinical decision-making and identification of priority interventions.

CRRN Practice Questions (SET 3)

Question 1: Which of the following is an appropriate nursing intervention to optimize a patient's elimination patterns?
A) Encouraging the patient to consume foods high in fiber
B) Administering laxatives on a regular basis
C) Limiting the patient's fluid intake
D) Discouraging the patient from engaging in physical activity

Question 2: When implementing a quality improvement model to improve patient care, which step involves identifying the specific needs and concerns of the patients and their families?
A) Plan
B) Do
C) Act
D) Study

Question 3: Mrs. Johnson is a 65-year-old female with a C6 spinal cord injury. She is admitted to the rehabilitation unit and is currently receiving enteral tube feeding due to dysphagia. The nurse performs an initial assessment of Mrs. Johnson's nutritional status. Which of the following findings would indicate a need for further intervention?
A) Weight loss of 2 pounds in the past week
B) Albumin level of 3.2 g/dL
C) Normal bowel sounds upon auscultation
D) Serum potassium level of 4.2 mEq/L

Question 4: Which intervention should a Certified Rehabilitation Registered Nurse (CRRN) prioritize when implementing and evaluating interventions for nutrition?
A) Assessing the patient's current nutritional status and needs
B) Administering enteral feedings without assessing the patient's preferences
C) Recommending parenteral nutrition without involving the dietitian
D) Restricting all oral intake for patients at risk of aspiration

Question 5: Mrs. Johnson, a 68-year-old patient with a history of depression and suicidal ideation, is admitted to the rehabilitation unit following a fall resulting in a fractured hip. During her time in the hospital, she becomes increasingly withdrawn and expresses feelings of hopelessness. Which of the following nursing interventions would be a priority in addressing Mrs. Johnson's safety concerns regarding harm to self?
A) Providing one-on-one supervision at all times during her hospital stay
B) Implementing suicide precautions, including removing any potential means for self-harm
C) Collaborating with the healthcare team to develop a comprehensive care plan addressing her psychosocial needs
D) Educating Mrs. Johnson on the importance of seeking help and providing a list of crisis hotlines

Question 6: You are a Certified Rehabilitation Registered Nurse (CRRN) working in a rehabilitation facility. A patient admitted to your unit, John, has a lower limb amputation and is scheduled for discharge in a few days. As part of your role, you need to ensure that the patient's care plan aligns with the rehabilitation scope of practice. Which of the following interventions demonstrates the correct application of the rehabilitation scope of practice for John?
A) Recommending the use of a wheelchair for all mobility activities to prevent falls.

B) Collaborating with the physical therapist to create an individualized exercise program focusing on upper body strength.
C) Scheduling regular follow-up appointments with a psychiatrist to monitor John's mental health.
D) Assisting John during therapy sessions to ensure he follows the prescribed exercises correctly.

Question 7: Which nursing theory emphasizes the importance of the nurse-client relationship in promoting holistic and individualized patient care in rehabilitation?
A) Roy's Adaptation Model
B) King's Theory of Goal Attainment
C) Neuman's Systems Model
D) Orem's Self-Care Deficit Theory

Question 8: Which standardized assessment tool is commonly used to measure functional independence in rehabilitation settings?
A) Mini-Mental State Examination (MMSE)
B) Glasgow Coma Scale (GCS)
C) Functional Independence Measure (FIM)
D) Barthel Index

Question 9: Mrs. Johnson, a 35-year-old female patient with paraplegia, has been admitted to the rehabilitation unit after sustaining a spinal cord injury in a car accident. The patient expresses concerns about her sexual and reproductive health post-injury. As a Certified Rehabilitation Registered Nurse (CRRN), which of the following is the most appropriate nursing action to assess the patient's goals related to sexuality and reproduction?
A) Provide the patient with brochures about sexual health and reproductive options.
B) Discuss the patient's concerns and offer to involve a sexuality counselor.
C) Ignore the patient's concerns as they may be influenced by her current emotional state.
D) Assure the patient that sexual and reproductive goals are irrelevant during rehabilitation.

Question 10: Mr. Johnson, a 58-year-old patient with a traumatic brain injury, is admitted to the rehabilitation unit. The patient is having difficulty communicating and is often frustrated with his inability to express himself. The nurse identifies the need to optimize the patient's ability to communicate effectively. Which intervention would be most appropriate for the nurse to implement?
A) Encouraging the patient to use hand gestures for communication
B) Assigning a communication board to the patient for written communication
C) Limiting visitor access to reduce distractions
D) Administering a sedative to calm the patient

Question 11: Which of the following is an instrumental activity of daily living (IADL)?
A) Bathing
B) Dressing
C) Cooking
D) Toileting

Question 12: Skill in promoting effective communication is crucial for a Certified Rehabilitation Registered Nurse (CRRN) to provide optimal psychosocial support to patients and their caregivers. Which of the following

strategies would be most effective in promoting effective communication?
A) Using medical jargon to facilitate understanding
B) Speaking quickly to save time during patient interactions
C) Listening actively and attentively to patients and caregivers
D) Interrupting patients and caregivers to provide immediate solutions

Question 13:   A patient, John, has been admitted to a rehabilitation facility following a stroke. He has been experiencing swallowing difficulties, known as dysphagia. The rehabilitation team is working on implementing teaching interventions to help John manage his swallowing deficits. The nurse is providing education to John and his family about specific techniques to improve safe swallowing. Which of the following interventions should the nurse recommend to John and his family?
A) Eating quickly to prevent aspiration
B) Consuming thin liquids to minimize choking risk
C) Eating large meals at once to reduce overall mealtime
D) Taking small bites and chewing thoroughly before swallowing

Question 14:   A patient with a spinal cord injury has been admitted to the rehabilitation unit. The patient is experiencing difficulty coping with the changes in their physical abilities and is feeling overwhelmed. The nurse is implementing coping strategies to promote psychosocial well-being. Which intervention is most appropriate for the nurse to implement?
A) Encouraging the patient to explore their feelings and emotions related to their injury
B) Recommending that the patient avoid discussing their injury with family and friends
C) Suggesting that the patient withdraw from participating in social activities
D) Ignoring the patient's emotional needs and focusing solely on physical rehabilitation

Question 15:   Mr. Johnson is a 55-year-old patient with multiple sclerosis (MS) who requires self-management techniques to cope with the challenges of his condition. Which technology intervention would be most effective for Mr. Johnson's self-management of MS?
A) Monitoring his blood pressure regularly
B) Using a smartphone application to track his medication schedule
C) Monitoring his blood glucose levels
D) Using a pedometer to track his daily steps

Question 16:   Nurse Sarah is providing care to a patient named Mr. Johnson, who has recently suffered a spinal cord injury resulting in paralysis. As part of the rehabilitation process, Mr. Johnson will require training in activities of daily living to promote independence. Which of the following skills is essential for Nurse Sarah to demonstrate while teaching Mr. Johnson?
A) Effective communication
B) Medication administration
C) Wound care
D) Intravenous line insertion

Question 17:   Mr. Johnson, a 65-year-old patient with a spinal cord injury, requires assistance with activities of daily living. He has limited upper body strength and cannot grasp objects effectively. Which adaptive equipment would be most appropriate for Mr. Johnson to facilitate his independence with eating?
A) Built-up utensils

B) Sippy cup
C) Plate guard
D) Bendable straws

Question 18:   Mr. Johnson is a 70-year-old male patient admitted to the rehabilitation unit following a stroke. He has dysphagia, limited physical activity, and a decreased appetite. As the rehabilitation nurse, you are responsible for assessing his nutritional needs. Which of the following would be the most appropriate intervention for Mr. Johnson?
A) Encourage Mr. Johnson to eat a regular diet without modifications.
B) Consult a dietician to place Mr. Johnson on a clear liquid diet.
C) Collaborate with the speech therapist to evaluate Mr. Johnson's swallowing function.
D) Offer Mr. Johnson a high-protein diet without modification.

Question 19:   Mrs. Johnson, a 65-year-old woman, is admitted to a rehabilitation facility following a stroke that has left her with right-sided weakness and difficulty in speaking. As a Certified Rehabilitation Registered Nurse (CRRN), what is your priority action to promote Mrs. Johnson's community reintegration or transition to the next level of care?
A) Assess Mrs. Johnson's cognitive function and communication abilities.
B) Coordinate a team meeting to discuss Mrs. Johnson's rehabilitation goals and progress.
C) Teach Mrs. Johnson's family about home modifications and assistive devices.
D) Collaborate with the social worker to arrange for transportation services.

Question 20:   According to the skill set required in the field of rehabilitation nursing, which of the following is included under the task of "Use the nursing process to deliver cost-effective patient-centered care"?
A) Analyzing insurance coverage for patients
B) Creating individualized care plans
C) Evaluating the cost-effectiveness of medications
D) Implementing evidence-based practice

Question 21:   What is the role of the Certified Rehabilitation Registered Nurse (CRRN) in the transition of care for patients?
A) Coordinating discharge planning and ensuring appropriate community resources are in place.
B) Conducting physical assessments and providing hands-on care during the rehabilitation process.
C) Collaborating with the physical therapist to design exercise programs for patients.
D) Administering medications and managing pain during the rehabilitation process.

Question 22:   Which nursing model focuses on the concept of the nurse-client relationship as the foundation of nursing practice?
A) Orem's Self-Care Model
B) Roy's Adaptation Model
C) Peplau's Interpersonal Relations Model
D) Neuman's Systems Model

Question 23:   According to the skill in 'Collaborate with the interdisciplinary team to achieve patient-centered goals,' which of the following is NOT a key component of effective collaboration in a rehabilitation setting?
A) Active listening and communication
B) Respecting and valuing each team member's expertise

C) Making decisions independently without seeking input from others

D) Sharing information and resources

Question 24: Sarah, a rehabilitation registered nurse, is assisting a patient with spinal cord injury to use assistive technology for communication. The patient is unable to verbally communicate due to paralysis. Sarah suggests using a device that translates eye movements into letters and words for communication purposes. Which assistive technology is Sarah referring to?

A) Mouthstick
B) Headpointer
C) Eye-gaze system
D) Gesture-based system

Question 25: Which healthcare professional is responsible for coordinating the rehabilitation team and facilitating care transitions for a patient in a rehabilitation setting?

A) Speech therapist
B) Physical therapist
C) Rehabilitation nurse
D) Social worker

Question 26: Which of the following factors may increase the risk of falls in a rehabilitation setting?

A) Dim lighting
B) Cluttered hallways
C) Slippery floors
D) All of the above

Question 27: Mr. Smith, a 64-year-old stroke patient, has been admitted to the rehabilitation unit following a left hemispheric stroke. He presents with expressive aphasia, making it difficult for him to express his thoughts and understand spoken language. As the Certified Rehabilitation Registered Nurse (CRRN), you are responsible for optimizing his ability to communicate effectively. Which of the following interventions is most appropriate to facilitate communication for Mr. Smith?

A) Speak louder and slower to help Mr. Smith understand.
B) Utilize nonverbal cues such as gestures and visual aids.
C) Encourage Mr. Smith to repeat words and sentences multiple times.
D) Limit social interactions to minimize frustration for Mr. Smith.

Question 28: Mrs. Smith, a 45-year-old patient with spinal cord injury, is preparing for discharge from the rehabilitation facility. The nurse is discussing the importance of self-advocacy with Mrs. Smith. Which statement made by Mrs. Smith indicates a correct understanding of self-advocacy?

A) "I will rely on my family to make decisions for me since they know me best."
B) "I will always follow the healthcare team's recommendations without question."
C) "I understand the importance of speaking up for my needs and preferences."
D) "I will delegate the responsibility of self-advocacy to the healthcare professionals."

Question 29: Which of the following is a key legislation that promotes a safe environment of care for patients and staff and minimizes risk?

A) The Occupational Safety and Health Act (OSHA)
B) The Americans with Disabilities Act (ADA)
C) The Health Insurance Portability and Accountability Act (HIPAA)

D) The Family and Medical Leave Act (FMLA)

Question 30: Nancy, a 62-year-old patient with multiple sclerosis, has been prescribed a baclofen pump for the management of her spasticity. The nurse assesses the patient's understanding of the device and its use. Which statement made by Nancy indicates a correct understanding of the baclofen pump?

A) "I will need to change the batteries in the pump every week."
B) "The catheter will be inserted into my spinal cord to deliver the medication."
C) "I can adjust the dosage of medication as needed by using the pump."
D) "The pump will send electrical impulses to my muscles to reduce spasticity."

Question 31: Which of the following resources would be most appropriate for assisting a patient with completing a living will?

A) Financial planner
B) Physical therapist
C) Hospice nurse
D) Attorney specializing in elder law

Question 32: Which of the following is an example of a legal issue related to promoting a safe environment of care?

A) Ensuring the availability of personal protective equipment (PPE) for staff
B) Implementing infection control measures to prevent the spread of communicable diseases
C) Conducting regular safety inspections of the physical environment
D) Maintaining accurate documentation of patient care and incidents

Question 33: What is the purpose of reporting healthcare-acquired pressure injuries in a rehabilitation facility?

A) To increase the facility's reputation and attract more patients.
B) To ensure compliance with legal regulations.
C) To track the facility's rate of readmissions.
D) To promote a culture of safety and quality improvement.

Question 34: Mrs. Johnson, a 54-year-old patient, has recently suffered a stroke and is admitted to a rehabilitation center. During the team meeting, a nurse asks about the philosophy of rehabilitation. Which statement best describes the philosophy of rehabilitation?

A) Rehabilitation is solely focused on curing the underlying medical condition.
B) Rehabilitation aims to optimize functional independence and quality of life.
C) Rehabilitation mainly involves the administration of medications and medical procedures.
D) Rehabilitation primarily focuses on providing emotional support to the patient and their family.

Question 35: Mr. Johnson, a 53-year-old patient with a history of hypertension, is admitted to the rehabilitation unit following a recent stroke. While providing care, the nurse observes that Mr. Johnson experiences shortness of breath, sweating, and increased heart rate during physical therapy sessions. These symptoms are consistent with the stress response. Which of the following hormones is primarily responsible for these physiological changes?

A) Epinephrine
B) Insulin
C) Estrogen
D) Growth hormone

Question 36: Mr. Johnson, a 55-year-old patient with multiple sclerosis, is admitted to the rehabilitation unit. He complains of difficulty falling asleep at night. The nurse understands that optimizing the patient's sleep and rest patterns is crucial for his recovery. Which of the following interventions should the nurse prioritize to help Mr. Johnson improve his sleep?
A) Encouraging Mr. Johnson to nap during the day
B) Administering a sedative medication at bedtime
C) Implementing a regular sleep schedule
D) Allowing Mr. Johnson to stay up late watching television

Question 37: Mr. Johnson, a 72-year-old patient, has undergone a hip replacement surgery and is now being transferred to the rehabilitation unit for further recovery. The nurse is assessing his self-care ability and mobility. Which intervention should the nurse prioritize to optimize Mr. Johnson's functional ability?
A) Encouraging Mr. Johnson to independently perform activities of daily living (ADLs) to promote self-care and independence.
B) Placing Mr. Johnson on a strict bed rest to prevent any potential complications.
C) Administering pain medication to ensure Mr. Johnson's comfort and encourage mobility.
D) Limiting Mr. Johnson's mobility to avoid any potential complications.

Question 38: Sarah, a Certified Rehabilitation Registered Nurse (CRRN), is working with a patient named John who has a spinal cord injury. John is interested in using technology and assistive devices to improve his mobility. Sarah provides education to John about various options available to him.
Question : Which of the following assistive devices would be most suitable for John to improve his mobility?
A) Communication board
B) Powered wheelchair
C) Hearing aids
D) Splints

Question 39: Emily, a 45-year-old woman, is being treated in a rehabilitation facility following a spinal cord injury. She is experiencing not only physical challenges but is also struggling with feelings of anxiety and depression. The healthcare team recognizes the need for psychological support and suggests a referral to a mental health professional. Which of the following statements is true regarding the referral process for Emily's psychological needs?
A) The rehabilitation facility should wait for Emily to request a referral.
B) The rehabilitation team should refer Emily to mental health services without her consent.
C) The rehabilitation team should assess Emily's psychological needs and discuss the possible benefits of a referral with her.
D) Emily should take the initiative to find a mental health professional on her own.

Question 40: Sarah, a rehabilitation nurse, is providing care to a patient who suffered a stroke and is experiencing difficulties with mobility. Which nursing model or theory would guide Sarah in her approach to care for this patient?

A) Adaptation Model by Sister Callista Roy
B) Health Promotion Model by Nola Pender
C) Transcultural Nursing Theory by Madeleine Leininger
D) Self-Care Deficit Nursing Theory by Dorothea Orem

Question 41: Which skill in the area of 'Skill in:' under the broad topic of 'Task 1: Apply the nursing process to optimize the restoration and preservation of the patient's health and holistic well-being across the lifespan, Functional Health Patterns' involves identifying and implementing appropriate interventions to promote functional independence and improve quality of life?
A) Assessment techniques
B) Rehabilitation planning
C) Patient education
D) Safety measures

Question 42: A rehabilitation unit is implementing a quality improvement model to improve patient care. The team decides to use the Plan-Do-Study-Act (PDSA) cycle for their improvement projects. Which of the following correctly describes the PDSA cycle?
A) Plan, Develop, Standardize, Analyze
B) Propose, Develop, Stimulate, Assist
C) Pilot, Document, Summarize, Analyze
D) Plan, Do, Study, Act

Question 43: A patient with a spinal cord injury has been admitted to a rehabilitation facility. The interdisciplinary team is discussing the patient's care plan, and the nurse team lead is considering delegation of responsibilities. Which task would be appropriate for the nurse team lead to delegate to a certified nursing assistant (CNA)?
A) Developing the patient's individualized plan of care.
B) Monitoring the patient's vital signs and pain levels.
C) Collaborating with the physical therapist to develop a mobility program.
D) Administering medications and providing wound care.

Question 44: A 45-year-old male patient has been admitted to a rehabilitation unit following a spinal cord injury. As a Certified Rehabilitation Registered Nurse (CRRN), you are responsible for documenting the services provided during the patient's stay. Which of the following statements regarding documenting services provided is true?
A) Documentation should be done at the end of each shift to ensure accuracy.
B) Documenting only the positive aspects of care is acceptable.
C) Abbreviations and acronyms should be used to save time and space in documentation.
D) Incomplete or illegible documentation can compromise patient care.

Question 45: A CRRN is assessing a patient's nutritional status. Which of the following findings would indicate a need for further intervention?
A) Adequate weight gain
B) Albumin level of 4.5 g/dL
C) Oral intake of less than 50% of meals
D) Normal bowel movements and digestion

Question 46: Which of the following statements about the use of technology for self-management is true?
A) Technology can replace the need for healthcare professionals in self-management.
B) Technology is not effective in promoting patient engagement and empowerment.

C) Technology cannot assist in monitoring and tracking health-related data.
D) Technology can provide real-time feedback and support for self-management.

Question 47: Mrs. Thompson, a 78-year-old patient, is admitted to a rehabilitation unit following a hip replacement surgery. The healthcare team is developing a plan of care for Mrs. Thompson and is reviewing clinical practice guidelines related to post-operative pain management. Which of the following statements regarding clinical practice guidelines is accurate?
A) Clinical practice guidelines are only applicable in acute-care settings.
B) Clinical practice guidelines are evidence-based recommendations to guide healthcare professionals in making decisions about patient care.
C) Clinical practice guidelines are exclusive to specific medical specialties.
D) Clinical practice guidelines are developed solely by individual healthcare providers.

Question 48: As a Certified Rehabilitation Registered Nurse (CRRN), you are responsible for promoting a safe environment of care for patients and staff to minimize risk. One aspect of this role involves understanding legislative, economic, ethical, and legal issues. Which legislative issue should a CRRN be particularly vigilant about when it comes to promoting a safe work environment for staff and minimizing risk?
A) Occupational Safety and Health Administration (OSH A) regulations
B) The Health Insurance Portability and Accountability Act (HIPAA)
C) The Americans with Disabilities Act (ADA)
D) The Affordable Care Act (ACA)

Question 49: Which factor is known to disrupt normal sleep patterns?
A) Consuming a diet high in caffeine
B) Engaging in regular exercise
C) Maintaining a consistent sleep schedule
D) Creating a calm sleep environment

Question 50: Mr. Johnson, a 54-year-old patient with a spinal cord injury at the T5 level, is admitted to the rehabilitation unit. The nurse is assessing Mr. Johnson's nutritional and metabolic patterns. Which finding would indicate the need for further intervention?
A) Mr. Johnson has a body mass index (BMI) of 26.
B) Mr. Johnson has a 3 cm pressure ulcer on his sacrum.
C) Mr. Johnson has a decreased appetite and is only eating half of his meals.
D) Mr. Johnson is maintaining a fluid intake of 2000 mL per day.

Question 51: As a Certified Rehabilitation Registered Nurse (CRRN), you are responsible for implementing safety prevention measures to promote a safe environment of care for patients and staff. Which of the following actions demonstrates an appropriate safety measure?
A) Providing a patient with a non-slip mat in the shower.
B) Placing a patient with decreased mobility near the exit door for easy access.
C) Administering medications without double-checking the patient's identification.
D) Leaving the bedrails down for a confused patient to prevent restriction.

Question 52: Mr. Johnson, a 50-year-old male, has recently suffered a stroke and is admitted to the rehabilitation unit. As a Certified Rehabilitation Registered Nurse (CRRN), you are responsible for optimizing his restoration and preservation of health. Which skill is most important for you to demonstrate in this situation?
A) Administering medications correctly
B) Performing physical assessment and monitoring vital signs
C) Assisting with activities of daily living (ADLs)
D) Providing emotional support and counseling

Question 53: Mrs. Johnson, a 75-year-old patient, was admitted to the rehabilitation unit for physical therapy following a stroke. As a Certified Rehabilitation Registered Nurse (CRRN), you understand the importance of federal quality measurement efforts in healthcare. Which of the following is an example of a federal quality measurement initiative?
A) Medicare Conditions of Participation (CoPs)
B) Hospital Consumer Assessment of Healthcare Providers and Systems (HCAHPS)
C) National Council Licensure Examination for Registered Nurses (NCLEX-RN)
D) American Nurses Credentialing Center (ANCC) Magnet Recognition Program

Question 54: What is the goal of rehabilitation nursing?
A) To provide direct care and treatment to individuals with disabilities or chronic illnesses
B) To promote independent functioning and improve quality of life for individuals with disabilities or chronic illnesses
C) To advocate for individuals with disabilities or chronic illnesses
D) To assist in the development of individualized care plans for individuals with disabilities or chronic illnesses

Question 55: Mrs. Smith is a 45-year-old patient who suffered a spinal cord injury resulting in quadriplegia. During the rehabilitation process, the healthcare team introduced her to various adaptive equipment to enhance her independence in daily activities. Which of the following electronic hand-held devices would be most beneficial for Mrs. Smith to assist with communication?
A) Electric wheelchair
B) Overhead lift system
C) Speech recognition software
D) Service animal

Question 56: Sarah is a Certified Rehabilitation Registered Nurse (CRRN) working in a rehabilitation center. She is caring for a patient named John who is undergoing physical therapy after a spinal cord injury. John is concerned about the cost of his rehabilitation treatments and asks Sarah about financial assistance programs that he may be eligible for. Question: Which legislation provides financial assistance for individuals with disabilities, such as John, to cover the cost of rehabilitation treatments?
A) HIPAA (Health Insurance Portability and Accountability Act)
B) IDEA (Individuals with Disabilities Education Act)
C) Affordable Care Act D) Medicare

Question 57: Which of the following is a potential complication of central lines, ports, and catheters?
A) Catheter dislodgement
B) Hypotension
C) Respiratory distress
D) Constipation

Question 58: Which adaptive equipment can be used to enhance activities of daily living for a patient with limited hand dexterity?
A) Service animal
B) Electronic hand-held device
C) Electrical stimulation
D) None of the above

Question 59: Which communication intervention would be most appropriate for a patient with dysarthria?
A) Providing written instructions
B) Using visual aids
C) Speaking slowly and clearly
D) Conducting a group therapy session

Question 60: A 35-year-old male patient with a spinal cord injury is admitted to the rehabilitation unit. He is experiencing difficulties in expressing his needs and emotions, often becoming frustrated and angry during therapy sessions. The patient's wife frequently accompanies him and tries to communicate on his behalf. The nurse recognizes the importance of effective communication and utilizes various techniques to facilitate understanding and promote positive interactions. Which communication technique would be most appropriate for the nurse to use when interacting with this patient?
A) Interrupting the patient to clarify his needs
B) Providing unsolicited advice to resolve his frustrations
C) Demonstrating empathy and active listening
D) Ignoring the patient's wife's attempts to communicate

Question 61: The use of the Transtheoretical Model (TTM) provides a framework for understanding and promoting behavioral change in rehabilitation patients. Which stage of the TTM involves the individual's awareness and consideration of making a change?
A) Precontemplation
B) Contemplation
C) Preparation
D) Action

Question 62: Which of the following is an essential step in incorporating evidence-based research into practice?
A) Conducting a literature review to identify relevant studies
B) Relying solely on clinical expertise and experience
C) Disregarding current research findings
D) Implementing outdated care practices

Question 63: Mr. Johnson is a 59-year-old patient who suffered a spinal cord injury and is currently receiving rehabilitation at a specialized facility. During the discharge planning process, the rehabilitation nurse realizes that Mr. Johnson may face financial barriers in accessing the resources needed for his community reintegration. Which of the following actions should the nurse take to identify financial barriers and provide appropriate resources for Mr. Johnson?
A) Assess Mr. Johnson's current financial situation and insurance coverage.
B) Assume that Mr. Johnson will be able to afford all necessary resources.
C) Suggest that Mr. Johnson take out a loan to cover any financial gaps.
D) Ignore the financial aspect and focus solely on the patient's medical needs.

Question 64: Which assistive device is most appropriate for a patient with limited mobility due to a spinal cord injury?
A) Cane
B) Walker
C) Manual wheelchair
D) Power wheelchair

Question 65: Which nursing model emphasizes the importance of the therapeutic nurse-patient relationship in rehabilitation nursing?
A) Roy's Adaptation Model
B) Orem's Self-Care Deficit Model
C) Watson's Human Caring Theory
D) Levine's Conservation Model

Question 66: What assessment technique can be used to evaluate a patient's ability to comprehend and retain information?
A) Observation of non-verbal cues
B) Checking blood pressure
C) Auscultating lung sounds
D) Measuring urine output

Question 67: A patient admitted to the rehabilitation unit has a newly placed central line for the administration of long-term antibiotics. The registered nurse is teaching the patient and caregiver about the purpose and caring for the central line. Which statement made by the patient indicates a need for further teaching?
A) "I should avoid touching the central line insertion site to prevent infection."
B) "I will clean the insertion site daily with alcohol swabs."
C) "If I notice any redness or discharge at the insertion site, I will contact the healthcare provider."
D) "I can take showers and get the central line wet without any problem."

Question 68: Which teaching intervention is most effective in promoting health and wellness among individuals with a chronic illness?
A) Providing printed educational materials
B) Conducting group education sessions
C) Utilizing multimedia presentations
D) Offering one-on-one counseling sessions

Question 69: Which of the following is an example of a Functional Health Pattern in rehabilitation nursing?
A) Medication administration techniques
B) Pain management strategies
C) Communication skills
D) Transfer and mobility techniques

Question 70: Mr. Jones, a 70-year-old patient with a history of diabetes and peripheral neuropathy, has been admitted to a rehabilitation unit after a below-the-knee amputation. The nurse is planning to assess the patient's safety risks. Which of the following would the nurse prioritize in the assessment?
A) Assessing the patient's knowledge regarding his condition and self-care management
B) Evaluating the patient's range of motion and muscle strength in the remaining leg
C) Identifying potential fall risks in the patient's environment
D) Reviewing the patient's medication history for potential adverse drug reactions

Question 71: Which nursing model was developed by Dorothea Orem and emphasizes the individual's ability to perform self-care tasks?

A) Roy's Adaptation Model
B) Neuman Systems Model
C) Orem's Self-Care Deficit Theory
D) Watson's Theory of Human Caring

Question 72: Mrs. Johnson, a 72-year-old patient with a history of chronic pain due to osteoarthritis, is admitted to the rehabilitation unit following a hip replacement surgery. She is currently experiencing severe pain postoperatively. The healthcare provider orders an analgesic medication to help manage her pain. Which of the following analgesics would be most appropriate for Mrs. Johnson in this situation?
A) Morphine sulfate
B) Ibuprofen
C) Acetaminophen
D) Codeine sulfate

Question 73: When implementing behavioral management strategies, which technique involves the establishment of clear guidelines and expectations?
A) Contracts
B) Positive reinforcement
C) Rule setting
D) Aversion therapy

Question 74: Mary, a Certified Rehabilitation Registered Nurse (CRRN), works at a rehabilitation facility that provides comprehensive care to individuals with disabilities. She ensures that the facility complies with all regulatory standards and regulations related to disability and rehabilitation. Mary recently attended a training session on regulatory agencies and their roles in healthcare. She learned about various agencies and their functions, including CARF, The Joint Commission, APS, CPS, CMS, SSA, and OSHA. Mary wants to test her knowledge about these agencies. Which agency is primarily responsible for accrediting rehabilitation facilities and ensuring they meet specific quality standards?
A) APS
B) SSA
C) CARF
D) OSHA

Question 75: A 55-year-old patient, Mr. Smith, is admitted to the rehabilitation unit following a stroke. During the initial assessment, the nurse identifies impaired mobility and muscle weakness on the affected side. The nurse formulates a nursing diagnosis of impaired physical mobility related to neuromuscular impairment. Which intervention should the nurse prioritize to optimize the restoration and preservation of the patient's health and holistic well-being?
A) Monitor vital signs every 4 hours
B) Administer pain medication as needed
C) Provide active range of motion exercises
D) Assess urine output every 2 hours

Question 76: John is a 55-year-old patient who suffered a traumatic brain injury in a car accident. He is now undergoing rehabilitation in a healthcare facility. The nurse is using a nursing model that emphasizes the patient's ability to adapt to their environment. Which nursing model is being utilized in this case?
A) King's Goal Attainment Theory
B) Rogers' Science of Unitary Human Beings
C) Neuman's Systems Model
D) Orem's Self-Care Deficit Theory

Question 77: Which skill is important for a Certified Rehabilitation Registered Nurse (CRRN) when applying the nursing process to promote optimal nutrition and hydration?
A) Assessing the client's dietary preferences and cultural beliefs.
B) Collaborating with the client's family regarding meal planning.
C) Planning and implementing individualized diet and fluid intake.
D) Administering enteral feedings and intravenous fluids.

Question 78: Which of the following medications is commonly used as an anticholinergic for the treatment of urinary incontinence?
A) Morphine
B) Omeprazole
C) Tolterodine
D) Gabapentin

Question 79: Jane is a registered nurse working in a rehabilitation center. She is familiar with various nursing models and theories that are used to guide patient care. One of her patients, Mr. Smith, sustained a traumatic brain injury and is currently undergoing cognitive rehabilitation. Jane wants to implement a model that focuses on the cognitive development of an individual. Which of the following models would be most appropriate for Mr. Smith's rehabilitation?
A) Freud's psychoanalytic theory
B) Erikson's psychosocial theory
C) Piaget's cognitive development theory
D) Skinner's behaviorism

Question 80: Which community resource can provide emotional support and a sense of belonging to individuals and families facing rehabilitation challenges?
A) Internet forums and chat groups
B) Respite care services
C) Face-to-face support groups
D) Clergy or religious leaders

Question 81: Mrs. Johnson, a 75-year-old female, was admitted to the rehabilitation facility after undergoing hip replacement surgery. The nurse is conducting a skin assessment using the Braden scale to evaluate Mrs. Johnson's risk for pressure ulcers. While assessing Mrs. Johnson's skin, the nurse notices a reddened area on the coccyx that does not blanch when pressure is applied. The nurse should interpret this finding as which stage of pressure ulcers?
A) Stage I
B) Stage II
C) Stage III
D) Stage IV

Question 82: Which communication technique is helpful in establishing rapport and building trust with patients?
A) Active listening and empathetic responses
B) Using medical jargon and abbreviations
C) Providing minimal responses and avoiding lengthy conversations
D) Interrupting patients to expedite the conversation

Question 83: Which of the following interventions will have the greatest impact on promoting self-efficacy in a patient undergoing rehabilitation?
A) Providing resources and educational materials on available community support groups.

B) Encouraging the patient to set realistic goals and praising their efforts towards achieving them.
C) Administering medication to manage the patient's pain and discomfort.
D) Assisting the patient with activities of daily living to ensure a safe and comfortable environment.

Question 84: Which of the following activities is a part of the regulatory agency audit process?
A) Assessing patient satisfaction
B) Developing a nursing care plan
C) Conducting staff education
D) Reviewing medical records for compliance

Question 85: Which technology is commonly used to treat sleep apnea by delivering a steady flow of air pressure to keep the airways open during sleep?
A) Sleep study
B) CPAP machine
C) BiPAP machine
D) Relaxation technology

Question 86: Sarah, a 6-year-old child, is brought to the rehabilitation center following a car accident. The accident has left her with a traumatic brain injury. As a certified rehabilitation registered nurse (CRRN), you assess Sarah's developmental factors to provide appropriate care. Question: Which of the following developmental factors is crucial to consider when caring for Sarah?
A) Social and emotional development
B) Fine motor skills development
C) Sensory development
D) Cognitive development

Question 87: Mr. Thompson, a 45-year-old patient with a history of a spinal cord injury, is experiencing increased levels of stress related to his disability. As a rehabilitation nurse, which coping strategy should you suggest to promote stress management?
A) Avoidance
B) Substance abuse
C) Problem-solving
D) Denial

Question 88: Which nursing intervention would be most effective in promoting sleep and rest patterns in a patient with insomnia?
A) Encouraging the patient to take a long nap during the day.
B) Providing the patient with a large cup of coffee before bedtime.
C) Implementing a quiet and soothing environment in the patient's room.
D) Administering a sedative medication without the patient's consent.

Question 89: Mrs. Johnson, a 78-year-old patient, is admitted to a rehabilitation facility following a stroke. As the nurse responsible for her care, you plan to use a standardized assessment tool to assess her functional capabilities. Which of the following tools would be most appropriate for assessing Mrs. Johnson's functional status?
A) Glasgow Coma Scale
B) Barthel Index
C) Epworth Sleepiness Scale
D) Geriatric Depression Scale

Question 90: Mr. Johnson, a 56-year-old male, has recently suffered a stroke and is admitted to the rehabilitation unit. His wife, Mrs. Johnson, has been constantly by his side, providing physical and emotional support. As the rehabilitation nurse, you recognize the importance of accessing supportive team resources and services to address the psychosocial needs of both Mr. Johnson and his wife. Which of the following resources would be most appropriate in this situation?
A) Physical therapist
B) Occupational therapist
C) Psychologist
D) Nutritionist

Question 91: Which of the following is a safety measure to minimize risk in a rehabilitation setting?
A) Encouraging patients to engage in physical activities as much as possible.
B) Providing patient education on proper medication administration.
C) Allowing visitors to bring in outside food for patients.
D) Keeping the environment clean and free of clutter.

Question 92: Which action is the most appropriate for the Certified Rehabilitation Registered Nurse (CRRN) to take in order to assess the self-care ability and mobility of a patient?
A) Observe the patient while performing activities of daily living (ADLs).
B) Provide the patient with a self-report questionnaire to complete.
C) Perform a physical examination focusing on range of motion.
D) Ask the patient's family or caregiver about the patient's self-care ability and mobility.

Question 93: When including the patient and caregiver in the plan of care, which of the following is the most important reason for their involvement?
A) To improve communication between healthcare providers and patients
B) To ensure that patients are compliant with their medications
C) To increase patient satisfaction and promote a sense of ownership in their own care
D) To decrease the workload for healthcare providers

Question 94: A 65-year-old patient with limited vision due to macular degeneration is admitted to the rehabilitation unit. The patient is experiencing difficulty reading and comprehending written material. Which of the following interventions would be most appropriate to optimize this patient's ability to communicate effectively?
A) Use small font size when providing written information to the patient.
B) Provide the patient with a magnifying glass to read written material.
C) Encourage the patient to rely solely on auditory communication.
D) Utilize large-print materials for written information.

Question 95: Mr. Johnson, a 65-year-old male, was admitted to the rehabilitation unit following a severe stroke that resulted in left-sided weakness. As his rehabilitation nurse, you are responsible for providing appropriate care to support his recovery. Which of the following interventions should be prioritized for Mr. Johnson?
A) Administering pain medication as needed
B) Promoting physical mobility and exercise
C) Providing emotional support and counseling
D) Monitoring vital signs regularly

Question 96: When using voice activated call systems as an adaptive equipment, which of the following should the certified rehabilitation registered nurse (CRRN) keep in mind?
A) Voice recognition technology may not be as accurate for individuals with speech impairments.
B) All voice activated call systems require the use of a personal computer.
C) Voice activated call systems are only suitable for use in rehabilitation settings.
D) Voice recognition technology is not widely available in the market.

Question 97: Ms. Johnson, a 42-year-old patient, sustained a spinal cord injury in a motor vehicle accident and has been admitted to a rehabilitation facility for comprehensive care. As a Certified Rehabilitation Registered Nurse (CRRN), you prioritize quality improvement processes in nursing practice. Which of the following actions aligns with this skill?
A) Adhering to ethical standards and principles
B) Advocating for patient rights
C) Implementing evidence-based practice
D) Documenting patient assessments accurately

Question 98: Mrs. Johnson, a 55-year-old patient, is admitted to the rehabilitation unit after a stroke. She is experiencing urinary incontinence and is embarrassed by her condition. The nurse explains the use of pharmacologic and non-pharmacological interventions to manage her symptoms. Which of the following interventions would be most appropriate for Mrs. Johnson?
A) Prescribing an anticholinergic medication to decrease bladder contractions
B) Teaching Mrs. Johnson to perform Kegel exercises to strengthen her pelvic floor muscles
C) Using a bladder training program to gradually increase the time between voiding
D) Encouraging Mrs. Johnson to wear adult diapers to manage her incontinence

Question 99: Which of the following is an example of an ethical consideration in nursing practice?
A) Ensuring patient confidentiality
B) Managing patient finances
C) Assigning patient care tasks
D) Obtaining informed consent for treatment

Question 100: Which nursing action demonstrates the implementation phase of the nursing process in rehabilitation nursing?
A) Assessing the patient's functional abilities and limitations
B) Developing an individualized care plan based on the patient's goals
C) Evaluating the effectiveness of interventions in achieving desired outcomes
D) Administering medication to manage pain and discomfort

Question 101: The CRRN is responsible for applying the nursing process to optimize the restoration and preservation of the patient's health and holistic well-being across the lifespan. Which of the following is a step in the nursing process?
A) Assessing the patient's vital signs
B) Administering medications to the patient
C) Scheduling follow-up appointments
D) Documenting the patient's medical history

Question 102: Which of the following is NOT a developmental factor to consider when caring for a patient as a certified rehabilitation registered nurse (CRRN)?
A) Cognitive development
B) Emotional development
C) Nutritional development
D) Physical development

Question 103: Which of the following actions best demonstrates a proper infection control practice for a Certified Rehabilitation Registered Nurse (CRRN) to minimize the risk of cross-contamination?
A) Wearing gloves while assisting with patient rehabilitation exercises.
B) Sharing stethoscopes between patients after cleaning with alcohol wipes.
C) Using the same thermometer for multiple patients after cleaning with soap and water.
D) Washing hands with soap and water before and after every patient interaction.

Question 104: Which of the following is an appropriate responsibility to delegate to a nursing assistant in the rehabilitation team?
A) Administering medications
B) Assessing the patient's readiness for discharge
C) Developing the patient's care plan
D) Assisting with activities of daily living

Question 105: Which of the following is an example of a non-pharmacological sleep aid?
A) Melatonin supplement
B) Zolpidem (Ambien)
C) Progressive muscle relaxation technique
D) Trazodone (Desyrel)

Question 106: Which nonpharmacological intervention is effective in managing pain and promoting comfort in patients?
A) Deep breathing exercises
B) Administering opioid medications
C) Applying heat packs to the affected area
D) Providing distraction techniques

Question 107: Mr. Johnson, a 65-year-old patient, is admitted to the rehabilitation unit following a stroke. The nurse is implementing the nursing process for Mr. Johnson's care. During the assessment phase, the nurse gathers data such as the patient's medical history, physical abilities, and functional limitations. In which step of the nursing process is the nurse actively gathering this information?
A) Diagnosis
B) Planning
C) Implementation
D) Assessment

Question 108: Which factor is most likely to contribute to alterations in sexual function and reproduction in individuals with spinal cord injuries (SCI)?
A) Increased muscle tone below the level of injury
B) Normal sexual desire and arousal
C) Increased motor control and coordination
D) Preservation of voluntary control over bladder and bowel function

Question 109: Which of the following skills is most important for a Certified Rehabilitation Registered Nurse (CRRN) to possess in the area of 'Skill in:'?

A) Assessment and evaluation of patients' functional health patterns
B) Administering medications
C) Performing complex medical procedures
D) Documentation of patients' medical history

Question 110:   Jane is a rehabilitation nurse working with patients who have neurological conditions. She is implementing behavioral management strategies to optimize the management of her patient's conditions. Today, Jane is working with a patient named Mark, who has suffered a traumatic brain injury and exhibits impulsive behavior. Mark often engages in risky activities without considering the consequences. Jane decides to use positive reinforcement as a behavioral management strategy to promote safer behaviors.   Which of the following actions by Jane would be an example of positive reinforcement in this scenario?
A) Giving a verbal warning to Mark every time he engages in risky behavior.
B) Ignoring Mark whenever he engages in impulsive behavior.
C) Providing a small reward to Mark whenever he makes a safe choice.
D) Restricting Mark's access to activities whenever he makes unsafe choices.

Question 111:   Which of the following medications is commonly used as an antispasmodic in the management of neurological conditions?
A) Amitriptyline
B) Morphine
C) Atropine
D) Ibuprofen

Question 112:   When facilitating appropriate referrals in the rehabilitation process, the Certified Rehabilitation Registered Nurse (CRRN) should consider which of the following?
A) The patient's financial status
B) The patient's social network
C) The patient's educational background
D) The patient's cultural beliefs and practices
and practices are taken into account is essential in facilitating appropriate referrals in the rehabilitation process.

Question 113:   In the context of rehabilitation nursing, skill in communication and collaboration includes:
A) Providing education to patients and their families about their condition and treatment plans.
B) Implementing and coordinating a multidisciplinary team approach to patient care.
C) Using therapeutic communication techniques to establish rapport and trust with patients.
D) All of the above.

Question 114:   Mrs. Johnson, a 65-year-old stroke survivor, is receiving rehabilitation therapy in a long-term care facility. She expresses concerns about updating her legal documents, such as her will and power of attorney. Which of the following would be an appropriate resource for Mrs. Johnson to assist with these legal documents?
A) A nutritionist
B) A physical therapist
C) A lawyer who specializes in elder law
D) A recreational therapist

Question 115:   A 45-year-old male patient with a history of spinal cord injury presents to the rehabilitation unit. The interdisciplinary team is discussing the patient's plan of care. The team is considering implementing electrical stimulation as a therapeutic intervention for the patient's lower extremity muscle strengthening. As the rehabilitation nurse, you suggest referring to evidence-based research to guide the decision-making process. Which of the following statements regarding evidence-based research is true?
A) Evidence-based research involves the use of anecdotal evidence and personal opinions.
B) Evidence-based research is not applicable to rehabilitation nursing.
C) Evidence-based research incorporates the best available evidence with clinical expertise and patient preferences.
D) Evidence-based research focuses solely on the healthcare professional's expertise.

Question 116:   Mrs. Anderson, a 65-year-old patient with a spinal cord injury, is preparing to be discharged from the acute care hospital to a rehabilitation center. The patient is uninsured and cannot afford the cost of the rehabilitation services. As a Certified Rehabilitation Registered Nurse (CRRN), you collaborate with various resources to ensure the patient's access to the required services. Which of the following would be the most appropriate course of action?
A) Discuss with the patient's family the option of taking Mrs. Anderson home and providing care without professional rehabilitation services.
B) Apply for Medicaid on behalf of the patient to cover the cost of rehabilitation services.
C) Inform the patient's family that the rehabilitation center has a financial assistance program for uninsured patients.
D) Advise the patient to seek private loan options to finance the rehabilitation services.

Question 117:   Which nursing model is commonly used as a framework for rehabilitation nursing practice?
A) Orem's Self-Care Deficit Theory
B) Roy's Adaptation Model
C) Neuman's Systems Model
D) Benner's Skill Acquisition Model

Question 118:   Which intervention can help prevent contractures in patients with musculoskeletal impairments?
A) Encouraging active range of motion exercises
B) Implementing strict bed rest
C) Applying ice packs to the affected area
D) Administering nonsteroidal anti-inflammatory drugs

Question 119:   A patient with a recent stroke is experiencing difficulty with daily activities such as dressing, bathing, and grooming. The nurse recognizes the need to assist the patient in improving these skills to enhance functional ability and independence. Which skill would be most appropriate for the nurse to focus on?
A) Cognitive skills
B) Mobility skills
C) Communication skills
D) Socialization skills

Question 120:   Ms. Johnson, a 62-year-old patient with dysphagia, is admitted to the rehabilitation unit following a stroke. The physician has ordered enteral nutrition via a nasogastric tube. The nurse is preparing to administer the feedings and is reviewing the plan of care. Which intervention should the nurse include in the plan to promote optimal enteral nutrition?
A) Flush the nasogastric tube with 60 mL of sterile water after each medication administration.

B) Elevate the head of the bed to at least 45 degrees during feedings and for at least one hour afterward.
C) Administer medications directly through the nasogastric tube without crushing or grinding them.
D) Maintain continuous enteral feedings at room temperature to prevent clogging of the feeding tube.

Question 121: Ms. Smith, a 65-year-old patient with a spinal cord injury, has been admitted to a rehabilitation unit following a recent fall. While reviewing her treatment plan, you notice that the nurse has failed to include any referrals for psychological counseling or support for Ms. Smith's emotional well-being. As a CRRN, what should be your next course of action?
A) Ignore the oversight since it is not directly related to the patient's physical rehabilitation.
B) Inform the nurse manager about the missing referrals and request for them to be added to the treatment plan.
C) Discuss the importance of psychological support with Ms. Smith and encourage her to advocate for herself.
D) Leave it to the patient's family to address the issue, as they are the primary caregivers.

Question 122: Ms. Johnson, a 45-year-old female patient with multiple sclerosis, is experiencing severe muscle spasms that are interfering with her daily activities. The healthcare provider prescribes a medication to manage these muscle spasms. Which medication would be most appropriate for Ms. Johnson to alleviate her symptoms?
A) A selective serotonin reuptake inhibitor (SSRI)
B) An anticholinergic agent
C) A nonsteroidal anti-inflammatory drug (NSAID)
D) A benzodiazepine

Question 123: Which of the following is not an example of a functional health pattern?
A) Activity and exercise
B) Nutrition and metabolism
C) Coping and stress tolerance
D) Communication and collaboration

Question 124: When using a nasogastric tube for enteral feeding, which action should the rehabilitation registered nurse take to ensure proper maintenance and patient safety?
A) Secure the tube loosely to allow for movement
B) Flush the tube with water before and after medication administration
C) Use smaller tube sizes for improved patient comfort
D) Change the tube position to the opposite nostril every shift

Question 125: A patient with a history of stroke is admitted to a rehabilitation unit. The patient has expressive aphasia and is unable to speak and express their thoughts verbally. Which intervention is most appropriate for the nurse to optimize the patient's ability to communicate effectively?
A) Encourage the patient to use written communication.
B) Provide the patient with a communication board.
C) Schedule the patient for speech therapy sessions.
D) Initiate a referral for augmentative and alternative communication systems.

Question 126: Which of the following is an example of a linguistic deficit?
A) Difficulty in understanding and producing speech sounds
B) Difficulty in coordinating muscle movements required for speech
C) Difficulty in using correct grammar and syntax

D) Difficulty in understanding and using written language

Question 127: Which of the following steps is NOT a part of the nursing process when optimizing the management of a patient's neurological and other complex medical conditions?
A) Assessment
B) Diagnosis
C) Implementation
D) Analysis

Question 128: Mrs. Smith, a 55-year-old stroke survivor, has recently been discharged from an inpatient rehabilitation facility and is transitioning back to her community. As her rehabilitation nurse, you are responsible for assisting her in accessing community resources. Which of the following community resources would be most appropriate to support Mrs. Smith's community reintegration?
A) A specialized stroke support group that meets weekly at the local community center.
B) An Alzheimer's disease support group that meets monthly at the senior center.
C) A yoga class offered at a nearby gym.
D) A daycare center for children with special needs.

Question 129: A patient with multiple sclerosis has difficulty with self-feeding due to hand tremors. The nurse decides to implement adaptive equipment to promote independence. Which adaptive equipment should the nurse recommend?
A) Built-up utensils
B) Long-handled shoe horn
C) Jar opener
D) Sock aid

Question 130: Which theory focuses on understanding how individuals and groups go through a process of change and adaptation?
A) Social cognitive theory
B) Transformational leadership theory
C) Transitions theory
D) Chaos theory

Question 131: Which of the following is an example of a key component of rehabilitation scope of practice?
A) Assessment and evaluation of patient condition and needs
B) Administration of medications
C) Performing surgical procedures
D) Customizing treatment plans for individuals based on personal preference

Question 132: Mr. Davis, a 53-year-old patient, is admitted to a rehabilitation unit following a stroke. The nurse is responsible for providing cost-effective patient-centered care. Which action by the nurse demonstrates adherence to ethical and legal standards?
A) Administering medication without verifying the patient's identification
B) Sharing the patient's confidential health information with other healthcare professionals
C) Collaborating with the interdisciplinary team to develop a comprehensive care plan
D) Implementing a treatment plan without obtaining informed consent

Question 133: Mr. Johnson, a 68-year-old patient with a history of dementia, has been admitted to the rehabilitation unit. Due to his cognitive impairment, he often gets disoriented and tries to wander around, putting

himself at risk for falls. The healthcare team is concerned about his safety and decides to implement appropriate safety devices. Which of the following safety devices would be most appropriate to address Mr. Johnson's risk of falls?
A) Physical restraints
B) Bed exit alarm
C) Chemical restraints
D) Patient education

Question 134: When implementing safety interventions to optimize a patient's functional ability, which intervention is considered non-behavioral restraint?
A) Placing the patient in a geriatric chair with a lap belt
B) Using restraints that limit the patient's movement
C) Encouraging physical activity to redirect excessive energy
D) Providing a private room with a calm environment

Question 135: You are a Certified Rehabilitation Registered Nurse (CRRN) working in a multidisciplinary healthcare team in a rehabilitation facility. Mr. Johnson, a 65-year-old patient, has been admitted following a stroke. His rehabilitation program involves physical therapy, occupational therapy, speech therapy, and nursing care. The team meets weekly to discuss and coordinate their efforts to provide comprehensive care for Mr. Johnson. During one of the team meetings, a nursing assistant suggests that the team should adopt a transdisciplinary approach instead of a multidisciplinary one. Which of the following best explains the difference between these two models of healthcare teams?
A) In a transdisciplinary team, healthcare professionals work independently and do not collaborate with one another.
B) In a transdisciplinary team, healthcare professionals work in segregated roles and do not share responsibilities.
C) In a multidisciplinary team, healthcare professionals work together but maintain their professional boundaries.
D) In a multidisciplinary team, healthcare professionals collaborate closely and share responsibilities.

Question 136: Which of the following is an important aspect of planning discharge for a rehabilitation patient?
A) Coordinating home visits for assessment and modifications
B) Teaching caregivers about the patient's condition and care needs
C) Ensuring the patient has access to necessary medical equipment and supplies
D) All of the above

Question 137: What nursing action should the Certified Rehabilitation Registered Nurse (CRRN) prioritize when assessing goals related to sexuality and reproduction in a patient?
A) Implementing interventions to promote sexual function and satisfaction
B) Providing education about contraception options
C) Assessing for psychological barriers to sexual activity
D) Encouraging patients to discuss sexual concerns with their partners

Question 138: Ms. Anderson, a 45-year-old patient with newly diagnosed obstructive sleep apnea (OSA), has been prescribed continuous positive airway pressure (CPAP) therapy. She expresses concern about using the CPAP machine and asks the nurse about alternative options. The nurse educates Ms. Anderson about various sleep apnea treatment options. Which alternative technology may be considered as a treatment option for obstructive sleep apnea (OSA) besides CPAP?
A) Aromatherapy

B) Meditation
C) Sound therapy
D) BiPAP machine

Question 139: When assessing a patient's cognition, which of the following techniques would be most appropriate?
A) Observing the patient's behavior and interactions
B) Conducting a neurological exam
C) Reviewing the patient's medical history
D) Performing a sensory evaluation

Question 140: Which nursing model/framework is commonly used in rehabilitation care to provide individualized patient-centered care?
A) Transtheoretical Model
B) Roy Adaptation Model
C) Biopsychosocial Model
D) Orem's Self-Care Deficit Nursing Theory

Question 141: Which intervention is most effective in promoting positive interaction among patients and caregivers?
A) Encouraging the caregiver to take breaks from their caregiving duties
B) Providing the caregiver with written instructions on patient care
C) Limiting the caregiver's involvement in the patient's care
D) Advising the patient to not rely on the caregiver for emotional support

Question 142: Which of the following is not a key component of quality improvement processes in nursing practice?
A) Collecting and analyzing data
B) Implementing evidence-based practices
C) Collaborating with interdisciplinary teams
D) Adhering to legislative and legal requirements

Question 143: Which of the following is an appropriate resource for a patient facing financial barriers to rehabilitation?
A) Social media support groups
B) Personal financial counseling
C) Access to a computer and internet
D) Pet therapy sessions

Question 144: A patient with dysphagia is receiving thickened liquids as a safety measure. Which intervention should the nurse implement to promote safe swallowing?
A) Elevate the head of the bed to 30 degrees during meals
B) Administering liquids at room temperature
C) Encouraging the patient to drink through a straw
D) Offering small, frequent sips of fluid

Question 145: Mr. Patel, a 68-year-old male patient, recently suffered a spinal cord injury resulting in lower limb paralysis. He is now experiencing difficulty with bladder emptying and requires intermittent catheterization. The nurse educates Mr. Patel about the different types of catheters available for his use. Which of the following types of catheters should the nurse recommend to Mr. Patel based on his condition?
A) Straight catheter
B) Indwelling (Foley) catheter
C) Condom (Texas) catheter
D) Suprapubic catheter

Question 146: Sarah is a nurse working in a rehabilitation center. She is implementing the Neuman Systems Model to provide holistic care to her patients. One of Sarah's patients, Mr. Anderson, recently had a stroke and is undergoing rehabilitation to regain his motor skills. According to the Neuman Systems Model, which of the following is a primary preventive intervention Sarah can implement for Mr. Anderson?
A) Administering medications to manage his pain
B) Providing physical therapy exercises to improve his mobility
C) Encouraging Mr. Anderson to participate in support groups
D) Educating Mr. Anderson about lifestyle modifications to reduce the risk of future strokes

Question 147: A 45-year-old patient with a history of chronic kidney disease is scheduled to undergo a renal biopsy to evaluate the progression of the disease. The nurse is explaining the procedure to the patient and is emphasizing the importance of diagnostic testing for accurate diagnosis and treatment. Which diagnostic test is performed to evaluate renal structure and function?
A) Electrocardiogram (ECG)
B) Magnetic Resonance Imaging (MRI)
C) Renal Angiography
D) Renal Ultrasound

Question 148: A patient with a spinal cord injury is admitted to the rehabilitation unit. The nurse is implementing the Rehabilitation Nursing Model in the care of this patient. Which of the following best represents the focus of this model?
A) Providing emotional support to the patient
B) Promoting independence and maximizing function

C) Administering medications for pain management
D) Educating the patient on wound care techniques

Question 149: Which legislation regulates the confidentiality and privacy of patient health information?
A) Americans with Disabilities Act (ADA)
B) Health Insurance Portability and Accountability Act (HIPAA)
C) Title VI of the Civil Rights Act of 1964
D) Occupational Safety and Health Act (OSHA)

Question 150: When communicating with a patient from a different cultural background, it is important for the Certified Rehabilitation Registered Nurse (CRRN) to:
A) Use medical jargon to demonstrate professional knowledge.
B) Avoid asking questions about the patient's cultural beliefs.
C) Use open-ended questions to encourage the patient to share their feelings and experiences.
D) Assume that the patient's cultural values and norms are similar to their own.

ANSWERS WITH DETAILED EXPLANATION (SET 3)

Question 1: Correct Answer: A) Encouraging the patient to consume foods high in fiber
Rationale: Encouraging the patient to consume foods high in fiber is an appropriate nursing intervention to optimize a patient's elimination patterns. Fiber adds bulk to the stool, promoting regular bowel movements and preventing constipation. It aids in softening the stool, making it easier to pass. Adequate fluid intake should accompany a high-fiber diet to ensure the fiber functions properly. Administering laxatives on a regular basis may lead to dependence and should only be used as a last resort. Limiting fluid intake can result in dehydration and further exacerbate elimination problems. Encouraging physical activity actually helps stimulate bowel motility and promotes regularity.

Question 2: Correct Answer: A) Plan
Rationale: The first step in implementing a quality improvement model is to plan. During this step, the specific needs and concerns of the patients and their families are identified. This helps to establish goals and objectives for improving patient care. By understanding the needs and concerns of the patients and their families, healthcare professionals can tailor interventions and strategies that are patient-centered and focused on enhancing the overall quality of care. Thus, the correct answer is A) Plan.

Question 3: Correct Answer: A) Weight loss of 2 pounds in the past week
Rationale: Weight loss is a concern in patients receiving enteral tube feeding, as it may indicate inadequate nutrition or complications related to feeding. A weight loss of 2 pounds in a week should raise concerns and warrant further intervention, such as increasing caloric intake or reassessing the enteral feeding plan. Albumin level, bowel sounds, and serum potassium level may provide additional information about the patient's nutritional status but are not specific indicators of the need for further intervention in this scenario.

Question 4: Correct Answer: A) Assessing the patient's current nutritional status and needs
Rationale: When implementing and evaluating interventions for nutrition, it is crucial for a CRRN to assess the patient's current nutritional status and needs. This assessment allows the nurse to identify if there are any deficiencies or excesses in the patient's nutritional intake. It helps to determine the appropriate interventions for the patient, such as dietary modifications, supplementation, or enteral or parenteral nutrition. Assessing preferences, allergies, and medical conditions is also important in developing an individualized nutrition plan. Administering enteral feedings without assessing the patient's preferences (option B), recommending parenteral nutrition without involving the dietitian (option C), or restricting all oral intake for patients at risk of aspiration (option D) may not be appropriate or beneficial for every patient and should be considered on a case-by-case basis.

Question 5: Correct Answer: B) Implementing suicide precautions, including removing any potential means for self-harm
Rationale: Given Mrs. Johnson's history of depression and suicidal ideation, implementing suicide precautions is crucial to ensure her safety. This includes removing any potential means for self-harm, such as belts or shoelaces, and maintaining a safe environment. While providing one-on-one supervision (option A) may be necessary in some cases, it is not always feasible due to limited staffing resources. Collaborating with the healthcare team (option C) and educating Mrs. Johnson (option D) are important interventions, but they are not the priority when addressing immediate safety concerns regarding harm to self.

Question 6: Correct Answer: B) Collaborating with the physical therapist to create an individualized exercise program focusing on upper body strength.
Rationale: The correct application of the rehabilitation scope of practice for a patient with a lower limb amputation, like John, involves collaborating with the physical therapist to create an individualized exercise program focusing on upper body strength. This intervention aligns with the goal of promoting optimum functional ability and independence in the patient's specific situation. Option A is incorrect because using a wheelchair for all mobility activities may hinder the patient's ability to adapt and learn to use prosthesis properly. Option C is incorrect as regular follow-up appointments with a psychiatrist are not directly related to the rehabilitation scope of practice for this specific patient scenario. Option D is incorrect because assisting the patient during therapy sessions should be the responsibility of the therapist rather than the nurse.

Question 7: Correct Answer: B) King's Theory of Goal Attainment
Rationale: King's Theory of Goal Attainment focuses on the nurse-client relationship and the mutual goal-setting process to achieve optimal health outcomes. This theory emphasizes the importance of active participation and collaboration between the nurse and the client to identify and achieve personalized goals. In rehabilitation, this approach is particularly relevant as it promotes holistic care by considering the physical, psychological, and social aspects of the client's well-being. By establishing a therapeutic partnership, the nurse can enhance the client's motivation, self-care abilities, and overall rehabilitation progress. Other nursing theories mentioned in the options, such as Roy's Adaptation Model, Neuman's Systems Model, and Orem's Self-Care Deficit Theory, focus on different aspects of care and may not prioritize the nurse-client relationship as strongly as King's Theory of Goal Attainment does.

Question 8: Correct Answer: C) Functional Independence Measure (FIM)
Rationale: The Functional Independence Measure (FIM) is a widely used standardized assessment tool in rehabilitation settings. It evaluates a patient's level of independence in performing activities of daily living (ADLs) and instrumental activities of daily living (IADLs). The FIM consists of 18 items, including self-care tasks, mobility, and cognitive functioning. Each item is rated on a scale of 1 to 7, with higher scores indicating greater independence. The FIM helps rehabilitation professionals measure a patient's progress, set goals, and develop appropriate intervention plans. The Mini-Mental State Examination (MMSE) and Glasgow Coma Scale (GCS) are tools used to assess cognitive function and level of consciousness, respectively, but they do not specifically evaluate functional independence. The Barthel Index is another ADL assessment tool but is not as comprehensive as the FIM.

Question 9: Correct Answer: B) Discuss the patient's concerns and offer to involve a sexuality counselor.
Rationale: It is essential for a CRRN to address the patient's concerns regarding sexuality and reproduction after a spinal cord injury. By discussing the patient's concerns and offering to involve a sexuality counselor, the nurse acknowledges the importance of these goals and provides the necessary support. Brochures can be provided, but a more comprehensive approach is needed, which involves open communication and collaboration with a specialized healthcare professional. Ignoring the patient's concerns or dismissing them as irrelevant is inappropriate and disregards the patient's holistic well-being.

Question 10: Correct Answer: B) Assigning a communication board to the patient for written communication
Rationale: Assigning a communication board to the patient for written communication would be the most appropriate intervention in this scenario. It allows the patient to communicate effectively by writing down his thoughts and needs. Hand gestures may not be sufficient or clear for proper communication. Limiting visitor access may not directly address the patient's communication difficulties. Administering a sedative is not an appropriate intervention as it does not address the patient's communication needs.

Question 11: Correct Answer: C) Cooking
Rationale: Instrumental activities of daily living (IADLs) are complex skills necessary for independent living. These activities include household chores, managing finances, taking medications, shopping, and meal preparation. Cooking is an example of an IADL because it requires cognitive and physical skills to plan, prepare, and cook meals. Other examples of IADLs include using transportation, managing personal and household communication, and managing finances. Bathing, dressing, and toileting are considered activities of daily living (ADLs) that relate to personal care and are essential for basic self-care.

Question 12: Correct Answer: C) Listening actively and attentively to patients and caregivers
Rationale: Effective communication plays a significant role in building trust and fostering a therapeutic relationship with patients and their caregivers. Listening actively and attentively allows the CRRN to understand their concerns, needs, and preferences, which in turn helps in tailoring individualized care plans. By actively listening, the CRRN can also identify non-verbal cues, such as body language and expressions, that may indicate unexpressed feelings or concerns. This approach promotes open dialogue, enhances patient satisfaction, and improves overall psychological well-being. The use of medical jargon, speaking quickly, and interrupting individuals can create barriers to effective communication and hinder the establishment of a therapeutic relationship.

Question 13: Correct Answer: D) Taking small bites and chewing thoroughly before swallowing
Rationale: Taking small bites and chewing thoroughly before swallowing is an important teaching intervention to promote safe swallowing in patients with dysphagia. This helps in reducing the risk of choking and aspiration. Eating quickly, consuming thin liquids, and eating large meals at once all increase the risk of choking and aspiration. Therefore, they are not appropriate interventions for John to manage his swallowing deficits effectively.

Question 14: Correct Answer: A) Encouraging the patient to explore their feelings and emotions related to their injury
Rationale: Encouraging the patient to explore their feelings and emotions related to their injury is an appropriate intervention to promote psychosocial well-being. Spinal cord injuries can have a profound impact on a patient's physical abilities and emotional state. Allowing the patient to express their emotions and providing a safe space for them to explore their feelings can contribute to their overall coping and adjustment process. This intervention facilitates the patient's ability to process their grief, frustration, and any other emotional challenges that may arise as a result of their injury. It also helps promote open communication between the patient and the healthcare team, which is essential for effective rehabilitation and psychosocial support.

Question 15: Correct Answer: B) Using a smartphone application to track his medication schedule
Rationale: For a patient with multiple sclerosis (MS), the use of a smartphone application to track medication schedules would be the most effective technology intervention for self-management. Multiple sclerosis is typically managed through the use of medications, and adherence to a strict medication schedule is crucial for optimal outcomes. Using a smartphone application to track medication schedules can help Mr. Johnson ensure that he takes the right medications at the right time, improving his ability to manage his condition effectively. Monitoring blood pressure, blood glucose levels, or daily steps may be relevant for other conditions but do not specifically address the self-management needs of a patient with MS.

Question 16: Correct Answer: A) Effective communication
Rationale: Effective communication is crucial for Nurse Sarah to teach Mr. Johnson the necessary skills for activities of daily living. By using clear and concise language, Nurse Sarah can explain and demonstrate each task in a way that Mr. Johnson can understand. Additionally, she can use visual aids and written instructions to enhance the teaching process. By promoting effective communication, Nurse Sarah can empower Mr. Johnson to participate actively in his own rehabilitation and promote his independence. Medication administration, wound care, and intravenous line insertion are important skills for nurses but not directly related to teaching activities of daily living.

Question 17: Correct Answer: A) Built-up utensils
Rationale: Built-up utensils are designed with thick handles that provide a comfortable grip for individuals with limited hand strength or dexterity. This adaptive equipment would be most appropriate for Mr. Johnson, allowing him to hold utensils securely and maintain independence while eating. A sippy cup is typically used for individuals with difficulty swallowing, but it may not be necessary for Mr. Johnson. A plate guard prevents food from falling off the plate, but it may not address Mr. Johnson's specific hand grip issue. Bendable straws are useful for individuals with limited neck mobility but may not be the most appropriate option for Mr. Johnson's situation.

Question 18: Correct Answer: C) Collaborate with the speech therapist to evaluate Mr. Johnson's swallowing function.
Rationale: Mr. Johnson has dysphagia, which puts him at risk for aspiration and malnutrition. By collaborating with the speech therapist, you can assess his swallowing function and determine the most appropriate diet modifications. This ensures the safety and nutritional needs of the patient are met, reducing the risk of complications and promoting optimal nutrition and hydration. A regular diet without modifications or a clear liquid diet may not address Mr. Johnson's specific needs, while offering a high-protein diet without modification does not address his swallowing difficulties.

Question 19: Correct Answer: A) Assess Mrs. Johnson's cognitive function and communication abilities.
Rationale: Assessing Mrs. Johnson's cognitive function and communication abilities is the priority action to address her specific rehabilitation needs. Understanding her cognitive status and communication abilities will guide the development of an appropriate care plan and interventions tailored to her individual situation. This assessment will help identify potential barriers to community reintegration and inform the team's decision-making process. While coordinating team meetings, teaching family members, and arranging transportation services are all important aspects of promoting community reintegration, none of these actions take precedence over assessing the patient's cognitive function and communication abilities as the initial step in the nursing process.

Question 20: Correct Answer: B) Creating individualized care plans
Rationale: One of the skills required in rehabilitation nursing is the ability to use the nursing process to deliver cost-effective patient-centered care. Creating individualized care plans is a key component of this skill set as it involves assessing the patient's unique needs, setting goals, and

implementing interventions that are specific to their rehabilitation needs. Analyzing insurance coverage for patients may be a relevant task, but it falls more under the broader topic of legislative, economic, ethical, and legal issues. Evaluating the cost-effectiveness of medications is important in healthcare management, but it is not specifically related to using the nursing process in rehabilitation nursing. Implementing evidence-based practice is a necessary skill, but it is not exclusive to the task of delivering cost-effective patient-centered care.

Question 21:   Correct Answer: A) Coordinating discharge planning and ensuring appropriate community resources are in place.

Rationale: The role of the CRRN in the transition of care is to coordinate the discharge planning process and ensure that appropriate community resources are in place for the patient's continued rehabilitation. This includes working closely with the interdisciplinary team, the patient, and their family to identify the patient's needs, develop a comprehensive plan of care, and facilitate a smooth transition from the rehabilitation setting to the patient's home or another level of care. The CRRN focuses on promoting community reintegration and helping the patient achieve independence and optimal functioning in their daily life activities. Option B is incorrect as hands-on care is typically provided by other healthcare professionals such as physical therapists. Option C is incorrect as designing exercise programs is typically the responsibility of the physical therapist, although the CRRN may collaborate with them. Option D is incorrect as medication administration and pain management are typically the responsibility of the nurse, but not specific to the CRRN role in the transition of care process.

Question 22:   Correct Answer: C) Peplau's Interpersonal Relations Model

Rationale: Peplau's Interpersonal Relations Model emphasizes the importance of the nurse-client relationship in promoting the client's well-being. This model focuses on the therapeutic use of communication and interpersonal skills to understand the client's needs, establish trust, and provide appropriate care. Peplau believed that through this relationship, nurses can help clients achieve personal growth and overcome health challenges. The model also emphasizes the roles of the nurse as a counselor, teacher, and resource person. Overall, Peplau's model highlights the significance of the interpersonal bond between the nurse and the client in achieving positive health outcomes.

Question 23:   Correct Answer: C) Making decisions independently without seeking input from others

Rationale: Effective collaboration in a rehabilitation setting requires active listening and communication, respecting and valuing each team member's expertise, and sharing information and resources. It is important to work together as a team, seeking input from others to make informed decisions that benefit the patient. Making decisions independently without considering the expertise and input of other team members can hinder effective collaboration and compromise patient-centered care. Therefore, option C is not a key component of effective collaboration in a rehabilitation setting.

Question 24:   Correct Answer: C) Eye-gaze system

Rationale: Sarah is recommending an eye-gaze system as an assistive technology for communication. This technology allows the patient with paralysis to use their eye movements as input to control the device and generate text or speech. A mouthstick is a device used by individuals with limited hand or arm function to perform tasks by holding the stick in the mouth. A headpointer is a device that allows individuals to control a computer cursor by using their head movements. A gesture-based system uses body movements or gestures to control devices, typically through sensors or cameras.

Question 25:   Correct Answer: C) Rehabilitation nurse

Rationale: The rehabilitation nurse plays a crucial role in coordinating the rehabilitation team and facilitating care transitions for patients in a rehabilitation setting. They collaborate with various healthcare professionals, including speech therapists, physical therapists, and social workers, to ensure a comprehensive and coordinated approach to patient care. Rehabilitation nurses assess and monitor patients, develop and implement care plans, provide patient and family education, and advocate for the patient's needs throughout their rehabilitation journey. With their specialized knowledge and skills, rehabilitation nurses promote effective communication and foster a smooth transition of care across different healthcare settings, thereby optimizing patient outcomes.

Question 26:   Correct Answer: D) All of the above

Rationale: Falls are a major safety concern in rehabilitation settings. Several factors contribute to the risk of falls, including dim lighting, cluttered hallways, and slippery floors. Dim lighting can impair visibility and make it difficult for patients to navigate their surroundings safely. Cluttered hallways increase the risk of tripping and falling. Slippery floors, especially when wet or recently cleaned, can cause patients to lose their footing. Understanding and addressing these risk factors can help prevent falls and improve patient safety in a rehabilitation setting.

Question 27:   Correct Answer: B) Utilize nonverbal cues such as gestures and visual aids.

Rationale: Expressive aphasia is characterized by difficulty expressing thoughts and understanding spoken language. Using nonverbal cues, such as gestures and visual aids, can help individuals with aphasia understand and convey information. Speaking louder and slower may not address the underlying deficits in language processing and could potentially cause frustration. While repetition can be helpful in some cases, it may not be effective for individuals with expressive aphasia. Social interactions should not be limited as they are an essential part of rehabilitation and communication therapy for aphasia patients. Utilizing nonverbal cues is the most appropriate intervention to optimize communication for Mr. Smith.

Question 28:   Correct Answer: C) "I understand the importance of speaking up for my needs and preferences."

Rationale: Self-advocacy is an essential skill for individuals with disabilities to advocate for their needs, preferences, and rights. It involves actively participating in decision-making, expressing concerns, and communicating with healthcare professionals. By stating that she understands the importance of speaking up for her needs and preferences, Mrs. Smith demonstrates a correct understanding of self-advocacy. Options A, B, and D indicate a lack of self-advocacy and reliance on others or healthcare professionals, which is not the desired outcome for promoting patient independence and community reintegration.

Question 29:   Correct Answer: A) The Occupational Safety and Health Act (OSHA)

Rationale: The Occupational Safety and Health Act (OSHA) is a federal legislation that ensures a safe and healthy working environment for employees. It establishes standards and regulations for workplace safety, including those specifically applicable to healthcare settings. OSHA regulations cover a wide range of areas such as infection control, handling hazardous materials, ergonomics, and preventing workplace violence. By complying with OSHA standards, healthcare organizations can minimize risks and create a safe environment for both patients and staff. The Americans with Disabilities Act (ADA) focuses on protecting the rights of individuals with disabilities, the Health Insurance Portability and Accountability Act (HIPAA) addresses privacy and security of health information, and the Family and Medical Leave Act (FMLA) provides job protection for eligible employees who need to take leave for specific reasons. While these legislations are important, they are not directly related to promoting a safe environment of care as OSHA is.

Question 30: Correct Answer: B) "The catheter will be inserted into my spinal cord to deliver the medication."
Rationale: The baclofen pump is an implantable device that delivers medication, typically baclofen, directly into the spinal cord. The catheter is surgically placed in the intrathecal space for targeted drug delivery. It is not battery-operated, so changing batteries is not necessary. The dosage of medication is adjusted by a healthcare professional, not the patient. Electrical impulses to the muscles are delivered by a TENS unit, which is a separate device used for pain management.

Question 31: Correct Answer: D) Attorney specializing in elder law
Rationale: When assisting a patient with completing a living will, it is important to involve an attorney specializing in elder law. These attorneys are knowledgeable about the legal requirements and intricacies of creating and implementing living wills. They can provide guidance and ensure that the document accurately reflects the patient's wishes and complies with applicable laws. Financial planners, physical therapists, and hospice nurses may have valuable roles in a patient's overall care, but they do not possess the expertise required to navigate the legal complexities of completing a living will.

Question 32: Correct Answer: D) Maintaining accurate documentation of patient care and incidents
Rationale: Maintaining accurate documentation of patient care and incidents is an essential legal requirement to promote a safe environment of care. Accurate documentation provides evidence of the care provided, helps in identifying potential risks or errors, and ensures compliance with legal standards. It serves as a crucial communication tool among healthcare professionals and can be used as legal evidence if needed. Option A refers to an ethical issue of ensuring staff safety, while Options B and C are examples of promoting a safe environment but do not specifically address legal issues.

Question 33: Correct Answer: D) To promote a culture of safety and quality improvement.
Rationale: The purpose of reporting healthcare-acquired pressure injuries in a rehabilitation facility is to promote a culture of safety and quality improvement. By reporting these injuries, the facility can identify trends, implement preventive measures, and continuously improve patient care. Reporting also helps in monitoring the effectiveness of interventions and identifying areas for staff education. It is crucial for healthcare facilities to prioritize patient safety and use reported data to make evidence-based decisions, reduce the incidence of such injuries, and ensure optimal outcomes for patients. Compliance with legal regulations is essential but not the primary purpose of reporting healthcare-acquired pressure injuries.

Question 34: Correct Answer: B) Rehabilitation aims to optimize functional independence and quality of life.
Rationale: The philosophy of rehabilitation is centered around helping individuals achieve the highest level of functional independence and quality of life possible, despite any physical or cognitive limitations they may have. Rehabilitation is not solely focused on curing the underlying medical condition but rather on maximizing the individual's abilities and promoting their overall well-being. While medical interventions and emotional support may be components of rehabilitation, they are not the primary focus.

Question 35: Correct Answer: A) Epinephrine
Rationale: Epinephrine, also known as adrenaline, is a hormone released in response to stress. It activates the sympathetic nervous system, leading to various physiological changes such as increased heart rate, sweating, and dilated airways. These changes prepare the body for a fight-or-flight response. Insulin, estrogen, and growth hormone do not have direct effects on the stress response. Insulin regulates blood sugar levels, estrogen is involved in female reproductive system function, and growth hormone promotes tissue growth and development. In Mr. Johnson's case, his symptoms during physical therapy sessions can be attributed to the release of epinephrine as part of his body's stress response.

Question 36: Correct Answer: C) Implementing a regular sleep schedule
Rationale: Implementing a regular sleep schedule is essential to optimize sleep and rest patterns. Establishing consistent times for going to bed and waking up helps regulate the body's internal clock and promotes better sleep quality. Napping during the day might interfere with nighttime sleep by disrupting the sleep-wake cycle. While sedative medications can be prescribed in certain situations, they are not the first-line intervention for improving sleep patterns. Allowing Mr. Johnson to stay up late watching television can further disrupt his sleep-wake cycle and hinder his sleep quality.

Question 37: Correct Answer: A) Encouraging Mr. Johnson to independently perform activities of daily living (ADLs) to promote self-care and independence.
Rationale: Encouraging independence and promoting self-care abilities are essential for optimizing a patient's functional ability. By encouraging Mr. Johnson to independently perform ADLs, the nurse can facilitate his recovery process, enhance his sense of control, and promote his overall well-being. This intervention will empower Mr. Johnson, enabling him to regain self-confidence, promote muscle strength, and improve mobility. It is crucial to assess and monitor his abilities while providing appropriate support and assistance as needed. Strict bed rest (option B) can lead to complications such as muscle atrophy and increased risk of blood clots. Administering pain medication (option C) is important, but it should not be the only priority. Limiting mobility (option D) can hinder the recovery process and potentially lead to further complications.

Question 38: Correct Answer: B) Powered wheelchair
Rationale: A powered wheelchair would be the most suitable assistive device for John to improve his mobility. It would provide him with independent mobility and enable him to move around without assistance. A communication board is typically used for individuals with communication difficulties, hearing aids are used for hearing impairments, and splints are used to support and immobilize joints. However, in John's case, a powered wheelchair would address his specific need for mobility assistance.

Question 39: Correct Answer: C) The rehabilitation team should assess Emily's psychological needs and discuss the possible benefits of a referral with her.
Rationale: In facilitating appropriate referrals for patients' psychological needs, it is important for the rehabilitation team to assess the individual's psychological needs and discuss the recommended referral with the patient. Collaboration and shared decision-making between the healthcare team and the patient are crucial to ensure the patient's understanding of the benefits of a mental health referral and to address any concerns they may have. This approach empowers the patient and respects their autonomy, promoting a patient-centered care approach in addressing their psychosocial needs during the rehabilitation process.

Question 40: Correct Answer: A) Adaptation Model by Sister Callista Roy
Rationale: The Adaptation Model by Sister Callista Roy focuses on assisting patients in adapting to altered physiological and psychological functioning. The stroke patient's mobility challenges require adaptation, and this model emphasizes the importance of individuality, environment, and the nurse's role in promoting the patient's

adaptation. The Health Promotion Model by Nola Pender focuses on promoting positive health behaviors but may not directly address the patient's mobility issues. The Transcultural Nursing Theory by Madeleine Leininger focuses on providing culturally congruent care and may not directly address the stroke patient's mobility concerns. The Self-Care Deficit Nursing Theory by Dorothea Orem focuses on enabling patients to meet their self-care needs and may not directly address the patient's need for mobility assistance.

Question 41: Correct Answer: B) Rehabilitation planning

Rationale: Rehabilitation planning is a crucial skill for a Certified Rehabilitation Registered Nurse (CRRN) as it involves developing and implementing individualized plans of care for patients. This skill focuses on identifying and addressing the specific needs and goals of patients, including promoting functional independence and improving their overall quality of life. By utilizing rehabilitation planning skills, nurses can collaborate with interdisciplinary teams to coordinate various interventions, therapies, and resources aimed at optimizing the restoration and preservation of the patient's health and holistic well-being. This skill plays a vital role in ensuring comprehensive care and supporting patients throughout their rehabilitation journey.

Question 42: Correct Answer: D) Plan, Do, Study, Act

Rationale: The PDSA cycle is a quality improvement model that consists of four stages: Plan, Do, Study, Act. During the planning stage, the team identifies the problem, establishes goals, and develops a plan for improvement. In the doing stage, the plan is implemented and data is collected. The study stage involves analyzing the data and evaluating the outcomes. Based on the study stage findings, the team then takes action in the act stage to make necessary changes and further improve the process. The PDSA cycle emphasizes iterative testing and continuous improvement.

Question 43: Correct Answer: B) Monitoring the patient's vital signs and pain levels.

Rationale: Monitoring the patient's vital signs and pain levels can be appropriately delegated to a certified nursing assistant (CNA) as it falls within their scope of practice. CNAs are trained to measure and document vital signs such as blood pressure, pulse, respirations, and temperature. They can also assist in assessing and documenting pain levels using appropriate pain scales. However, developing the patient's individualized plan of care requires advanced nursing knowledge and should be performed by a registered nurse. Collaborating with the physical therapist and administering medications and wound care are tasks that also require specialized knowledge and should be performed by licensed professionals such as physical therapists and registered nurses, respectively.

Question 44: Correct Answer: D) Incomplete or illegible documentation can compromise patient care.

Rationale: Incomplete or illegible documentation can compromise patient care as it may lead to miscommunication or confusion among healthcare providers. Accurate and complete documentation is essential for continuity of care, legal purposes, and reimbursement. Documentation should be done in a timely manner, reflecting the care provided during each shift. It is important to document both positive and negative aspects of care to provide an accurate representation of the patient's condition. Avoid using abbreviations and acronyms unless they are standardized and easily understood. Patient care and safety should always be prioritized when documenting services provided.

Question 45: Correct Answer: C) Oral intake of less than 50% of meals

Rationale: Oral intake of less than 50% of meals indicates inadequate nutritional intake and may require further intervention to ensure the patient's nutritional needs are met. Adequate weight gain (Option A) and normal bowel movements and digestion (Option D) are positive findings that suggest good nutritional status. Albumin level of 4.5 g/dL (Option B) within the normal range also indicates appropriate nutrition. Therefore, these options do not require immediate intervention as compared to the option of oral intake less than 50% of meals.

Question 46: Correct Answer: D) Technology can provide real-time feedback and support for self-management.

Rationale: Technology plays a crucial role in self-management by providing real-time feedback and support to patients. It helps individuals monitor their health-related data, track progress, and make informed decisions. Although technology is not intended to replace healthcare professionals, it can enhance patient engagement and empowerment by enabling them to take an active role in their care. By leveraging various applications, wearables, and telehealth platforms, patients can access personalized education, reminders, and assistance whenever needed. Therefore, incorporating technology in self-management strategies can significantly improve patient outcomes and facilitate a proactive approach to healthcare.

Question 47: Correct Answer: B) Clinical practice guidelines are evidence-based recommendations to guide healthcare professionals in making decisions about patient care.

Rationale: Clinical practice guidelines are evidence-based recommendations that provide guidance to healthcare professionals in the delivery of patient care. They are developed by multidisciplinary teams of experts and are aimed at improving the quality and consistency of care across different settings. Clinical practice guidelines are not exclusive to specific medical specialties; they can be applicable across a wide range of healthcare settings, including rehabilitation units. These guidelines are used to inform decision-making and promote patient-centered care that is based on the best available evidence.

Question 48: Correct Answer: A) Occupational Safety and Health Administration (OSHA) regulations

Rationale: Occupational Safety and Health Administration (OSHA) regulations play a crucial role in ensuring a safe work environment for healthcare staff. CRRNs must be knowledgeable about OSHA's guidelines, which cover topics such as safe handling of hazardous materials, prevention of workplace injuries, and protocols for reporting and documenting incidents. By complying with OSHA regulations, CRRNs can effectively minimize risks for staff and promote a safe environment of care. While HIPAA, ADA, and ACA are important legislations in healthcare, they primarily address patient- and policy-related issues rather than staff safety in the workplace.

Question 49: Correct Answer: A) Consuming a diet high in caffeine

Rationale: Consuming a diet high in caffeine, such as drinking coffee or energy drinks, can disrupt normal sleep patterns and result in difficulty falling asleep or staying asleep. Caffeine is a stimulant that increases alertness and can interfere with the body's natural sleep-wake cycle. It is recommended to limit caffeine intake, especially in the evening, to promote better sleep. Engaging in regular exercise, maintaining a consistent sleep schedule, and creating a calm sleep environment are factors that can enhance sleep quality rather than disrupt it.

Question 50: Correct Answer: C) Mr. Johnson has a decreased appetite and is only eating half of his meals.

Rationale: The finding that Mr. Johnson has a decreased appetite and is only eating half of his meals indicates a potential nutritional deficit. This may lead to inadequate intake of essential nutrients needed for wound healing and optimal recovery. It is important for the nurse to further assess Mr. Johnson's nutritional needs and collaborate with the interdisciplinary team, including a dietitian, to develop a plan to improve his nutritional intake. While the BMI and presence of a pressure ulcer are important assessment findings, they do not directly indicate the need for further intervention related to nutritional and metabolic patterns. Mr. Johnson's fluid intake of 2000 mL per day is within the normal range and does not require further intervention.

Question 51: Correct Answer: A) Providing a patient with a non-slip mat in the shower.

Rationale: When implementing safety prevention measures, it is important to consider patient needs and potential risks. Providing a patient with a non-slip mat in the shower reduces the risk of falls and promotes safety in the bathroom environment. Placing a patient with decreased mobility near the exit door may compromise the patient's safety in case of an emergency and should be avoided. Administering medications without double-checking the patient's identification increases the risk of medication errors. Leaving the bedrails down for a confused patient may result in falls and should be avoided to ensure patient safety.

Question 52: Correct Answer: B) Performing physical assessment and monitoring vital signs

Rationale: Performing physical assessments and monitoring vital signs is a crucial skill for a CRRN to possess in order to effectively evaluate the patient's condition and progress during rehabilitation. By closely monitoring vital signs such as blood pressure, heart rate, and respiratory rate, the nurse can identify any changes or complications that may arise and take appropriate actions. Additionally, physical assessments provide valuable information about the patient's functional abilities and potential areas of improvement. This skill ensures the safety and well-being of the patient throughout the rehabilitation process.

Question 53: Correct Answer: B) Hospital Consumer Assessment of Healthcare Providers and Systems (HCAHPS)

Rationale: The Hospital Consumer Assessment of Healthcare Providers and Systems (HCAHPS) is a federal quality measurement initiative that assesses patients' perspectives on their hospital experiences. It is a standardized survey used to measure the quality of care provided by hospitals. Medicare Conditions of Participation (CoPs) are federal regulations that healthcare facilities must meet to participate in the Medicare program. The National Council Licensure Examination for Registered Nurses (NCLEX-RN) is a standardized exam for nursing licensure. The American Nurses Credentialing Center (ANCC) Magnet Recognition Program recognizes healthcare organizations that demonstrate nursing excellence. While important, these options are not specific to federal quality measurement efforts.

Question 54: Correct Answer: B) To promote independent functioning and improve quality of life for individuals with disabilities or chronic illnesses

Rationale: The goal of rehabilitation nursing is to promote independent functioning and improve the quality of life for individuals with disabilities or chronic illnesses. This includes providing direct care and treatment, advocating for patients, and assisting in the development of individualized care plans. Rehabilitation nurses focus on empowering patients to reach their maximum potential in physical, cognitive, emotional, and social functioning. By providing comprehensive care, education, and support, rehabilitation nurses help individuals regain or maintain their independence and enhance their overall well-being.

Question 55: Correct Answer: C) Speech recognition software

Rationale: Speech recognition software would be the most beneficial electronic hand-held device to assist Mrs. Smith with communication. With quadriplegia, Mrs. Smith may have limited or no movement in her arms and hands to operate traditional communication devices. Speech recognition software allows her to communicate using her voice, converting spoken words into written text. This technology enables her to interact with others, access information, and participate in daily activities, promoting her community reintegration and independence. Electric wheelchairs, overhead lift systems, and service animals are not electronic hand-held devices specifically designed for communication purposes.

Question 56: Correct Answer: D) Medicare

Rationale: Medicare is a federal program in the United States that provides health insurance coverage for individuals who are 65 years or older, individuals with certain disabilities, and individuals with end-stage renal disease. Part A of Medicare covers inpatient hospital stays, which can include rehabilitation treatments. John, being a patient with a spinal cord injury, may be eligible for Medicare benefits to help cover the cost of his rehabilitation treatments.

Question 57: Correct Answer: A) Catheter dislodgement

Rationale: Central lines, ports, and catheters can pose potential complications. One of the common complications is catheter dislodgement, which can occur due to patient movement or accidental removal. This can result in the loss of access and potential damage to the vessel. Hypotension and respiratory distress are not directly related to central lines, ports, and catheters. Constipation may be a side effect of certain medications or conditions but is not specifically associated with these devices. It is important for the rehabilitation nurse to monitor central lines, ports, and catheters closely to prevent complications such as dislodgement and promptly intervene if any issues arise.

Question 58: Correct Answer: B) Electronic hand-held device

Rationale: An electronic hand-held device, such as a tablet or smartphone, can be particularly useful for individuals with limited hand dexterity. These devices often have touch screen capabilities, allowing patients to control functions with just a simple tap or swipe. They can be customized with various accessibility features to accommodate the individual's specific needs, such as larger buttons or voice activation. Service animals are trained to assist with specific tasks but may not directly address hand dexterity limitations. Electrical stimulation, on the other hand, is a therapeutic modality used to improve muscle function and is not specifically considered an adaptive equipment for activities of daily living.

Question 59: Correct Answer: C) Speaking slowly and clearly

Rationale: Dysarthria is a motor speech disorder that affects muscle control, making speech difficult to understand. Speaking slowly and clearly can help improve the patient's comprehension of verbal communication. Providing written instructions may not be effective as the patient may have difficulty reading due to their condition. Using visual aids may not address the specific speech impairment. Conducting a group therapy session may not be helpful since the patient's speech may be difficult to understand and may not contribute effectively to the group communication dynamics. Therefore, speaking slowly and clearly is the most appropriate communication intervention for a patient with dysarthria.

Question 60: Correct Answer: C) Demonstrating empathy and active listening

Rationale: In this scenario, the most appropriate communication technique for the nurse to use when interacting with the patient is demonstrating empathy and active listening. This technique involves understanding and validating the patient's feelings, which can help build trust and enhance therapeutic communication. It is important for the nurse to create a safe space for the patient to express his needs and frustrations without interruption or judgment. Interrupting the patient or providing unsolicited advice may further frustrate the patient and hinder effective communication. Additionally, the nurse should acknowledge the patient's wife's attempts to communicate as she plays a crucial role in assisting the patient.

Question 61: Correct Answer: B) Contemplation

Rationale: The Transtheoretical Model (TTM) proposes that behavior change occurs in a series of stages: precontemplation, contemplation, preparation, action, and maintenance. In the contemplation stage, individuals are aware of the need for change and are considering taking action within the next six months. It is during this stage that the rehabilitation team can provide education, advice, and information to help the patient evaluate the pros and cons of making the change. By understanding the stage of contemplation, rehabilitation professionals can tailor their interventions to effectively promote behavioral change and improve patient outcomes.

Question 62: Correct Answer: A) Conducting a literature review to identify relevant studies

Rationale: When incorporating evidence-based research into practice, it is crucial to conduct a thorough literature review to identify relevant studies. This process allows healthcare professionals to stay updated with current research findings and ensure that their practice aligns with the most up-to-date evidence. Relying solely on clinical expertise and experience (option B) may not be sufficient as it can be subjective and may not incorporate the latest research. Disregarding current research findings (option C) and implementing outdated care practices (option D) can be detrimental to patient outcomes and quality of care. Therefore, conducting a literature review is vital for evidence-based practice.

Question 63: Correct Answer: A) Assess Mr. Johnson's current financial situation and insurance coverage.

Rationale: It is essential for rehabilitation nurses to identify financial barriers that may impede a patient's community reintegration. By assessing Mr. Johnson's current financial situation and insurance coverage, the nurse can understand if there are any potential challenges in accessing the necessary resources. This assessment can help the nurse develop an appropriate plan and explore available financial assistance options, such as insurance coverage, grants, or community programs. Ignoring the financial aspect or assuming that the patient can afford everything may lead to inadequate resource provision and hinder the patient's successful transition.

Question 64: Correct Answer: D) Power wheelchair

Rationale: A power wheelchair would be the most appropriate assistive device for a patient with limited mobility due to a spinal cord injury. Power wheelchairs allow for independent mobility and can be controlled by the patient, providing greater freedom and independence. Canes and walkers are generally used for patients with mild mobility impairments, while a manual wheelchair requires upper body strength and may not be suitable for patients with limited upper body function. Therefore, a power wheelchair is the best option for maximizing functional ability and independence for a patient with limited mobility due to a spinal cord injury.

Question 65: Correct Answer: C) Watson's Human Caring Theory

Rationale: Watson's Human Caring Theory is a nursing model that focuses on the significance of the nurse-patient relationship. It emphasizes the nurse's role in promoting healing, facilitating personal growth, and providing holistic care. In rehabilitation nursing, building a therapeutic relationship is vital as it establishes trust, enhances communication, and fosters a supportive environment for patients to achieve their rehabilitation goals. This model encourages nurses to view patients as holistic beings and to incorporate compassion, empathy, and active listening into their practice. By embracing Watson's Human Caring Theory,

rehabilitation nurses can enhance patient outcomes and promote overall well-being during the rehabilitation process.

Question 66: Correct Answer: A) Observation of non-verbal cues

Rationale: Assessing a patient's ability to comprehend and retain information requires observation of non-verbal cues, such as body language, facial expressions, and gestures. Non-verbal cues can provide valuable insights into a patient's level of understanding and their ability to retain information. Blood pressure, lung sounds, and urine output are unrelated to assessing comprehension and communication. By observing non-verbal cues, the nurse can make appropriate adjustments to the communication approach, ensuring the patient receives the necessary information effectively and efficiently.

Question 67: Correct Answer: D) "I can take showers and get the central line wet without any problem."

Rationale: It is important to teach patients and caregivers about appropriate care and maintenance of central lines. However, it is essential to stress that central lines should be kept dry and protected from water to minimize the risk of infection. Moisture can provide a breeding ground for bacteria and increase the chances of infection. Patients should be advised to cover the central line insertion site securely during showers or baths to avoid getting it wet.

Question 68: Correct Answer: D) Offering one-on-one counseling sessions

Rationale: While all the options can be valuable teaching interventions, offering one-on-one counseling sessions is the most effective in promoting health and wellness among individuals with a chronic illness. Individual counseling allows for personalized education tailored to the specific needs of the patient, addressing their unique concerns and providing the opportunity for in-depth discussions. This approach provides a safe and confidential environment for patients to ask questions, express fears or doubts, and receive individualized guidance and support, enhancing their understanding and empowering them to actively participate in managing their health and wellness.

Question 69: Correct Answer: D) Transfer and mobility techniques

Rationale: Transfer and mobility techniques are part of the Activity and Exercise Functional Health Pattern in rehabilitation nursing. In this pattern, the nurse assesses the client's ability to perform activities of daily living, including transferring from one surface to another and maintaining mobility. Medication administration techniques, pain management strategies, and communication skills are important aspects of nursing care but they fall under different Functional Health Patterns such as Coping-Stress Tolerance, Comfort, and Role-Relationship patterns, respectively. It is crucial for rehabilitation nurses to assess and promote the client's functional ability in the area of transfer and mobility to ensure optimal rehabilitation outcomes.

Question 70: Correct Answer: C) Identifying potential fall risks in the patient's environment

Rationale: Assessing and identifying potential fall risks in the patient's environment is crucial for promoting a safe environment of care. Given the patient's medical history of peripheral neuropathy and recent amputation, he may be at a higher risk of falling. By identifying potential hazards in the patient's environment, the nurse can take appropriate measures to minimize the risk of falls and ensure a safe rehabilitation process. While assessing the patient's knowledge, evaluating range of motion and muscle strength, and reviewing medication history are also important aspects of care, in this scenario, the priority is to address safety risks to prevent falls.

Question 71: Correct Answer: C) Orem's Self-Care Deficit Theory

Rationale: Orem's Self-Care Deficit Theory promotes the concept that individuals have the ability to perform self-care activities to maintain their health and wellbeing. This theory emphasizes that nursing should aim to assist individuals in meeting their self-care needs when they are unable to do so independently due to a self-care deficit. The theory focuses on identifying and meeting the patient's self-care requirements to enhance their ability to manage their health. Other nursing models, such as Roy's Adaptation Model, Neuman Systems Model, and Watson's Theory of Human Caring, have different focuses and concepts but do not specifically address the individual's self-care abilities as emphasized in Orem's Self-Care Deficit Theory.

Question 72: Correct Answer: A) Morphine sulfate

Rationale: In this scenario, Mrs. Johnson is experiencing severe pain postoperatively, making a potent analgesic necessary. Morphine sulfate is a strong opioid analgesic that is commonly used to manage severe pain. Ibuprofen and acetaminophen are both non-opioid analgesics and may not provide adequate pain relief for Mrs. Johnson's condition. Codeine sulfate is a weaker opioid analgesic compared to morphine sulfate and may not be as effective in managing severe pain. Therefore, morphine sulfate would be the most appropriate choice in this situation.

Question 73: Correct Answer: C) Rule setting

Rationale: Rule setting is a technique used in behavioral management strategies to establish clear guidelines and expectations for the individual. It involves setting specific rules and boundaries that the individual needs to follow. This helps in promoting positive behavior and establishing a structured environment. Contracts (option A) are written agreements between the individual and healthcare provider, outlining specific goals and rewards for achieving them. Positive reinforcement (option B) involves rewarding desired behavior to encourage its repetition. Aversion therapy (option D) is a technique that pairs an unpleasant stimulus with an undesirable behavior to discourage its occurrence. While all strategies have their own significance, the technique involved in establishing clear guidelines and expectations is rule setting.

Question 74: Correct Answer: C) CARF

Rationale: CARF (Commission on Accreditation of Rehabilitation Facilities) is an international, nonprofit organization that accredits various healthcare facilities, including rehabilitation centers. CARF sets quality and safety standards that rehabilitation facilities must meet to provide high-quality care to individuals with disabilities. CARF's accreditation process ensures that facilities adhere to best practices and continuously improve their services. By choosing option C) CARF, the nurse demonstrates an understanding of the agency responsible for accrediting rehabilitation facilities and promoting quality standards in the field of rehabilitation.

Question 75: Correct Answer: C) Provide active range of motion exercises

Rationale: Providing active range of motion exercises is essential in optimizing physical mobility and preventing complications such as muscle contractures and joint stiffness. Monitoring vital signs, administering pain medication, and assessing urine output are important aspects of nursing care but do not directly address the nursing diagnosis of impaired physical mobility.

Question 76: Correct Answer: C) Neuman's Systems Model

Rationale: Neuman's Systems Model is based on the belief that stressors can affect an individual's balance and stability. In the case of John, who has suffered a traumatic brain injury, this model focuses on understanding the impact of the injury on his body's stability and providing interventions to restore and maintain his stability. This model emphasizes the importance of considering the patient's environment and its influence on their ability to adapt. By using Neuman's Systems Model, the nurse aims to promote John's adaptation and restore his balance and stability during the rehabilitation process.

Question 77: Correct Answer: C) Planning and implementing individualized diet and fluid intake.

Rationale: As a CRRN, having the skill to plan and implement individualized diet and fluid intake is critical. This involves assessing the client's nutritional needs, considering any dietary restrictions or preferences, and creating a tailored plan to optimize nutrition and hydration. Activities such as assessing dietary preferences and cultural beliefs (option A), collaborating with the client's family regarding meal planning (option B), and administering enteral feedings and intravenous fluids (option D) may be part of the overall care plan but do not specifically focus on the skill of planning and implementing individualized diet and fluid intake.

Question 78: Correct Answer: C) Tolterodine

Rationale: Tolterodine is a commonly prescribed anticholinergic medication for the treatment of urinary incontinence. It works by blocking the action of acetylcholine on the smooth muscles of the bladder, resulting in reduced bladder contractions and increased bladder capacity. Morphine is an analgesic used for moderate to severe pain, while omeprazole is a proton pump inhibitor used to reduce stomach acid production. Gabapentin is an anticonvulsant primarily used for neuropathic pain. Therefore, the correct option for an anticholinergic medication for urinary incontinence is Tolterodine (Option C).

Question 79: Correct Answer: C) Piaget's cognitive development theory

Rationale: Piaget's cognitive development theory is the most appropriate model for Mr. Smith's cognitive rehabilitation. This theory focuses on how individuals think, understand, and perceive the world around them. It emphasizes the importance of cognitive processes in learning and development. In Mr. Smith's case, understanding his cognitive abilities and limitations will help in devising appropriate rehabilitation strategies. Freud's psychoanalytic theory focuses on the unconscious mind, Erikson's psychosocial theory emphasizes social and emotional development, and Skinner's behaviorism focuses on observable behavior. These models may not be directly relevant to Mr. Smith's cognitive rehabilitation.

Question 80: Correct Answer: C) Face-to-face support groups

Rationale: Face-to-face support groups are valuable community resources that provide individuals and families with emotional support and a sense of belonging during their rehabilitation process. These groups offer opportunities to connect with others who are facing similar challenges, share experiences, and learn coping strategies. Unlike internet forums and chat groups (Option A), face-to-face support groups allow for in-person interactions and deeper connections. Respite care services (Option B) provide short-term relief for caregivers but may not directly address the need for emotional support. While clergy and religious leaders (Option D) can offer spiritual guidance and support, face-to-face support groups specifically focus on rehabilitation challenges and provide a unique peer support system.

Question 81: Correct Answer: B) Stage II

Rationale: The Braden scale is a commonly used tool to assess the risk for pressure ulcers. Stage II pressure ulcers are characterized by partial-thickness skin loss or blister formation. The reddened area on the coccyx that does not blanch indicates tissue damage and is consistent with a Stage II pressure ulcer. Stage I pressure ulcers typically present as intact skin with localized redness. Stage III pressure ulcers involve full-thickness skin loss with visible subcutaneous tissue. Stage IV pressure ulcers are the most severe, with extensive tissue damage that extends to muscle, bone, or supporting structures.

Question 82: Correct Answer: A) Active listening and empathetic responses

Rationale: Active listening and empathetic responses are essential communication techniques that contribute to establishing rapport and building trust with patients. By actively listening to patients, nurses can demonstrate empathy, validate their concerns, and show respect for their feelings. This approach helps in developing a therapeutic relationship, promoting effective communication, and enhancing patient satisfaction. On the other hand, using medical jargon and abbreviations can lead to miscommunication and confusion. Providing minimal responses may diminish patients' ability to express themselves fully, while interrupting patients can hinder dialogue and make them feel unheard. Therefore, choosing active listening and empathetic responses promotes open communication and better understanding between nurses and patients.

Question 83: Correct Answer: B) Encouraging the patient to set realistic goals and praising their efforts towards achieving them.

Rationale: Promoting self-efficacy involves helping the patient build confidence in their ability to perform specific tasks or achieve desired outcomes. By encouraging the patient to set realistic goals and acknowledging their efforts towards attaining them, the nurse reinforces and enhances their sense of self-efficacy. Providing resources and educational materials on community support groups (option A) may enhance self-care and social support, but it may not directly promote self-efficacy. Administering medication to manage pain (option C) and assisting with activities of daily living (option D) are important interventions but are not specifically aimed at promoting self-efficacy.

Question 84: Correct Answer: D) Reviewing medical records for compliance

Rationale: During the regulatory agency audit process, one of the essential activities is the review of medical records for compliance with established standards and regulations. This process ensures that documentation is accurate, complete, and meets the necessary requirements. Assessing patient satisfaction (Option A) is a part of quality improvement initiatives but not specifically related to the regulatory agency audit process. Developing a nursing care plan (Option B) and conducting staff education (Option C) are important aspects of patient-centered care delivery, but they are not direct activities within the regulatory agency audit process. The primary focus of the audit process is to evaluate adherence to regulatory standards through the review of medical records.

Question 85: Correct Answer: B) CPAP machine

Rationale: A CPAP (Continuous Positive Airway Pressure) machine is commonly used to treat sleep apnea by delivering a steady flow of air pressure to the airways. This airflow helps to keep the airways open during sleep, reducing episodes of breathing cessation and improving overall sleep quality. A sleep study, on the other hand, is a diagnostic test used to evaluate sleep patterns and identify sleep disorders such as sleep apnea. BiPAP (Bilevel Positive Airway Pressure) machines are also used in some cases, but they provide different levels of pressure for inhalation and exhalation. Relaxation technology, although beneficial for promoting sleep and relaxation, is not directly used to treat sleep apnea. Therefore, the correct answer is B) CPAP machine.

Question 86: Correct Answer: D) Cognitive development

Rationale: When caring for a child like Sarah with a traumatic brain injury, it is important to consider their cognitive development. Traumatic brain injuries can affect cognitive functions such as attention, memory, problem-solving, and learning. By understanding Sarah's cognitive abilities and limitations, the CRRN can tailor interventions and therapies to promote optimal recovery and rehabilitation. This includes implementing cognitive rehabilitation strategies, fostering a conducive learning environment, and engaging Sarah in activities to enhance her cognitive abilities. Monitoring and addressing cognitive development are crucial in helping Sarah regain her optimal level of function and improve her overall quality of life.

Question 87: Correct Answer: C) Problem-solving

Rationale: When assisting patients in coping with stress, it is important to promote effective coping strategies. Problem-solving is a constructive and adaptive coping strategy that involves identifying the problem, analyzing potential solutions, and implementing the most appropriate course of action. By engaging in problem-solving, patients like Mr. Thompson can actively address the challenges associated with their disability, which can lead to improved stress management and overall well-being. Options A, B, and D (avoidance, substance abuse, and denial, respectively) are maladaptive strategies that can perpetuate stress and hinder the patient's ability to effectively cope with his condition.

Question 88: Correct Answer: C) Implementing a quiet and soothing environment in the patient's room.

Rationale: Implementing a quiet and soothing environment in the patient's room is an effective nursing intervention to promote sleep and rest patterns in a patient with insomnia. This includes reducing noise levels, ensuring dim lighting, and promoting a calm and peaceful atmosphere. Taking a long nap during the day (option A) may interfere with the patient's ability to fall asleep at night, while consuming caffeine (option B) close to bedtime can worsen insomnia symptoms. Administering sedative medication without the patient's consent (option D) is unethical and disregards patient autonomy. Therefore, option C is the most appropriate and effective intervention for enhancing the patient's sleep and rest patterns.

Question 89: Correct Answer: B) Barthel Index

Rationale: The Barthel Index is a commonly used standardized assessment tool that measures a patient's ability to carry out activities of daily living (ADLs). As a rehabilitation nurse, assessing Mrs. Johnson's functional capabilities is crucial to develop an effective care plan. The Glasgow Coma Scale is used to assess neurological function, the Epworth Sleepiness Scale evaluates excessive daytime sleepiness, and the Geriatric Depression Scale assesses depressive symptoms. However, in this case, the most appropriate tool to assess Mrs. Johnson's functional status is the Barthel Index, which evaluates her ability to perform ADLs such as bathing, dressing, and toileting.

Question 90: Correct Answer: C) Psychologist

Rationale: After a traumatic event like a stroke, both the patient and their caregiver may experience various psychological challenges, such as anxiety, depression, and adjustment difficulties. A psychologist can provide counseling, emotional support, and coping strategies to help them navigate through these challenges. Physical and occupational therapists focus on the physical aspect of rehabilitation, while a nutritionist specializes in providing dietary guidance. Therefore, the most appropriate resource in this situation is a psychologist who can address the psychosocial needs of both the patient and caregiver.

Question 91: Correct Answer: D) Keeping the environment clean and free of clutter.

Rationale: Keeping the environment clean and free of clutter is essential in promoting a safe environment for patients and staff. Clutter can increase the risk of falls and accidents. This measure ensures that pathways are clear and accessible, reducing the likelihood of tripping or bumping into objects. Encouraging patients to engage in physical activities is important, but it may not directly address safety measures.

Providing education on medication administration is crucial, but it pertains more to the proper use of medications rather than environmental safety. Allowing visitors to bring in outside food may pose risks related to food allergies or contamination.

Question 92: Correct Answer: A) Observe the patient while performing activities of daily living (ADLs).

Rationale: Observing the patient while performing ADLs is the most appropriate action to assess their self-care ability and mobility. This allows the nurse to directly observe the patient's abilities, limitations, and any difficulties they may encounter during self-care activities. It provides valuable information about the patient's functional status and helps in identifying areas that require intervention or assistance. Self-report questionnaires are subjective and may not accurately reflect the patient's actual abilities. Performing a physical examination focusing on range of motion is important but may not provide a comprehensive assessment of self-care ability and mobility. Although involving the patient's family or caregiver in the assessment can provide additional information, direct observation of the patient remains the most reliable method for evaluation in this context.

Question 93: Correct Answer: C) To increase patient satisfaction and promote a sense of ownership in their own care

Rationale: Including the patient and caregiver in the plan of care is important to increase patient satisfaction and promote a sense of ownership in their own care. When patients are actively involved in decision-making and goal-setting, they are more likely to feel engaged and motivated to follow the plan. This involvement leads to better adherence to treatment regimens, improved outcomes, and a sense of control over their own health. In addition, including patients and caregivers in the plan of care fosters effective communication between healthcare providers and patients, which further enhances collaboration and mutual understanding. The involvement of patients and caregivers is not primarily aimed at ensuring medication compliance or decreasing the workload for healthcare providers, although these may be additional benefits.

Question 94: Correct Answer: D) Utilize large-print materials for written information.

Rationale: Since the patient has limited vision and difficulty reading, utilizing large-print materials for written information would be the most appropriate intervention. This would help enhance the patient's ability to see and comprehend written material more effectively. Options A and B would further impede the patient's ability to read due to the small font size or reliance on a magnifying glass. Option C would not address the patient's visual impairment and would not be sufficient for effective communication.

Question 95: Correct Answer: B) Promoting physical mobility and exercise

Rationale: Promoting physical mobility and exercise should be prioritized for Mr. Johnson as it plays a crucial role in his recovery from stroke-induced left-sided weakness. Regular physical activity and mobility exercises can help improve muscle strength, prevent joint contractures, enhance balance, and foster independence. By focusing on physical mobility, the nurse can facilitate Mr. Johnson's ability to perform activities of daily living, regain functional abilities, and achieve optimum quality of life. While administering pain medication, providing emotional support, and monitoring vital signs are important aspects of care, promoting physical mobility takes precedence in this scenario as it directly contributes to Mr. Johnson's rehabilitation and overall well-being.

Question 96: Correct Answer: A) Voice recognition technology may not be as accurate for individuals with speech impairments.

Rationale: When utilizing voice activated call systems as an adaptive equipment, it is important for the CRRN to consider that voice recognition technology may not be as accurate for individuals with speech impairments. While voice recognition technology has advanced significantly, it may still have difficulty accurately interpreting speech for individuals with speech impairments, leading to inaccurate commands or frustration. Therefore, alternative methods or technologies may need to be explored for these individuals to ensure effective communication and use of adaptive equipment.

Question 97: Correct Answer: C) Implementing evidence-based practice

Rationale: Implementing evidence-based practice is a crucial aspect of integrating quality improvement processes into nursing practice. A CRRN should strive to use the most current and relevant evidence to guide patient care decisions. By staying updated with research and best practices, the nurse can provide the most effective and efficient care to promote positive patient outcomes. Adhering to ethical standards, advocating for patient rights, and documenting patient assessments accurately are also important aspects of nursing practice but do not specifically address the skill of integrating quality improvement processes.

Question 98: Correct Answer: C) Using a bladder training program to gradually increase the time between voiding

Rationale: Bladder training is a non-pharmacological intervention that can be effective in managing urinary incontinence. It involves gradually increasing the time between voiding to allow the bladder to relearn and regain control. Anticholinergic medications may be used in some cases to decrease bladder contractions, but they have side effects and should be used cautiously. Kegel exercises can help strengthen pelvic floor muscles and may be beneficial in preventing incontinence, but they are not the most appropriate intervention for someone who is already experiencing incontinence. Using adult diapers should be a last resort and should not be the first choice for managing urinary incontinence.

Question 99: Correct Answer: A) Ensuring patient confidentiality

Rationale: Ensuring patient confidentiality is an ethical consideration in nursing practice. Nurses are responsible for maintaining the privacy and confidentiality of patient information, which includes protecting patient records and not disclosing personal health information without patient consent. This ethical principle is essential for building trust with patients and upholding their rights to privacy and autonomy. Managing patient finances (option B) falls more under the economic aspect, while assigning patient care tasks (option C) relates to task delegation. Obtaining informed consent for treatment (option D) is a legal obligation rather than an ethical consideration.

Question 100: Correct Answer: B) Developing an individualized care plan based on the patient's goals

Rationale: During the implementation phase of the nursing process, the nurse translates the care plan into action and provides nursing interventions to promote the patient's restoration and preservation of health. Developing an individualized care plan based on the patient's goals is a key nursing action in rehabilitation nursing during this phase. This involves collaborating with the patient, their family, and the interdisciplinary team to identify specific interventions that will help the patient achieve their rehabilitation goals. Assessing the patient's functional abilities and limitations is part of the assessment phase, evaluating the effectiveness of interventions is part of the evaluation phase, and administering medication is part of the intervention phase.

Question 101: Correct Answer: A) Assessing the patient's vital signs

Rationale: Assessing the patient's vital signs is a critical step in the nursing process. This involves obtaining baseline measurements such as temperature, blood pressure, pulse rate, and respiratory rate. Vital signs provide important information about the patient's current health status and can help in identifying any abnormalities or changes that may require further assessment or intervention. Administering medications, scheduling follow-up appointments, and documenting the patient's medical history are also important aspects of nursing care but are not specific steps in the nursing process.

Question 102: Correct Answer: C) Nutritional development

Rationale: As a certified rehabilitation registered nurse (CRRN), it is important to consider various developmental factors when caring for patients. Cognitive development refers to the patient's thinking and learning abilities, emotional development relates to their emotional well-being and regulation, and physical development involves their physical growth and abilities. However, nutritional development is not a typical developmental factor to consider as it does not directly relate to the patient's overall development. While proper nutrition is important for optimal health, it does not fall under the developmental factors that a CRRN would typically assess and address during patient care.

Question 103: Correct Answer: D) Washing hands with soap and water before and after every patient interaction.

Rationale: Proper hand hygiene is one of the crucial infection control practices to prevent the spread of infections. Washing hands with soap and water is essential before and after patient interactions to minimize the risk of cross-contamination. Wearing gloves is recommended during specific patient care activities to protect against direct contact with bodily fluids, but it does not replace proper hand hygiene. Sharing stethoscopes or using the same thermometer without proper disinfection promotes the transmission of infectious pathogens between patients. Therefore, option D is the most appropriate and effective infection control practice.

Question 104: Correct Answer: D) Assisting with activities of daily living

Rationale: Delegating appropriate responsibilities to team members is crucial for efficient and effective patient care. Assisting with activities of daily living, such as bathing, dressing, and feeding, is within the scope of practice for a nursing assistant. They are trained to provide direct patient care and support with these tasks. However, administering medications requires specialized knowledge and should be performed by a licensed nurse. Assessing the patient's readiness for discharge and developing the care plan require higher-level decision-making skills, typically performed by registered nurses or other healthcare professionals. It is important to delegate tasks appropriately to ensure patient safety and optimize the team's efficiency.

Question 105: Correct Answer: C) Progressive muscle relaxation technique

Rationale: Non-pharmacological sleep aids are interventions that do not involve the use of medications. Progressive muscle relaxation is a technique that involves tensing and then relaxing different muscle groups in the body to promote physical and mental relaxation, which can help improve sleep. This technique can be used to relieve muscle tension and promote sleep by reducing anxiety and stress, making it an effective non-pharmacological sleep aid. Melatonin, Zolpidem, and Trazodone, on the other hand, are examples of pharmacological sleep aids as they involve the use of medications to treat sleep disturbances.

Question 106: Correct Answer: A) Deep breathing exercises

Rationale: Deep breathing exercises are an effective nonpharmacological intervention for managing pain and promoting comfort in patients. When patients practice deep breathing, it helps to trigger the relaxation response in the body and reduce stress and anxiety, which can worsen pain perception. Deep breathing also increases oxygen saturation, improves lung function, and promotes a sense of well-being.

Administering opioid medications (option B) is a pharmacological intervention rather than a nonpharmacological one. Applying heat packs (option C) may provide temporary relief but may not be suitable for all patients. Providing distraction techniques (option D) can be helpful, but deep breathing exercises are a more direct and focused approach to pain management.

Question 107: Correct Answer: D) Assessment

Rationale: During the assessment phase of the nursing process, the nurse collects data about the patient's medical history, physical abilities, and functional limitations. This step involves the systematic gathering of information to identify the patient's needs, problems, and current health status. By conducting a thorough assessment, the nurse can obtain a comprehensive understanding of the patient's condition and develop an individualized care plan. The data gathered in the assessment phase serves as a foundation for subsequent steps in the nursing process, such as diagnosis, planning, implementation, and evaluation. Thus, option D is the correct answer.

Question 108: Correct Answer: A) Increased muscle tone below the level of injury

Rationale: Alterations in sexual function and reproduction are common in individuals with SCI. Increased muscle tone below the level of injury can lead to spasticity, which may interfere with sexual activity and impair the ability to achieve or maintain an erection. Normal sexual desire and arousal (Option B) may not be affected, but the ability to physically engage in sexual activity can be limited. Increased motor control and coordination (Option C) are not associated with alterations in sexual function and reproduction. Preservation of voluntary control over bladder and bowel function (Option D) can be beneficial but is not directly related to sexual function and reproduction.

Question 109: Correct Answer: A) Assessment and evaluation of patients' functional health patterns

Rationale: A CRRN plays a vital role in assessing and evaluating patients' functional health patterns in order to optimize their rehabilitation process. This assessment allows the nurse to identify the patient's strengths, weaknesses, and needs, thus providing a foundation for individualized care planning and goal setting. By applying the nursing process and conducting a thorough assessment, the CRRN can gain a comprehensive understanding of the patient's condition and develop appropriate interventions to enhance their functional abilities. Other options such as administering medications, performing complex medical procedures, and documentation are important components of nursing care, but the assessment and evaluation of functional health patterns take precedence in the rehabilitation setting.

Question 110: Correct Answer: C) Providing a small reward to Mark whenever he makes a safe choice.

Rationale: Positive reinforcement involves providing a reward or incentive to promote desired behaviors. In this scenario, Jane aims to promote safer behaviors in Mark. By providing a small reward whenever Mark makes a safe choice, Jane is using positive reinforcement to increase the likelihood of him making safer choices in the future. The other options, such as giving a verbal warning (A), ignoring the behavior (B), or restricting access to activities (D), do not involve the use of positive reinforcement and may not be as effective in promoting safer behaviors.

Question 111: Correct Answer: C) Atropine

Rationale: Atropine is a commonly used medication as an antispasmodic in the management of neurological conditions. It acts by inhibiting the action of acetylcholine, thereby reducing excessive muscle contractions and spasms. Amitriptyline is an antidepressant medication, Morphine is an opioid analgesic, and Ibuprofen is a nonsteroidal anti-inflammatory drug (NSAID), none of which possess significant antispasmodic properties. As a rehabilitation registered nurse, it is important to have knowledge of the different medications used for symptom management in neurological conditions to optimize patient care and outcomes.

Question 112: Correct Answer: D) The patient's cultural beliefs and practices

Rationale: When facilitating appropriate referrals for patients in the rehabilitation process, it is crucial for the CRRN to consider the patient's cultural beliefs and practices. Cultural factors can significantly impact a patient's acceptance of and participation in healthcare interventions. By understanding the patient's cultural background, the CRRN can tailor their approach to ensure that referrals align with the patient's beliefs and preferences. This consideration promotes patient-centered care and enhances the effectiveness of rehabilitation interventions by addressing any potential cultural barriers or disparities that may hinder the patient's progress. Therefore, ensuring that cultural beliefs and practices are taken into account is essential in facilitating appropriate referrals in the rehabilitation process.

Question 113: Correct Answer: D) All of the above.

Rationale: Skill in communication and collaboration is essential for rehabilitation nurses. Providing education to patients and their families helps to increase their understanding of the condition and treatment plans, empowering them to actively participate in their rehabilitation. Implementing and coordinating a multidisciplinary team approach ensures that all healthcare professionals involved in the patient's care work together towards common goals. Using therapeutic communication techniques, such as active listening and empathy, helps to establish rapport and trust, enhancing the nurse-patient relationship. Therefore, all the options mentioned in the question are correct and reflect the various aspects of communication and collaboration in rehabilitation nursing.

Question 114: Correct Answer: C) A lawyer who specializes in elder law

Rationale: When addressing legal issues, it is essential to involve professionals who specialize in the respective field. In this case, Mrs. Johnson's concerns can be best addressed by a lawyer who specializes in elder law. These attorneys possess the expertise and knowledge necessary to assist older adults with their legal documents, ensuring that they are updated and legally binding. A nutritionist, physical therapist, and recreational therapist do not possess the specific expertise needed to address Mrs. Johnson's concerns related to her legal documents.

Question 115: Correct Answer: C) Evidence-based research incorporates the best available evidence with clinical expertise and patient preferences.

Rationale: Evidence-based research in healthcare, including rehabilitation nursing, involves the integration of the best available evidence from scientific studies, clinical expertise, and patient preferences. It goes beyond anecdotal evidence or personal opinions and seeks to provide the most effective and individualized care for patients. By incorporating evidence-based research, the interdisciplinary team can make informed decisions regarding interventions such as electrical stimulation for lower extremity muscle strengthening in this patient with a spinal cord injury.

Question 116: Correct Answer: B) Apply for Medicaid on behalf of the patient to cover the cost of rehabilitation services.

Rationale: Medicaid is a government program that provides health coverage to individuals with low income, including those with disabilities. As a CRRN, it is essential to explore options such as Medicaid to ensure access to rehabilitation services for uninsured patients. By applying for Medicaid on behalf of the patient, the cost of rehabilitation services can be covered, thereby facilitating the patient's recovery and improving their quality of life. Options A, C, and D are not the most appropriate courses of action as they do not address the financial constraint faced by the patient or provide viable solutions for accessing the required services.

Question 117: Correct Answer: B) Roy's Adaptation Model

Rationale: Roy's Adaptation Model is commonly used as a framework for rehabilitation nursing practice. This model focuses on the individual's adaptation to their environment and the steps they take to meet their needs and achieve optimal health. It emphasizes the importance of assessment, intervention, and evaluation in facilitating adaptation. Orem's Self-Care Deficit Theory focuses on self-care needs and the nurse's role in assisting individuals to meet these needs. Neuman's Systems Model focuses on the individual as a dynamic system in interaction with their environment. Benner's Skill Acquisition Model focuses on the stages of skill development in nursing practice. While these models are important in nursing practice, Roy's Adaptation Model is specifically used in rehabilitation nursing.

Question 118: Correct Answer: A) Encouraging active range of motion exercises

Rationale: Contractures are one of the complications that can arise in patients with musculoskeletal impairments. To prevent contractures, it is important to encourage active range of motion exercises. These exercises help maintain joint mobility and prevent the shortening of muscles and tendons. Implementing strict bed rest (option B) can actually contribute to muscle weakness and the development of contractures. Applying ice packs (option C) may help alleviate pain and inflammation, but it does not directly prevent contractures. Administering nonsteroidal anti-inflammatory drugs (option D) may provide pain relief, but it does not address the underlying issue of contracture prevention. Therefore, option A is the correct approach for preventing contractures in patients with musculoskeletal impairments.

Question 119: Correct Answer: B) Mobility skills

Rationale: Given that the patient is having difficulty with activities such as dressing, bathing, and grooming, the most appropriate skill for the nurse to focus on would be mobility. By improving mobility skills, the patient will be able to move more freely and independently, allowing for greater participation in daily activities and improved functional ability. Cognitive skills refer to mental processes such as memory and problem-solving, which may not directly address the patient's difficulty with daily activities. Communication skills and socialization skills may be important for overall patient well-being but may not directly address the issue of difficulty with dressing, bathing, and grooming.

Question 120: Correct Answer: B) Elevate the head of the bed to at least 45 degrees during feedings and for at least one hour afterward.

Rationale: Elevating the head of the bed to at least 45 degrees during feedings and for at least one hour afterward helps to minimize the risk of aspiration and reflux, which are common issues in patients receiving enteral nutrition. Flush the nasogastric tube with water before and after each medication administration (Option A) helps to prevent medication interactions. Administering medications directly through the nasogastric tube without crushing or grinding them (Option C) may not always be suitable as some medications are not meant to be given via the enteral route. Continuous enteral feedings should be maintained at room temperature or at the recommended temperature by the manufacturer (Option D) to prevent bacterial growth, but preventing clogging of the feeding tube is not the primary reason for this practice.

Question 121: Correct Answer: B) Inform the nurse manager about the missing referrals and request for them to be added to the treatment plan.

Rationale: As a CRRN, it is your ethical responsibility to advocate for the patient's overall well-being, which includes addressing their emotional needs. By notifying the nurse manager about the oversight and requesting the addition of psychological referrals, you ensure that the patient receives comprehensive care that encompasses both physical and emotional rehabilitation. Ignoring the oversight or leaving it to the patient's family would be a disservice to the patient's holistic recovery. While discussing the importance of psychological support with the patient is important, it is necessary to involve the nurse manager to make appropriate changes to the treatment plan.

Question 122: Correct Answer: B) An anticholinergic agent

Rationale: Anticholinergic agents are commonly used to manage muscle spasms in patients with conditions such as multiple sclerosis. These medications work by blocking the action of acetylcholine, a neurotransmitter involved in muscle contraction. By inhibiting acetylcholine, anticholinergic agents help relax muscles and reduce spasms. Selective serotonin reuptake inhibitors (SSRIs) are primarily used to treat depression and anxiety disorders, and would not be effective in managing muscle spasms. Nonsteroidal anti-inflammatory drugs (NSAIDs) are commonly used to manage pain and inflammation, but they do not directly target muscle spasms. Benzodiazepines are central nervous system depressants and may be used to manage anxiety or promote sleep, but they are not specifically indicated for muscle spasms.

Question 123: Correct Answer: D) Communication and collaboration

Rationale: The functional health patterns are a framework used to assess an individual's health status. They include the following categories: health perception and health management, nutrition and metabolism, elimination, activity and exercise, sleep and rest, cognition and perception, self-perception and self-concept, roles and relationships, coping and stress tolerance, and sexuality and reproduction. Communication and collaboration is not considered a functional health pattern, but rather an important aspect of nursing practice that enhances patient care. Therefore, option D is the correct answer.

Question 124: Correct Answer: B) Flush the tube with water before and after medication administration

Rationale: Proper maintenance and patient safety are essential when using a nasogastric tube for enteral feeding. Flushing the tube with water before and after medication administration helps prevent medication residue from clogging the tube and ensures proper medication absorption. This action also helps maintain tube patency and reduces the risk of complications such as clogging or blockage. Therefore, the correct answer is to flush the tube with water before and after medication administration. Securing the tube loosely can lead to displacement, using smaller tube sizes may compromise delivery efficiency, and changing the tube position every shift can cause discomfort and mucosal trauma.

Question 125: Correct Answer: D) Initiate a referral for augmentative and alternative communication systems.

Rationale: In cases where patients have expressive aphasia and are unable to speak, initiating a referral for augmentative and alternative communication systems is the most appropriate intervention to optimize their ability to communicate effectively. These systems include tools and strategies such as electronic devices, sign language, and gestures that can be used to supplement or replace verbal communication. Encouraging the patient to use written communication (Option A) may be difficult or impossible for someone with expressive aphasia. While providing a communication board (Option B) can be helpful, it may not fully address the patient's communication needs. Although speech therapy sessions (Option C) may be beneficial, it may not be sufficient to address the patient's expressive aphasia. Hence, the most appropriate intervention is to initiate a referral for augmentative and alternative communication systems (Option D).

Question 126: Correct Answer: A) Difficulty in understanding and producing speech sounds

Rationale: Linguistic deficits refer to impairments in language abilities. One common example of a linguistic deficit is difficulty in understanding and producing speech sounds, known as dysarthria. Dysarthria is characterized by weakness or paralysis of the muscles used for speech, leading to slurred or unintelligible speech. It can result from neurological conditions such as stroke or brain injury. Options B, C, and D describe other language disorders but not specifically linguistic deficits.

Question 127: Correct Answer: D) Analysis

Rationale: The nursing process consists of five steps: Assessment, Diagnosis, Planning, Implementation, and Evaluation. The step not included in the nursing process for optimizing the management of a patient's neurological and other complex medical conditions is Analysis. Analysis is not a separate step but is integrated into the other steps of the nursing process. Assessment involves gathering information about the patient's condition, Diagnosis involves identifying the patient's problems or needs, Planning involves setting goals and developing a plan of care, Implementation involves carrying out the plan of care, and Evaluation involves assessing the effectiveness of the plan of care.

Question 128: Correct Answer: A) A specialized stroke support group that meets weekly at the local community center. **Rationale:** The most appropriate community resource to support Mrs. Smith's community reintegration after a stroke would be a specialized stroke support group that meets weekly at the local community center. This resource will provide Mrs. Smith with an opportunity to connect with other individuals who have experienced a stroke, share their experiences, and learn from one another. The support group can also offer emotional support, information, and practical strategies for managing post-stroke challenges. It is specifically tailored to address the needs and concerns of stroke survivors, making it the most relevant and beneficial resource for Mrs. Smith's situation. The other options, such as an Alzheimer's disease support group, yoga class, or daycare center, do not align with Mrs. Smith's needs as a stroke survivor.

Question 129: Correct Answer: A) Built-up utensils

Rationale: Built-up utensils are specifically designed to assist individuals with hand tremors. They have larger handles that provide a better grip and control, making it easier for the patient to feed themselves. Long-handled shoe horns are used to help individuals put on shoes without bending over, and in this scenario, it does not address the patient's difficulty with self-feeding. Jar openers and sock aids are also not relevant to the patient's specific needs in this case. Therefore, built-up utensils are the most appropriate adaptive equipment for this patient to enhance their independence with self-feeding.

Question 130: Correct Answer: C) Transitions theory

Rationale: Transitions theory, developed by Dr. Afaf Meleis, focuses on understanding how individuals and groups go through a process of change and adaptation. It explores the impact of various transitions, such as health-related changes, on individuals' well-being and emphasizes the importance of providing appropriate support during these transitions. This theory is particularly relevant in the field of rehabilitation nursing as patients often undergo significant physical and emotional changes during their recovery process. Understanding transitions theory helps rehabilitation nurses in developing effective interventions and promoting patient-centered care that facilitates successful adjustment and adaptation to new circumstances. Social cognitive theory focuses on the reciprocal interaction between an individual's cognitive processes, behavior, and environment. Transformational leadership theory relates to leadership style that inspires and motivates followers. Chaos theory explores complex systems and their behavior.

Question 131: Correct Answer: A) Assessment and evaluation of patient condition and needs

Rationale: Rehabilitation nurses have a key role in assessing and evaluating the condition and needs of patients undergoing rehabilitation. This involves conducting comprehensive assessments, identifying strengths and limitations, and formulating individualized plans of care. By understanding the patient's condition and needs, rehabilitation nurses can provide appropriate interventions and ensure effective rehabilitation outcomes. Administration of medications and performing surgical procedures are not within the scope of practice for rehabilitation nurses. Customizing treatment plans based on personal preference may be considered, but it should always be supported by evidence-based practice and clinical guidelines, ensuring patient safety and optimal outcomes.

Question 132: Correct Answer: C) Collaborating with the interdisciplinary team to develop a comprehensive care plan

Rationale: Ethical and legal standards in nursing practice require collaboration with the interdisciplinary team to provide comprehensive care. By involving other healthcare professionals, such as physical therapists, occupational therapists, and social workers, the nurse ensures that all aspects of the patient's rehabilitation and well-being are addressed. This contributes to the provision of cost-effective and patient-centered care. Administering medication without verifying the patient's identification is a violation of patient safety protocols and may lead to medication errors. Sharing confidential health information without the patient's consent is a breach of privacy and violates HIPAA regulations. Implementing a treatment plan without obtaining informed consent disregards the patient's autonomy and rights.

Question 133: Correct Answer: B) Bed exit alarm

Rationale: The use of physical restraints and chemical restraints should be avoided whenever possible, as they can cause physical and psychological harm to the patient. Patient education alone may not be effective in preventing falls for a cognitively impaired patient like Mr. Johnson. The most appropriate safety device in this scenario would be a bed exit alarm. This device alerts the healthcare team when a patient attempts to get out of bed, allowing for timely intervention and prevention of falls.

Question 134: Correct Answer: D) Providing a private room with a calm environment

Rationale: Non-behavioral restraints refer to interventions that do not physically restrict a patient's movement. These interventions aim to create a safe environment and promote patient well-being without restricting their freedom. Providing a private room with a calm environment falls under this category as it focuses on optimizing the patient's functional ability by reducing external stimuli and promoting a peaceful atmosphere. Placing the patient in a geriatric chair with a lap belt (option A) and using restraints that limit the patient's movement (option B) are examples of physical restraints. Encouraging physical activity to redirect excessive energy (option C) is a behavioral intervention.

Question 135: Correct Answer: C) In a multidisciplinary team, healthcare professionals work together but maintain their professional boundaries.

Rationale: In a multidisciplinary team, healthcare professionals work together but maintain their professional boundaries. Each discipline has its own goals and plans of care for the patient. In this model, collaboration occurs, but decision-making and responsibilities remain within each discipline's scope of practice. On the other hand, in a transdisciplinary team, healthcare professionals work

collaboratively and share responsibilities. They work together to develop shared goals and plans of care, breaking down professional boundaries. Hence, the suggestion to adopt a transdisciplinary approach would imply a shift towards a more integrated and collaborative model where professionals work across disciplines to provide holistic care. However, in the given scenario, the nursing assistant's suggestion is incorrect as the team is already following a multidisciplinary approach.

Question 136: Correct Answer: D) All of the above

Rationale: When planning discharge for a rehabilitation patient, it is crucial to consider various aspects to promote a successful transition to the community. Coordinating home visits allows healthcare professionals to assess the patient's living environment and make any necessary modifications to ensure safety and accessibility. Teaching caregivers about the patient's condition and care needs enables them to provide appropriate support and assistance once the patient returns home. Finally, ensuring the patient has access to necessary medical equipment and supplies is essential for their continued rehabilitation and well-being. Therefore, all of the options listed are important aspects of planning discharge for a rehabilitation patient.

Question 137: Correct Answer: C) Assessing for psychological barriers to sexual activity

Rationale: When assessing goals related to sexuality and reproduction in a patient, the CRRN should prioritize assessing for psychological barriers to sexual activity. This includes evaluating the patient's beliefs, attitudes, cultural influences, and emotional well-being related to sexuality and reproduction. By identifying any psychological barriers, the nurse can develop appropriate interventions and provide resources to address these issues, ultimately promoting the patient's sexual health and well-being. While implementing interventions to promote sexual function and satisfaction, providing education about contraception options, and encouraging patients to discuss sexual concerns with their partners are all important aspects of care, assessing for psychological barriers should be the initial priority to guide holistic care planning.

Question 138: Correct Answer: D) BiPAP machine

Rationale: While aromatherapy, meditation, and sound therapy may promote relaxation and improve sleep quality, they are not considered as primary treatment options for obstructive sleep apnea (OSA). BiPAP (Bilevel Positive Airway Pressure) therapy is a suitable alternative for patients who are unable to tolerate CPAP or require additional support during the expiratory phase of breathing. BiPAP therapy provides different pressure levels for inhalation and exhalation, making it more comfortable for some patients with sleep apnea. It is essential to assess and consider individual patient needs and preferences when recommending alternative treatments for OSA.

Question 139: Correct Answer: A) Observing the patient's behavior and interactions

Rationale: When assessing a patient's cognition, observing their behavior and interactions is the most appropriate technique. This allows the nurse to gather information about the patient's cognitive abilities, attention, memory, and problem-solving skills. It provides valuable insights into their level of consciousness, alertness, and orientation to time, place, and person. Conducting a neurological exam, reviewing the patient's medical history, and performing a sensory evaluation are important, but they focus on different aspects of the assessment and may not provide a complete picture of the patient's cognition. Observing the patient's behavior and interactions allows for a comprehensive evaluation of their cognitive function in real-life situations.

Question 140: Correct Answer: C) Biopsychosocial Model

Rationale: The Biopsychosocial Model is commonly used in rehabilitation care to provide individualized patient-centered care. This model takes into account the biological, psychological, and social factors that influence a patient's health and well-being. It recognizes that rehabilitation care should not only focus on the physical aspect, but also consider the patient's psychological and social needs. By incorporating all these factors, the Biopsychosocial Model helps healthcare professionals develop individualized care plans that address the holistic needs of the patient. This model is widely accepted and used in the field of rehabilitation nursing to promote patient-centered care and facilitate the recovery process.

Question 141: Correct Answer: A) Encouraging the caregiver to take breaks from their caregiving duties

Rationale: Encouraging the caregiver to take breaks from their caregiving duties is an effective intervention for promoting positive interaction among patients and caregivers. Caregivers often experience high levels of stress and burnout, which can impact their ability to provide proper care and create a positive environment. By encouraging and supporting caregivers to take regular breaks, they can recharge and have time for self-care, reducing stress and enhancing their ability to interact positively with the patient. This intervention also helps to prevent caregiver burden and allows them to maintain their own physical and mental well-being. Providing written instructions or limiting the caregiver's involvement may not address the emotional and relational aspects of positive interaction, while advising the patient to not rely on the caregiver for emotional support can undermine the caregiver-patient relationship.

Question 142: Correct Answer: D) Adhering to legislative and legal requirements

Rationale: Quality improvement processes in nursing practice involve various components, such as collecting and analyzing data to identify areas for improvement, implementing evidence-based practices to enhance patient outcomes, and collaborating with interdisciplinary teams for effective care coordination. However, adhering to legislative and legal requirements is not specifically focused on quality improvement processes. While it is essential for nurses to abide by laws and regulations, it does not fall under the direct scope of quality improvement.

Question 143: Correct Answer: B) Personal financial counseling

Rationale: When a patient is facing financial barriers to rehabilitation, one appropriate resource to address this issue is personal financial counseling. This service can help patients develop an understanding of their financial situation, explore options for financial assistance, and create a plan to manage their expenses during the rehabilitation process. Social media support groups and access to a computer and internet can provide emotional support, but they may not directly address the financial barriers. Pet therapy sessions, while beneficial for emotional well-being, are not directly related to financial resource management. Therefore, personal financial counseling is the most suitable resource to assist patients in overcoming financial barriers to rehabilitation.

Question 144: Correct Answer: A) Elevate the head of the bed to 30 degrees during meals

Rationale: Elevating the head of the bed to 30 degrees during meals helps in reducing the risk of aspiration while swallowing. This position allows gravity to assist in the movement of the liquid down the esophagus rather than into the trachea. Administering liquids at room temperature, encouraging the patient to drink through a straw, and offering small, frequent sips of fluid are not directly related to promoting safe swallowing in a patient with dysphagia.

Question 145: Correct Answer: A) Straight catheter

Rationale: In patients with lower limb paralysis, intermittent catheterization is commonly performed to facilitate bladder emptying. Straight catheters are recommended for this purpose as they are single-use catheters inserted through the urethra to drain the bladder and then removed. Indwelling (Foley) catheters are not suitable for long-term use as they increase the risk of urinary tract infections. Condom (Texas) catheters are external catheters used in male patients who are unable to self-catheterize or are contraindicated for indwelling catheters. Suprapubic catheters are surgically inserted through the abdominal wall directly into the bladder and are typically used in cases of long-term bladder dysfunction.

Question 146: Correct Answer: D) Educating Mr. Anderson about lifestyle modifications to reduce the risk of future strokes.

Rationale: The Neuman Systems Model emphasizes primary prevention, which focuses on interventions to prevent potential threats to an individual's well-being. In this case, educating Mr. Anderson about lifestyle modifications, such as healthy diet, exercise, and stress management, can reduce the risk of future strokes. Administering medications (option A) and providing physical therapy exercises (option B) are examples of secondary prevention, which aim to minimize the impact of an existing health problem. Support groups (option C) are part of the Neuman Systems Model's tertiary prevention, which focuses on the restoration and rehabilitation of the patient's optimal wellness.

Question 147: Correct Answer: D) Renal Ultrasound

Rationale: A renal ultrasound is a non-invasive diagnostic test that uses sound waves to produce images of the kidneys. It is commonly performed to evaluate renal structure and function, including the size, shape, and presence of any abnormalities such as cysts or tumors. This test provides valuable information to healthcare providers for accurate diagnosis and treatment planning for patients with renal diseases, including chronic kidney disease. Electrocardiogram (ECG) is used to evaluate cardiac function, Magnetic Resonance Imaging (MRI) is used to visualize soft tissues and organs, and Renal Angiography is used to assess blood flow in the renal arteries. Therefore, these options are incorrect in this context.

Question 148: Correct Answer: B) Promoting independence and maximizing function

Rationale: The Rehabilitation Nursing Model focuses on promoting independence and maximizing function in individuals with disabilities or chronic illness. This model emphasizes the holistic care of patients, addressing physical, psychosocial, and environmental aspects of their lives. While emotional support (option A) is an essential component of nursing care, it is not the primary focus of the Rehabilitation Nursing Model. Administering medications (option C) and educating patients on wound care (option D) are important tasks but do not encompass the comprehensive approach of the Rehabilitation Nursing Model.

Question 149: **Rationale:** The Health Insurance Portability and Accountability Act (HIPAA) regulates the confidentiality and privacy of patient health information. It ensures that healthcare providers protect the privacy and security of patients' health information. HIPAA outlines requirements for safeguards, electronic transactions, privacy notices, and the handling of protected health information (PHI). Complying with HIPAA standards is crucial in maintaining patient confidentiality and privacy, as it establishes guidelines for healthcare professionals to follow when dealing with sensitive patient data. The other options mentioned in the question are related to different legislations but are not specifically focused on patient health information confidentiality and privacy.

Question 150: Correct Answer: C) Use open-ended questions to encourage the patient to share their feelings and experiences.

Rationale: When communicating with a patient from a different cultural background, it is essential for the CRRN to create a safe and inclusive environment. One way to achieve this is by using open-ended questions that allow the patient to express their thoughts, feelings, and experiences. This approach fosters effective communication and helps the CRRN gain valuable insights into the patient's cultural beliefs and practices that may impact their rehabilitation journey. It is important to avoid making assumptions about the patient's cultural values and norms, as cultural diversity requires individualized and culturally sensitive care.

Made in the USA
Las Vegas, NV
12 September 2024

95202309R00083